Diagnosis and Treatment of Large Animal Diseases

Diagnosis and Treatment of Large Animal Diseases

**Thomas John Doherty, MVB, MSc,
Diplomate ACVA, MRCVS**
Atlantic Veterinary College
University of Prince Edward Island
Charlottetown, Prince Edward Island
Canada

J. Paul Mulville, MVB, MRCVS
Department of Large Animal Clinical Studies
University College Dublin
Veterinary College of Ireland
Dublin, Ireland

W. B. SAUNDERS COMPANY
Harcourt Brace Jovanovich, Inc.
Philadelphia   London   Toronto   Montreal   Sydney   Tokyo

W. B. SAUNDERS COMPANY
Harcourt Brace Jovanovich, Inc.

The Curtis Center
Independence Square West
Philadelphia, Pennsylvania 19106

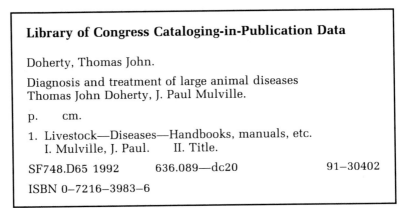

Library of Congress Cataloging-in-Publication Data

Doherty, Thomas John.

Diagnosis and treatment of large animal diseases
Thomas John Doherty, J. Paul Mulville.

p.   cm.

1. Livestock—Diseases—Handbooks, manuals, etc.
   I. Mulville, J. Paul.   II. Title.

SF748.D65 1992   636.089—dc20   91–30402

ISBN 0–7216–3983–6

Diagnosis and Treatment of Large Animal Diseases   ISBN 0–7216–3983–6

Printed in Mexico.

Last digit is the print number: 9   8   7   6   5   4   3   2   1

Preface

Now, what I want is Facts . . .
Facts alone are wanted in life.

Charles Dickens: *Hard Times*

This book is intended to be used as a quick reference for those involved in large animal care. The primary objective is to present a list of differential diagnoses for the conditions encountered by the practicing veterinarian; however, we anticipate that the book will also be helpful to students of animal science, animal health technicians, and stock owners.

Clearly, this book is not meant to be an all-inclusive reference text on large animal diseases; rather, it should be used as an *aide-memoire*. We have taken the unusual approach of presenting data on the basis of clinical signs, a concept that we expect will be popular with students and new graduates.

The book is arranged in two parts. Part I deals with the body systems, listing and briefly discussing common signs associated with diseases of each system. Species included are horses, cattle, sheep, goats, pigs, and New World Camelids (llamas, alpacas). In general, the diseases are not listed according to the frequency of their occurrence; instead, they are grouped on the basis of etiology. Some body systems are given more complete coverage than others. This is not intended to overemphasize their importance, but instead to ensure that adequate background information is provided. For example, Chapter 8, "Nervous System," includes a discussion of basic neuroanatomy and diagnostic guidelines. Part II deals with broad topics such as fluid therapy, shock, sudden death, and vaccination and parasite control programs.

Our thanks are extended to Myrna Pringle, who typed the manuscript. Finally, we thank the staff of W. B. Saunders, especially Linda Mills, for their guidance.

Thomas J. Doherty
Prince Edward Island, Canada

J. Paul Mulville
Dublin, Ireland

Contents

PART I

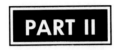

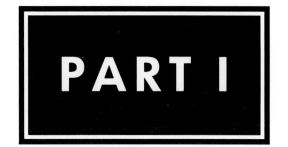

DISEASES OF THE BODY SYSTEMS

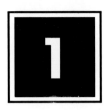

Integument

"The last thing one discovers in writing a book is what to put first."

Blaise Pascal

HORSES

Parasitic Skin Diseases

PEDICULOSIS: LOUSE INFESTATIONS. (*Haematopinus asini*—sucking louse; *Damalinia equi*—biting louse) Both biting and sucking lice occur in horses. Lice are distributed over dorsum, tailhead, and mane. Signs more common in winter and include pruritus.
  T R E A T M E N T: Topical organophosphates or ivermectin (0.2 mg/kg).

MANGE
Sarcoptic. *(Sarcoptes scabiei)* Signs include marked pruritus, alopecia and scabs. Lesions occur mainly over head and neck.
  T R E A T M E N T: Topical amitraz washes or ivermectin (0.2 mg/kg).

Psoroptic. *(Psoroptes equi, Psoroptes cuniculi)* Signs include pruritus and thick crusting of skin, especially along mane and root of tail. *P. cuniculi* may infest ear, causing head shaking.
  T R E A T M E N T: Topical organophosphates, lime sulfur, amitraz, or ivermectin (0.2 mg/kg).

Chorioptic. *(Chorioptes equi)* Stamping and kicking are common. Lesions include encrustations on palmar/plantar surface of fetlocks and are pruritic.
  T R E A T M E N T: As for psoroptic mange.

HORSE/DEER FLIES. (*Tabanus* spp., *Chrysops* spp.) These are blood-sucking flies that inflict painful bites.
  T R E A T M E N T: Topical repellents may be helpful.

STABLE FLIES. *(Stomoxys calcitrans)* Stable flies are an intermediate host for *Habronema* spp. and inflict a painful bite.
  T R E A T M E N T: Topical repellents may be helpful.

MIDGES. (*Culicoides* spp.) Midges are common and may cause "Queensland itch"/"sweet itch," the result of hypersensitivity to midges. Summer disease. Lesions occur especially over tailhead and flanks; extent depends on severity of hypersensitivity. Keep horses away from heavily infested areas.

T R E A T M E N T: Topical or systemic corticosteroids may be indicated.

CUTANEOUS HABRONEMIASIS. (*Habronema* spp.) Also known as "summer sores" and "swamp cancer." Larvae deposited on skin by flies cause local irritation and large granulomatous lesions, especially on face, midline, limbs, and prepuce.

T R E A T M E N T: Ivermectin (0.2 mg/kg) may be effective.

ONCHOCERCIASIS. (*Onchocerca* spp.) Common. Signs include ventral alopecia and scaliness associated with hypersensitivity to larvae (*O. cervicalis*). There may be pruritus as well as swelling and edema around suspensory ligament from O. reticulata.

T R E A T M E N T: Ivermectin (0.2 mg/kg).

OXYURIASIS. (*Oxyuris equi*) Common. Signs include pruritus of perineum. *O. equi* lays eggs on perineal area; irritation (and scratching) leads to loss of tail hairs.

T R E A T M E N T: Broad-spectrum anthelmintics, e.g., benzimidazoles, ivermectin, organophosphates, febantel.

TROMBICULIASIS. (*Trombicula* spp., chigger mites) Signs include pruritus and scaly skin. Autumnal occurrence. Affects face and lower limbs.

T R E A T M E N T: Topical solutions of organophosphates or lime sulfur.

Infections

Fungal

RINGWORM. (*Trichophyton* spp., *Microsporum* spp.) Common and nonpruritic. Signs include crusty scabs and alopecia, which may be localized or diffuse. Commonly occurs over areas where tack is applied.

T R E A T M E N T: Topical dilute iodine solutions, oral griseofulvin (10 mg/kg orally, once daily: not for pregnant mares).

MYCOTIC DERMATITIS: RAIN SCALD. (*Dermatophilus congolensis*) Common and nonpruritic. Wetting of skin predisposes to disease. Signs include matted hair with underlying scab; raw lesion if scab removed.

T R E A T M E N T: Topical dilute iodine solutions or parenteral penicillin may be used.

EPIZOOTIC LYMPHANGITIS, BLASTOMYCOSIS. *(Histoplasma farciminosus)* Occurs in Asia, Africa, and Mediterranean area.
Cutaneous Form. Chronic ulceration develops at the site of infection, followed by thickening of lymphatics.
T R E A T M E N T: Surgical excision and topical therapy, or parenteral iodides may be helpful.

SPOROTRICHOSIS. *(Sporotrichum* spp.) Occurs in USA, Europe, and India. May enter through wounds, causing formation of nodules on lower limb, rupture and drainage of purulent material. Lymphatic cording may occur.
T R E A T M E N T: Parenteral iodides or topical natamycin.

Bacterial

STAPHYLOCOCCAL DERMATITIS. *(Staphylococcus aureus)* Nodules up to 5 mm in diameter occur especially where harness contacts skin. Painful.
T R E A T M E N T: Topical ointments in combination with parenteral antibiotics may be indicated.

ULCERATIVE LYMPHANGITIS. *(Corynebacterium pseudotuberculosis)* Nonpruritic. Skin wounds become infected. Nodules form in lower limb, rupturing and discharging purulent matter. Other areas may also be affected.
T R E A T M E N T: Parenteral antibiotics, e.g., penicillin, are indicated.

CANADIAN HORSE POX. *(C. pseudotuberculosis)* Rare and nonpruritic. Painful papules and pustules occur in areas where harness or tack contacts skin.
T R E A T M E N T: Parenteral antibiotics, e.g., penicillin, or topical therapy.

GLANDERS. *(Actinobacillus mallei)* Occurs mainly in Europe, Middle East, and North Africa.
Acute. Signs include fever, cough, nasal discharge, and nodules on skin of lower limbs and on ventrum. Death is due to septicemia.

Chronic. Characteristic subcutaneous nodules ulcerate and discharge a dark, tenacious exudate. Medial aspect of the hock is commonly affected.
T R E A T M E N T: Sulfonamides are effective.

Viral

HORSEPOX. Rare. Vesicles appear with scabs and pustules on back of pastern; a buccal form occurs infrequently.

T R E A T M E N T: Topical ointments may be indicated.

PAPULAR DERMATITIS. (viral etiology) Nonpruritic. Signs include fever and multiple papules over body surface. Disease occurs in summer/autumn and regresses over several weeks. May occur in outbreaks.

T R E A T M E N T: Topical ointments.

Neoplasia

MELANOMA. Common in old gray horses, usually in perineal region.

T R E A T M E N T: Usually does not require therapy. In severe cases, surgical excision or long-term oral cimetidine therapy may be indicated.

SQUAMOUS CELL CARCINOMA. Rare. May be encountered in older males, especially on prepuce.

T R E A T M E N T: Surgical excision.

Miscellaneous Conditions

SARCOID. Common. May occur in groups or as single lesions. May be wartlike, sessile, or pedunculated, or may resemble granulation tissue. Commonly affected sites include lower limbs, head, and prepuce.

T R E A T M E N T: Cryosurgery, BCG vaccine injected into lesion, or local hyperthermia.

PHOTOSENSITIZATION. Uncommon, pruritic. Primary and secondary forms occur. (See Miscellaneous Conditions in Cattle, p. 10.)

T R E A T M E N T: Supportive care, remove animals from ultraviolet light. Corticosteroids may be indicated.

AMYLOIDOSIS. Rare condition. Signs include firm nodules, especially on the head, neck, and shoulders, which are usually multiple, nonpainful, and nonpruritic. Overlying skin is normal.

T R E A T M E N T: May regress spontaneously. Corticosteroids may be effective.

URTICARIA. Immunological or nonimmunological in origin. Commonly seen in horses. Signs include wheals or hives, which may be localized or generalized. They may occur in association with infection (e.g., strangles), drug reactions, toxins, biologicals (e.g., vaccines), therapeutic agents, or insect bites. May be transient or prolonged.

T R E A T M E N T: Depends on causes. Remove inciting factor(s) if possible. Corticosteroids may be indicated.

PEMPHIGUS FOLIACEUS. Rare autoimmune disease. Autoantibodies form to glycocalyx of keratinocytes. Lesions appear on head or limbs initially and may spread over the body. Coronitis is a feature of the disease in some horses. Vesicles and crusting occur initially, with scaling and erosions later. Skin biopsy may aid in diagnosis.

T R E A T M E N T: Glucocorticoids, e.g., dexamethasone. Gold salts, e.g., aurothioglucose, may be effective in refractory cases.

GREASY HEEL. (possibly viral etiology) Sporadic. Associated with poor hygiene. Signs include cracks in pastern (flexor surface).

T R E A T M E N T: Topical astringents.

EOSINOPHILIC GASTROENTERITIS AND DERMATITIS. Rare, often fatal disease of unknown cause. This is a multisystem disorder, commonly involving intestinal tract, pancreas, and skin. Signs include facial excoriation and alopecia, circumferential coronitis, laminitis, and thimbling of hoof in severe cases.

T R E A T M E N T: Some cases repond to corticosteroid therapy.

CATTLE

Congenital Dermatoses

IODINE DEFICIENCY. Iodine deficiency produces weak calves and stillbirths. Goiter and alopecia are common. Pregnant animals should receive approximately 1 mg/kg of iodine daily in the diet to prevent deficiency in fetus.

BALDY CALF SYNDROME. Affects Holstein heifers. Although normal at birth, the calves later develop scaliness and alopecia, and their horns fail to grow. Constant slobbering is a feature. The disease is familial.

INHERITED SYMMETRICAL ALOPECIA. Rare disease. Affects Holsteins.

INHERITED PARAKERATOSIS. Lethal disease affecting Black Pied Danish cattle and possibly some other breeds.

EPITHELIOGENESIS IMPERFECTA. Rare.

EPIDERMOLYSIS BULLOSA. Rare.

CONGENITAL ICHTHYOSIS. Rare. Affects Holsteins and some other breeds. The skin takes on a fish-scale appearance.

FAMILIAL ACANTHOLYSIS. Rare. Affects Aberdeen Angus.

Teat Lesions

Viral

PSEUDOCOWPOX. (poxvirus) Signs include erythema, with vesicle formation, leading to ring- or horseshoe-shaped lesions. Heals in 7 days. Usually affects whole herd eventually. Spreads to milker's hands, causing nodule formation.
  T R E A T M E N T: Topical astringents for ulcerated areas may be helpful.

BOVINE ULCERATIVE MAMMILLITIS. (herpesvirus) Signs include swollen, painful teat with serum exuding from raw surface. May also affect udder of recently calved cows. Usually occurs in autumn. Generally a herd outbreak. Infection may recur.
  T R E A T M E N T: Topical astringents for ulcerated areas may be helpful.

COWPOX. (orthopoxvirus) Rare. Occurs in Western Europe. Signs include erythema and edema of teats. Later, vesicles occur and develop into pustules, which rupture, producing pus. Thick scabs or ulcers develop. May involve udder. Slow to heal.
  T R E A T M E N T: Ointments and other soothing agents may be used but are only palliative.

BOVINE VACCINIA MAMMILLITIS. (vaccinia virus) Rare. Animals are infected by humans recently vaccinated with smallpox virus. Signs are similar to those of cowpox. Smallpox is now eradicated worldwide.
  T R E A T M E N T: Topical astringents for ulcerated areas may be helpful.

WARTS. (papovavirus) Common. May involve teats, occasionally become secondarily infected. Can cause mechanical difficulty with use of milking equipment. Usually regress spontaneously.
  T R E A T M E N T: None specific.

VESICULAR STOMATITIS. (rhabdovirus) Signs include fever, anorexia, salivation, lameness, and vesicles in mouth, on teats, and on coronary band. Occurs mainly in the summer and fall. May affect man.
  T R E A T M E N T: None specific. Quarantine of affected animals is essential for control.

Bacterial

UDDER IMPETIGO. *(Staphylococcus aureus)* Signs include small pustules and occasionally boils, often occurring at base of teats. It may be causally associated with mastitis.
T R E A T M E N T :   Topical antiseptic creams are usually helpful. Parenteral antibiotics may be indicated in persistent cases. Strictly attend to hygiene.

BLACK SPOT. *(Fusobacterium necrophorum, Staphylococcus aureus)* Occurrence is confined to tip of teat. May predispose to mastitis. Painful.
T R E A T M E N T :   Topical antiseptic ointments, salicylates, or iodophors may be helpful.

Miscellaneous Conditions

FROSTBITE. Common in conditions of severe cold.
T R E A T M E N T :   None specific.

TRAUMA. Associated with treading by other cows and inadequate stall size. Barbed-wire fencing is also a common cause.
T R E A T M E N T :   Surgical repair of damaged teats is indicated.

Pruritic Skin Diseases

Parasitic

MANGE
Sarcoptic. *(Sarcoptes scabiei* var. *bovis)* Occurs most commonly under poor nutritional and housing conditions, with a higher incidence in winter. Signs include pruritus, edema of affected area, and wrinkling and cracking of skin.
T R E A T M E N T :   Ivermectin (0.2 mg/kg). Not to be used in lactating animals.

Chorioptic. *(Chorioptes bovis)* The perineum and escutcheon are often involved in milder cases. In severe cases, hindlimbs are primarily affected. Moderate pruritus may be noted.
T R E A T M E N T :   Topical dressings, e.g., 2% lime sulfur.

Psoroptic. *(Psoroptes bovis)* Withers, neck, and base of tail are affected. Signs include intense pruritus. Begins as a papule, later developing into scabs, which may coalesce to form large lesions.
T R E A T M E N T :   Lime sulfur, benzyl benzoate, and organophosphate solutions are useful. Ivermectin is also effective.

FLY INFESTATIONS
Black Flies. (*Simulium* spp.) Bites occur on legs, belly, and head area, causing wheals. May transmit filarial stage of *Onchocerca* spp.
T R E A T M E N T: Insect repellents may be effective.

Midges. (*Culicoides* spp.) Midges inflict painful bites and wheals and are potential carriers for bluetongue virus and *Onchocerca* spp.
T R E A T M E N T: Insect repellents may be effective.

Tabanids. (Horse fly, deer fly) Inflict painful, irritating bites. Mainly affects legs and ventral abdomen.
T R E A T M E N T: Insect repellents may be effective.

PEDICULOSIS
Louse Infestation. Sucking lice (*Haematopinus* spp., *Linognathus* spp.) and biting lice (*Bovicola* spp.). Signs include irritation of skin and anemia. Overcrowding and malnutrition may aggravate signs. Mainly a winter disease.
T R E A T M E N T: Topical dressings and dusting may be effective. Ivermectin (0.2 mg/kg) is effective against sucking lice.

MYIASIS
Screwworms. (*Cochliomyia* spp.) Occurs in subtropical North and South America. Flies are attracted to wounds, where they lay their eggs. Maggots attack affected area. Toxemia may result in death. Reportable disease.
Blow Fly. (*Lucilia, Calliphora* spp.) Wounds or wet skin attract blow fly. Maggots may cause skin damage. Death in severe cases.
T R E A T M E N T: Clipping of affected area, proper wound care, and topical insecticides are indicated.

Miscellaneous Conditions

PHOTOSENSITIZATION
Primary. Caused by ingestion of photodynamic agents in certain plants, e.g., St. Johnswort, buckwheat, perennial ryegrass. Congenital porphyria is also a rare cause.
Secondary. Hepatitis due to toxic plants (e.g., *Senecio jacobea, Tribulus terrestris*), or other agents (e.g., sporidesmin, *Pithomyces chartarum*) may lead to photosensitization. Prevention of exposure to toxic plants is important.
T R E A T M E N T: Remove animals from source, protect from ultraviolet light, supportive treatment if hepatitis is present. Corticosteroids may be indicated.

URTICARIA. There are multiple causes, both immunological and nonimmunological, e.g., drug reactions, insect bites. Signs include wheals, or hives, localized (more common) or generalized. Milk allergy is an autoallergic disease resulting in edema.

T R E A T M E N T: Clipping of affected area, proper wound care, and topical insecticides are indicated.

Nonpruritic Skin Diseases

Parasitic

DEMODICOSIS. (*Demodex bovis*) Signs include small nodules and pustules containing caseous material. Neck and shoulder are frequently affected. Often minimal or no clinical signs.

T R E A T M E N T: Ivermectin (0.2 mg/kg: except in lactating cows); topical amitraz is also effective.

WARBLES. (*Hypoderma* spp.) Signs include lumps with associated skin perforations along dorsum and over thoracolumbar region. Rarely, warbles may cause spinal paralysis during migration or following treatment.

T R E A T M E N T: Systemic pour-on organophosphates are effective.

ONCHOCERCIASIS. (*Onchocerca* spp.) Worldwide distribution. Signs include subcutaneous nodules along the brisket, lateral thigh area.

T R E A T M E N T: Ivermectin (0.2 mg/kg) may be effective. Do not use in lactating animals.

Fungal

DERMATOMYCOSES: RINGWORM. (usually *Trichophyton verrucosum*) Common. Signs include circular lesions, with thickening of skin, and alopecia. Regresses in 10–14 weeks. More common in younger animals. Rarely, oral lesions may interfere with food intake.

T R E A T M E N T: Topical dilute iodine or Captan solutions. Calves may be treated with griseofulvin orally.

Viral

PAPILLOMATOSIS. (papovavirus) Signs include single or multiple, slow-growing warts on skin—often on head, neck, teats. Associated with skin abrasions. Spontaneous regression is usual.

T R E A T M E N T: Autogenous vaccines may be used in severe cases. Large warts may require surgical intervention.

VESICULAR LESIONS*

Vesicular Stomatitis. (rhabdovirus) Arthropod transmission suspected. Occurs in North and South America. Affects all large animal species. Vesicles develop on lips, in oral cavity, at coronary band, in interdigital spaces and near teat orifice. Rupture produces ulcerative lesions; fever, anorexia, weight loss, drooling, and lameness occur. Long course, 3–4 weeks.

T R E A T M E N T: Palliative. Isolation of affected animals important for control.

Foot and Mouth Disease. (picornavirus) Signs are similar to vesicular stomatitis and include rapid spread, severe weight loss, fever, and oral and foot lesions. Does not affect horses. Isolation of affected cases is essential to prevent spread. Slaughter policy usually used to eliminate disease.

T R E A T M E N T: None. Vaccines are available in enzootic areas.

Bluetongue. (orbivirus) Mainly a disease of sheep. Usually subclinical in cattle. Signs include fever, ulceration of mouth, necrosis of dental pad, coronitis, thimbling of hoof, and occasionally, teat lesions.

T R E A T M E N T: None specific. Topical treatment of skin lesions.

Lumpy Skin Disease. (poxvirus) Africa. Multiple cutaneous nodules.
T R E A T M E N T: None specific.

Bacterial

SKIN TUBERCULOSIS. (etiology uncertain) Role of acid-fast organisms in skin tuberculosis is unclear. Discrete subcutaneous swellings on distal forelimb is most common presentation.

T R E A T M E N T: None specific.

BOVINE FARCY. (*Mycobacterium farcinogens, Nocardia farcinica*) Tropical disease and chronic. Signs include purulent discharge from lymphatic tissue, especially in lower limbs.

T R E A T M E N T: Parenteral sodium iodide may effect some improvement.

ULCERATIVE LYMPHANGITIS. (*Corynebacterium pseudotuberculosis*) Uncommon. Signs include subcutaneous lymph node enlargement,

---

*Note: Important differential diagnoses for the vesicular diseases include *mucosal disease, infectious bovine rhinotracheitis, malignant catarrhal fever, rinderpest.*

with cording of lymphatics. Lymph nodes may rupture to discharge yellow-green pus.

T R E A T M E N T: Parenteral penicillin and local treatment are indicated.

Miscellaneous Conditions

GANGRENE. Potential causes include ergot poisoning (*Claviceps purpurea*), chronic salmonellosis in calves, mastitis (udder gangrene) (*Staphylococcus aureus*), bovine ulcerative mammillitis (udder gangrene), frostbite injury, and fescue poisoning.

T R E A T M E N T: None effective.

NEOPLASIA. Rare. Skin form of bovine leukosis. Squamous cell carcinoma of vulva, mastocytoma, and melanoma are potential causes.

T R E A T M E N T: Surgical excision in selected cases.

ZINC DEFICIENCY. Uncommon. Signs include cracking and wrinkling of skin, alopecia, and coronitis.

T R E A T M E N T: Supplemental zinc sulfate in diet is protective; parenteral form may be used in clinical cases.

SHEEP

Pruritic Skin Diseases

Parasitic

SHEEP SCAB. (*Psoroptes ovis,* nonburrowing mite) Signs include nibbling at affected area, pruritus, loss of wool (mainly over flank). Primarily a fall/winter disease. Notifiable disease.

T R E A T M E N T: Isolation, dipping of affected animals with solutions containing gamma hexachlorocyclohexane (lindane), diazinon, or propetamphos.

SCABIES. (*Sarcoptes scabiei*) Mainly affects face. Signs include intense pruritus and thick scabs over affected areas.

T R E A T M E N T: Ivermectin (0.2 mg/kg/s.c.) or topical organophosphates repeated at weekly intervals for two to three treatments.

TICK INFESTATION. Common. Heavy infestations may cause weight loss. The major importance of ticks is their involvement in disease transmission.

T R E A T M E N T: Topical acaracides as sprays or dips, or as medicated ear tags. Ivermectin (0.2 mg/kg).

HEAD FLY INFESTATION. (*Hydrotaea irritans*) Occurs in Europe and U.K. Bites cause irritation, self-inflicted trauma, and "broken heads" (damaged skin).

T R E A T M E N T: Topical insecticides and spraying of insect breeding grounds. See under Control and Treatment of External Parasitism, pp. 298–299.

SHEEP KED INFESTATION. (*Melophagus ovinus*) Keds are bloodsuckers whose bites cause intense irritation. Live their entire life cycle on host. Wool staining by keds is a significant problem.

T R E A T M E N T: Dipping of all animals in herd.

MYIASIS: BLOW-FLY STRIKE. (*Phormia* spp., *Lucilia* spp., *Calliphora* spp.) Flies are attracted to soiled or dead tissue. Larvae develop in the fleece, creating intense pruritus, and debilitation. The sheep may develop toxemia in severe cases and some may die.

T R E A T M E N T: Clipping of affected area, wound care, topical insecticides.

PEDICULOSIS: LOUSE INFESTATION. (*Damalinia* spp., *Linognathus* spp.) Signs include irritation and broken, yellow-stained fleece.

T R E A T M E N T: Topical insecticides or ivermectin (0.2 mg/kg s.c.).

Fungal

DERMATOMYCOSES: RINGWORM. (*Trichophyton* spp., *Microsporum* spp.) Signs include circumscribed, scaly, or encrusted lesions, pruritus, and loss of wool.

T R E A T M E N T: Topical Captan or iodine solution, oral griseofulvin. Isolate severely affected animals.

Bacterial

STAPHYLOCOCCAL DERMATITIS. (*Staphylococcus aureus*) Multiple small pustules are common over facial area.

T R E A T M E N T: Topical and/or parenteral antibiotics may be indicated.

Viral

SCRAPIE. Slow virus disease. Agent not fully identified. Only adults are affected. Signs include sporadic neurologic involvement with excitability, muscle tremors, pruritus, incoordination, and recumbency. Reported in many countries. Death occurs in all cases. Wool loss is extensive due to scratching.

T R E A T M E N T: None.

Miscellaneous Conditions

PHOTOSENSITIZATION
Primary. Due to ingestion of photodynamic agents (e.g., hypericin from St. Johnswort, fagopyrum from buckwheat.)

Secondary. Liver damage results from failure to excrete phylloerythrin. Signs include edema and erythema of nonpigmented areas, such as face, ears, eyelids, and coronary bands. Sloughing and pruritus may follow.

T R E A T M E N T: Identify and remove inciting cause. House animals to prevent exposure to ultraviolet light. Corticosteroids may be indicated.

Nonpruritic Skin Diseases

Parasitic

CHORIOPTIC MANGE. (*Chorioptes* spp.) Signs include thickened, wrinkled skin, affecting primarily the scrotum and hindlimbs. Not common.

T R E A T M E N T: Topical solutions, e.g., 2% lime sulfur, or ivermectin (0.2 mg/kg s.c.).

DEMODICOSIS. (*Demodex* spp.) Rare in sheep. Signs include pustules on nose, around eyes, and on coronet. Usually subclinical.

T R E A T M E N T: Topical rotenone, amitraz, or ivermectin (0.2 mg/kg s.c.).

Bacterial

DERMATOPHILOSIS: LUMPY WOOL DISEASE. (*Dermatophilus congolensis*) Also known as "strawberry foot rot." Common. Wetting of skin predisposes to infection. Signs include wool loss or ulcerative pododermatitis with scab formation (strawberry foot rot). Rarely pruritic.

T R E A T M E N T: Topical alum or 0.5% zinc sulfate may be useful. Systemic antibiotics may be indicated.

CASEOUS LYMPHADENITIS. (*Corynebacterium pseudotuberculosis*) Secondary to contamination of skin wounds, e.g., at shearing, abscessation of regional lymph nodes, rupture and contamination of environment.

T R E A T M E N T: None specific. Surgical excision feasible in selected cases. Isolate or cull affected animals.

FOOT ROT. (*Bacteroides nodosus, Fusobacterium necrophorum*) Common. Varying degrees of severity.

Benign Foot Rot: Scald. Associated with mild underrunning of horn and mild dermatitis.

Virulent Foot Rot. Signs include marked interdigital dermatitis, necrosis of skin, fetid odor, severe underrunning of sole, and lameness. Outbreaks occur.

T R E A T M E N T: Individual cases may be treated with parenteral (penicillin or tetracycline) or topical antibiotics (e.g., tetracycline) and trimming of underrun horn. Footbaths (5% formalin or 10% zinc sulfate) are helpful in treatment and prevention. Vaccination is an effective means of control. Chronically affected animals should be culled.

INFECTIOUS BULBAR NECROSIS. (*Fusobacterium necrophorum, Actinomyces pyogenes*) Foot abscesses in adult sheep.

T R E A T M E N T: Local treatment and parenteral pencillin or sulfonamides are effective.

Viral

CONTAGIOUS ECTHYMA: SORE MOUTH, ORF. (parapoxvirus) Common. Direct transmission. Signs include scabby proliferative lesions, predominantly on lips, but also on eyelids. Feet can be affected. More severe in lambs. Low mortality.

T R E A T M E N T: None effective. Self-limiting disease. Vaccination seems to be protective.

ULCERATIVE DERMATOSIS: "LIP AND LEG." Similar to orf. Signs include lesions on philtrum of lips, on coronary bands, and in interdigital spaces. Self-limiting.

T R E A T M E N T: None specific.

BLUETONGUE. (orbivirus) Signs include fever, anorexia, depression, and cracking and fissuring of skin of lips and muzzle (ears may also be affected). Coronitis and sloughing of hoof may occur. Diarrhea and pneumonia are common.

T R E A T M E N T: Treatment with systemic antibiotics is helpful to control secondary infections. Vaccination may be used in enzootic areas for control of disease.

Miscellaneous Conditions

GANGRENE. Result of fescue poisoning, frostbite, ergotism. May affect distal limbs and tip of ears.

T R E A T M E N T: None specific.

REDFOOT DISEASE. (suspected hereditary etiology) Rare. Affects

Scottish Blackface sheep. Signs include sloughing of skin of lower limbs and buccal mucosa, and separation of hoof from coronary band. There may also be corneal lesions. Signs develop within a few days of birth.

T R E A T M E N T: None specific.

Abnormalities of the Fleece

BORDER DISEASE: "HAIRY SHAKERS." In utero infection with border disease virus. Halo hairs are prominent over the neck, dorsum, flanks, and rump. There may also be abnormal pigmentation of the wool.

T R E A T M E N T: None specific.

COPPER DEFICIENCY/MOLYBDENOSIS. Wool loses its crimp. Fine wool becomes steely; dark wool becomes depigmented or shows bands of discoloration. Anemia, diarrhea, and a history of swayback in herd may be noted.

T R E A T M E N T: Copper sulfate (5 g per week p.o. or 5 mg/kg in feed) is recommended for treatment. Mineral licks may be helpful.

WOOL SLIP. Cause unknown, but increased cortisol levels have been implicated. Affects housed sheep. Signs include loss of wool over hindquarters, often after shearing in winter.

T R E A T M E N T: None specific.

DERMATOPHILOSIS: LUMPY WOOL DISEASE. (*Dermatophilus congolensis*) See similar entry under Nonpruritic Skin Diseases, p. 16.

FLEECE ROT. (*Pseudomonas aeruginosa*) Signs include dermatitis, with matting of overlying wool. Withers and dorsum are commonly affected. Wool is easily removed in severe cases and may be discolored. Wet weather predisposes to the disease.

T R E A T M E N T: Similar to dermatophilosis. Vaccination may reduce the incidence of disease.

ZINC DEFICIENCY. Signs include wool loss and wrinkling and thickening of skin. Pica may be seen, with affected lambs eating their wool. There is a decrease in growth rate and fertility.

T R E A T M E N T: Zinc sulfate may be added to feed or free-choice mineral licks may be provided.

DEBILITATION. Chronic diseases, e.g., paratuberculosis (Johne's disease), cobalt deficiency, and caseous lymphadenitis, may lead to wool loss.

T R E A T M E N T: Correct underlying problem.

GOATS

Pruritic Skin Diseases

Parasitic

MANGE
Sarcoptic. (*Sarcoptes scabiei*) Signs include intense pruritus, self-mutilation, and severe crusting and fissuring of skin. Periorbital skin and ears are affected initially. Then crusting spreads to neck, withers, axillae, perineum, and groin.

T R E A T M E N T: Ivermectin (0.2 mg/kg s.c.) or two or three weekly treatments with topical organophosphates.

Chorioptic. (*Chorioptes caprae*) Signs include intense pruritus, involving neck, base of tail, and flank. Infection may involve face, scrotum, and feet. Skin is scaly and thickened; crusts develop later. Crusts occur on plantar/palmar surface of fetlocks.

T R E A T M E N T: Topical lime sulfur, organophosphates, or ivermectin (0.2 mg/kg s.c.).

LOUSE INFESTATION. (*Damalinia* spp.—biting, *Linognathus* spp.—sucking) Signs include pruritus and localized alopecia, possibly accompanied by anemia. Parasites are visible on examination of the coat.

T R E A T M E N T: See Mange, Sarcoptic, above.

KED INFESTATION. (*Melophagus ovinus*) Bites cause intense irritation, pruritus, and damage to hair. Spread by direct contact.

T R E A T M E N T: Annual dipping of herd is recommended for control.

BLOW-FLY STRIKE. (*Lucilia* spp., *Calliphora* spp.) Common. Many species of fly may cause "strike." Skin wounds and contamination of perineum with diarrhea predispose to infection. Larvae are seen in large numbers over affected area.

T R E A T M E N T: Perineum should be kept clean and wounds appropriately cared for.

BESNOITIOSIS: "DIMPLE." (*Besnoitia besnoiti*) Signs include chronic dermatitis of ventral abdomen and legs, with dry seborrhea and multiple, crusty lesions. Cracked skin may ooze serum. Fetlocks may have severe lesions. Occurs in southern USA, Africa, and parts of Europe. Zoonotic.

T R E A T M E N T: None effective.

Fungal

DERMATOMYCOSES: RINGWORM. (*Trichophyton verrucosum*) Signs include circumscribed, scaly, or encrusted area with alopecia and possibly pruritus. Ears, face, and neck are most commonly affected.

T R E A T M E N T: Oral griseofulvin or topical iodine solutions are effective.

Viral

SCRAPIE. Slow virus disease. Causes chronic wasting, pruritus, and death.

T R E A T M E N T: None specific.

PSEUDORABIES. (porcine herpesvirus) Pigs act as a source of infection. Signs include neurologic signs, pyrexia, pruritus, and depression. Disease has a short course and high mortality.

T R E A T M E N T: None specific.

Miscellaneous Conditions

PEMPHIGUS FOLIACEUS. Rare. Signs include crusty, pruritic lesions of ventral abdomen, scrotum, and tail.

T R E A T M E N T: Parenteral or oral corticosteroids.

PHOTOSENSITIZATION
Primary. Caused by ingestion of St. Johnswort or buckwheat.
Secondary. Due to liver damage, e.g., by pyrrolizidine alkaloids.

T R E A T M E N T: Remove animals from source and protect them from exposure to ultraviolet light. Corticosteroids may be indicated.

Nonpruritic Skin Diseases

PARASITIC DEMODICOSIS. (*Demodex caprae*) Signs include skin nodules 1–2 cm in diameter, containing mites. Caseous material exudes after rupture of nodule. Face, neck, shoulders, and sides of trunk are affected.

T R E A T M E N T: Topical rotenone or amitraz or ivermectin (0.2 mg/kg s.c.).

PSOROPTIC MANGE. (*Psoroptes cuniculi*) Scaliness develops on inner surface of ear and head shaking is common.

T R E A T M E N T: Topical organophosphates, lime sulfur, or ivermectin (0.2 mg/kg s.c.).

Bacterial

DERMATOPHILOSIS. (*Dermatophilus congolensis*) This disease is a superficial exudative dermatitis associated with skin damage by wetting or insect damage. Secondary staphylococcal or other infections may be superimposed.

TREATMENT: Remove cause. Topical iodine solutions or lime sulfur is effective, if applied daily for 1 week and subsequently once weekly until resolved. Parenteral antibiotics may be helpful.

STAPHYLOCOCCAL DERMATITIS. (*Staphylococcus aureus*) Signs include nodular lesions on dorsum or udder.

TREATMENT: Administer antiseptics, e.g., iodophors or chlorhexidine, or parenteral penicillin.

Viral

CONTAGIOUS ECTHYMA: ORF, SORE MOUTH. (parapoxvirus) Signs include scabby lesions, predominantly on lips. Primarily, young goats are affected, but adults can get severe disease. In kids, death may occur from debilitation.

TREATMENT: None specific. Vaccination may be useful for control in endemic areas.

PAPILLOMATOSIS: WARTS. Papovavirus warts are firmly attached to skin and usually occur on head and neck. May also involve lips. Resembles orf. Usually self-limiting. Herd outbreaks may occur.

TREATMENT: Usually not necessary.

GOATPOX. Occurs in Middle East and Africa. Signs include anorexia, pyrexia, rhinitis, and conjunctivitis. Widespread papules are seen. High morbidity.

TREATMENT: None specific.

FOOT AND MOUTH DISEASE. (picornavirus) Signs include vesicular lesions in oral cavity, on coronary band, in interdigital spaces, and on teats. Highly contagious. Reportable disease.

TREATMENT: Supportive care, if in enzootic area.

Miscellaneous Conditions

ZINC DEFICIENCY. May be a cause of alopecia.

TREATMENT: Supplementation with 0.5–1.0 g of zinc sulfate daily is effective in prevention.

URINE SCALD. May be seen in bucks in breeding season and affects head region and back of forelimbs.

TREATMENT: None specific.

IODINE DEFICIENCY. Goiter, alopecia, and high mortality of newborn kids is associated with iodine deficiency.

T R E A T M E N T: Iodine in fertilizers or mineral licks will help prevent disease.

SELENIUM DEFICIENCY. Signs include periorbital alopecia with seborrhea.
T R E A T M E N T: May be responsive to dietary selenium supplementation.

MYCETOMAS: FUNGAL TUMOR. Single lesions, usually occur on limbs. Very rare.
T R E A T M E N T: Surgical excision.

NEOPLASIA. Quite rare. Occurs as fibroma, squamous cell carcinoma, or melanoma.
T R E A T M E N T: Surgical excision in selected cases.

STICKY KID SYNDROME. Thought to be due to a recessive gene. Affects Golden Guernsey goats. Signs include matted, sticky coat, which fails to dry normally after birth.
T R E A T M E N T: Provide supportive care. May resolve spontaneously.

Swellings of the Neck and Head

CASEOUS LYMPHADENITIS. (*Corynebacterium pseudotuberculosis*) Common and contagious. Signs include abscesses, often in head and neck region, usually in lymph nodes. Believed to enter through skin abrasions.
T R E A T M E N T: None effective. Surgical excision in selected cases.

SALIVARY CYSTS. The cysts resemble cheek abscesses and are usually fluctuant. Aspiration will confirm diagnosis.
T R E A T M E N T: Surgical removal.

CHEEK ABSCESSATION. Trauma to mucosa (thorns, etc.) may cause cheek abscess, which can develop a sinus tract to the exterior.
T R E A T M E N T: Surgical drainage.

IMPACTION OF CUD. Cud may become impacted between molars and cheek. Oral cavity examination confirms diagnosis.
T R E A T M E N T: Remove impaction.

BRANCHIAL CYSTS. Cysts occur at base of wattles and contain thin fluid. They are usually apparent at birth but may not be noticed until later.

T R E A T M E N T: Surgical drainage or excision.

SOFT TISSUE ABSCESSES. (*Staphylococcus* spp., *Actinomyces pyogenes*) Sporadic.
T R E A T M E N T: Surgical drainage or excision.

GOITER. Results from severe iodine deficiency. Marked symmetric swelling in throatlatch area due to thyroid gland enlargement. Goiter develops over a few months.
T R E A T M E N T: Add supplemental iodine to diet.

WARBLES. (*Hypoderma* spp.) Similar to disease in cattle. Exotic in goats. Occurs in Middle East and Eastern Europe.
T R E A T M E N T: Topical rotenone or organophosphates.

NEOPLASIA. Rare.
T R E A T M E N T: Surgical excision in selected cases.

PIGS

Preweaning Piglets

Congenital Conditions

DERMATOSIS VEGETANS. (inherited) Uncommon. Signs may be present at birth or develop later. Raised pink swellings on ventrum become encrusted. Occurs within first 4 weeks of life.
T R E A T M E N T: None specific.

PITYRIASIS ROSEA. (possibly inherited) Signs include small flat plaques of erythema on flanks and groin. Appears to be self-limiting.
T R E A T M E N T: None. Resolves spontaneously within a few weeks.

EPITHELIOGENESIS IMPERFECTA. Uncommon. Whole patches of skin are absent over various areas of body. May be confused with wounds.
T R E A T M E N T: None. Affected piglets die.

Bacterial Skin Diseases

EXUDATIVE EPIDERMITIS: GREASY PIG DISEASE. (*Staphylococcus hyicus*) Occurs most commonly in pigs under 6 weeks old. Signs include listlessness, crusty and greasy skin, increasing size of scabs, and matting of hair. Death may occur in severely affected pigs.
T R E A T M E N T: Administer parenteral antibiotics or topical

antiseptic washes. Clipping of teeth and preventing abrasions due to rough flooring will reduce the incidence.

FACIAL DERMATITIS. (possibly staphylococcal) High incidence in litters. Associated with trauma and fighting. Signs include scabs, with underlying ulcers.
T R E A T M E N T: Administer local or parenteral antibiotic therapy in severe cases.

ERYSIPELAS. (*Erysipelothrix rhusiopathiae*) Nonpruritic. Signs include diamond-shaped lesions of skin, which are raised and gradually become red. Associated fever, anorexia, and depression may be severe. Death may occur.
T R E A T M E N T: Parenteral penicillin is the drug of choice. Vaccination is effective in preventing the disease. Mortality is high if condition is untreated.

Viral Skin Diseases

SWINEPOX. (possible link with ectoparasitism) Common in young pigs. Signs include fever and development of small red papules, which later rupture and become crusty. Lesions are distributed over ventral abdomen and sometimes involve oral region.
T R E A T M E N T: Topical solutions for ectoparasite control are recommended (see Ectoparasites, p. 301).

Miscellaneous Conditions

TRAUMA. Common. Teat and vulval lesions may result from hard or abrasive flooring.
T R E A T M E N T: Remove inciting causes. Administer topical ointments and care for wound.

Postweaning and Adult Pigs

Parasitic Skin Diseases

SCABIES. (*Sarcoptes scabiei* var. *suis*) Very common. Signs include alopecia, and excoriations covered by thick brown scabs. Hair loss over flanks occurs, and head shaking from irritation may lead to aural hematomas. Contagious.
T R E A T M E N T: Topical organophosphates, 2% lime sulfur solution, or ivermectin (0.2 mg/kg).

DEMODICOSIS. (*Demodex phylloides*) Nonpruritic. Signs include small nodules and pustules, and lesions on face, neck, and abdomen. Often subclinical.

TREATMENT: Topical rotenone, amitraz, or ivermectin (0.2 mg/kg).

PEDICULOSIS: LOUSE INFESTATION. (*Haematopinus suis*) Pruritic. Spread by direct contact. Skin damage may result from constant scratching. Potential vector of swinepox.

TREATMENT: See Scabies.

Fungal Skin Diseases

RINGWORM. (*Trichophyton* spp., *Microsporum* spp.) Nonpruritic. Signs include circular, raised lesions, commonly behind ears or on dorsum. Usually seen in weaners.

TREATMENT: Treat with topical copper salts or dilute iodine; administer oral griseofulvin (10 mg/kg).

Bacterial Skin Diseases

EXUDATIVE EPIDERMITIS: GREASY PIG DISEASE. (*Staphylococcus hyicus*) Pruritic. More common in preweaning pigs. Ear necrosis may occur in some cases.

TREATMENT: Parenteral antibiotics are indicated. Antiseptic washes may be helpful. See also under Preweaning Piglets, p. 23.

ERYSIPELAS. (*Erysipelothrix rhusiopathiae*)
Acute Form. Signs include fever, depression, and the development of raised erythematous diamond-shaped lesions on the skin. Death may occur.

TREATMENT: Administer parenteral penicillin.

Viral Skin Diseases

SWINEPOX. See Preweaning Piglets, p. 23.
SWINE VESICULAR DISEASE. (enterovirus) Nonpruritic. Affects swine only. Primarily causes vesicular lesions of interdigital area and coronary band, skin of limbs, teats, and occasionally tongue. Other signs include fever, and severe lameness. Clinical presentation is very similar to that in foot and mouth disease.

TREATMENT: Provide supportive care. No specific therapy.

FOOT AND MOUTH DISEASE. (picornavirus) Nonpruritic. Lesions are indistinguishable from swine vesicular disease. Reportable disease. Also affects ruminants.

TREATMENT: Provide supportive care. No specific therapy.

VESICULAR STOMATITIS. (calicivirus) Nonpruritic. Rare in pigs. Horses and ruminants affected.

T R E A T M E N T: Provide supportive care. No specific therapy.

Miscellaneous Conditions

PARAKERATOSIS. Due to zinc deficiency. Nonpruritic. Clinical disease is rare. Usually growing pigs are affected. Papules develop from erythematous areas on ventral abdomen and spread to limbs. Skin cracks may develop. Symmetric distribution.

T R E A T M E N T: Oral zinc supplementation and topical astringents are indicated.

NICOTINIC ACID DEFICIENCY. Signs include dermatitis, with diarrhea and anorexia.

T R E A T M E N T: Supplementation of diet with nicotinic acid or tryptophan is indicated.

BIOTIN DEFICIENCY. Nonpruritic. Signs include crusty dermatitis with cracking of hooves.

T R E A T M E N T: Dietary supplementation is indicated.

TRAUMA. Dermal lesions may result from biting or fighting, scratching (lice), tail or flank sucking, tethering chains or pen elements.

T R E A T M E N T: Topical ointments and supportive care are indicated.

SUNBURN. Heat stroke may occur in white-skinned pigs kept outdoors without shade.

T R E A T M E N T: Provide supportive care and administer topical ointments on affected areas.

ABSCESSES. (*Actinobacillus suis*) Abscesses may occur in subcutis.

T R E A T M E N T: May require surgical drainage or excision.

NEW WORLD CAMELIDS

Parasitic Skin Diseases

SCABIES. (*Sarcoptes scabiei*) Signs include severe pruritus, diffuse crusting with alopecia, and hyperpigmentation. Eruptions generally occur on perineum and limbs, but may be generalized.

T R E A T M E N T: Ivermectin (0.2 mg/kg).

DEMODICOSIS. (*Demodex* spp.) Nonpruritic. Usually localized, draining tracts may be present.
T R E A T M E N T: Administer topical rotenone, amitraz, or ivermectin (0.2 mg/kg).

CHORIOPTIC MANGE. (*Chorioptes bovis*) Signs include pruritus, alopecia and crusting on the feet and interdigital areas.
T R E A T M E N T: Topical dressings may be useful, e.g., 2% lime sulfur or 50% methoxychlor powder. Ivermectin (0.2 mg/kg) is also effective.

PEDICULOSIS: LOUSE INFESTATION. (*Damalinia* spp., *Microthoracis* spp.) Pruritus is usually absent. Signs include alopecia and excoriation in pruritic cases, otherwise subclinical.
T R E A T M E N T: Ivermectin (0.2 mg/kg) is effective against *Microthoracis*. Pour-on solutions of fenthion are effective.

MYIASIS. Larvae of various flies may lay eggs on hair, leading to myiasis. See similar entry under Sheep, p. 15.
T R E A T M E N T: Clipping of affected area and application of dilute organophosphate solutions are usually effective.

TICK INFESTATION. Nonpruritic. Signs include reddening and macule formation at site of attachment. Spinose ear tick lives in the ear and may cause head shaking.
T R E A T M E N T: Difficult to control. Application of insecticides/acaricides as spray may be efficacious.

Fungal Infections

RINGWORM. (*Trichophyton* spp.) Nonpruritic. Signs include circular lesions with thick crusting.
T R E A T M E N T: Topical application of dilute iodine or Captan solution is recommended. Repeat treatments as necessary.

COCCIDIOIDOMYCOSIS. (*Coccidioides immitis*) The skin form is always accompanied ultimately by systemic involvement, such as pneumonia, osteomyelitis, and neurologic signs. Skin signs include large crusty or ulcerative nodular lesions or smaller dermal/epidermal nodules.
T R E A T M E N T: None effective.

Viral Infections

CONTAGIOUS ECTHYMA: ORF, SORE-MOUTH. Nonpruritic. Signs include crusty, proliferative lesion on lips, around eyes, and at other mucocutaneous junctions. Cracking of affected area may occur.

T R E A T M E N T: No specific treatments. Topical antiseptics may prevent secondary infection.

PAPILLOMATOSIS: WARTS. Nonpruritic. May occur anywhere on body, but happens more frequently around head. Spontaneous regression.
T R E A T M E N T: None specific. Autogenous vaccines might be considered in severe cases.

VESICULAR DISEASE. Not reported in North America. Potential causes include vesicular stomatitis and foot and mouth disease.
T R E A T M E N T: None specific.

Bacterial Infections

DERMATOPHILOSIS. (*Dermatophilus congolensis*) Nonpruritic. Damage to skin is associated with chronic wetting. Crusting and fiber matting are common.
T R E A T M E N T: Parenteral penicillin or tetracyclines are effective.

FURUNCULOSIS: BOILS. (*Staphylococcus* spp.) Nonpruritic. Alopecia and crustiness reflect purulent inflammation of the hair follicles. Facial area and limbs are affected.
T R E A T M E N T: Parenteral administration of antibiotics is indicated. Surgical drainage may be necessary for large boils.

ULCERATIVE PODODERMATITIS. (*Bacteroides* spp., *Fusobacterium* spp., *Actinomyces pyogenes*, other *Actinomyces* spp.) Nonpruritic. Signs include abscessation and ulceration of solar aspect of foot pads.
T R E A T M E N T: Local foot care and parenteral antibiotics are indicated, but prognosis is guarded.

Miscellaneous Conditions

CERVICAL ALOPECIA. Nonpruritic. Occurs in 2-year-olds in springtime and may be a normal pattern of fiber shedding. Skin appears normal and the hair usually regrows.
T R E A T M E N T: None effective or necessary.

ZINC-RESPONSIVE DERMATOSIS. Nonpruritic. Usually seen between 1 and 2 years of age. Signs include large areas of alopecia, scaling, and thickening of skin. Most obvious in head region, ventrum, and groin area.

T R E A T M E N T: Zinc sulfate (1 g/day orally) in combination with topical antiseborrheic creams.

DARK NOSE SYNDROME. (etiology unknown) Pruritic. Involves dorsum of nose. More common in dark-faced animals.

T R E A T M E N T: Corticosteroids may elicit some improvement.

STEROID-RESPONSIVE DERMATITIS. Pruritic and idiopathic. Seen in younger animals. Signs include scaling and hair loss due to scratching.

T R E A T M E N T: Oral prednisone may be useful caution, but may cause abortion in pregnant animals.

Gastrointestinal System

DIARRHEA

PATHOGENESIS

The intestinal mucosa has three major functions: secretion, digestion, and absorption. Mature cells specialize in the digestive and absorption processes, and immature cells are primarily involved in secretion.

Infectious agents (e.g., rotaviruses) that damage only the mature cells impair digestion and absorption, but secretion is unaffected. Agents (e.g., coronaviruses) that damage all epithelial cells lead, in addition, to secretory derangement. Enterotoxigenic *Escherichia coli* (ETEC) causes no structural damage, but activates the cellular secretory mechanisms of the immature epithelial cells, leading to massive fluid loss. Other agents, including *Clostridium perfringens*, *Salmonella* spp., and *Coccidia* spp., may cause more extensive damage, leading to bloody diarrhea (dysentery).

Neonates

NEONATAL DIARRHEA. Neonatal diarrhea results from an interaction between *agent*, *host*, and *environment*. Neonates depend on passive acquisition of immunoglobulins via colostrum, in the immediate postnatal period (within 12 h) to protect them against pathogenic organisms.

Factors that inhibit adequate ingestion of colostrum include

1. weak or abnormal neonate that is unable to stand or suckle
2. inadequate colostrum quality or quantity, e.g., as from a first-calf heifer, from premilking, or from leakage
3. maternal illness resulting in recumbency, e.g., hypocalcemia, mastitis, birth trauma
4. poor mothering, i.e., rejection of neonate
5. poor udder conformation.

Environmental factors leading to increased disease incidence:

1. overcrowding
2. failure to isolate infected animals
3. fluctuations in environmental temperature leading to stress (e.g., in piglets a decrease in environmental temperature leads to an increase of E. coli colonization of the gut).

Agents associated with neonatal diarrhea include

1. bacteria
2. viruses
3. protozoa
4. fungi
5. parasites.

Foals

SEPTICEMIA. Primarily due to gram-negative organisms (e.g., E. coli, Klebsiella pneumoniae, Salmonella spp., and Actinobacillus equuli); Inadequate colostrum intake predisposes to disease. Diarrhea may be a feature.

COLIBACILLOSIS. (enterotoxigenic Escherichia coli) Not common. Signs include profuse, watery diarrhea, rapid dehydration, and severe depression.

SALMONELLOSIS

Acute Form. Signs include watery diarrhea, colic, fever, dehydration, anorexia, and depression.

Chronic Form. Not common. Mild, persistent diarrhea.

CLOSTRIDIAL ENTEROTOXEMIA. (Clostridia spp.: C. perfringens types A, B, C; C. sordellii, C. difficile) Sporadic occurrence. Peracute or acute, hemorrhagic, necrotizing enteritis. Signs include severe dehydration, toxemia, diarrhea, and depression. High mortality.

RHODOCOCCUS EQUI INFECTION. Primarily a respiratory disease. In the intestinal form diarrhea may be acute, intermittent, or chronic. Affects foals 1–6 months of age.

ROTAVIRUS INFECTION. Uncomplicated infection probably causes mild to moderate diarrhea. Secondary bacterial complications may lead to fever, severe diarrhea, depression, and death.

CORONAVIRUS INFECTION. Has been isolated from diarrheic foals. Role of agent unclear.

CRYPTOSPORIDIOSIS. (*Cryptosporidium* spp.) Agent has been isolated from foals with diarrhea. Significance uncertain.

THREADWORM INFECTION. (*Strongyloides westeri*) Small nematode. Transferred in mare's milk. Heavy infection may cause mild diarrhea.

ASCARIASIS. (*Parascaris equorum*) Large roundworm. Causes ill-thrift, diarrhea, and a pot-bellied appearance. Usually affects older foals (4–10 months).

NUTRITIONAL ABNORMALITIES

Excessive Intake. Occurs especially under conditions of artificial rearing. Foal is afebrile and alert.

Mechanical Irritation. Ingesting sand or other debris has been suggested as a factor in foal diarrhea.

FOAL HEAT DIARRHEA. Affects foals between 4–14 days of age. Signs include lack of fever, alertness, and good appetite. Self-limiting.

Adult Horses

MONOCYTIC EHRLICHIOSIS: POTOMAC HORSE FEVER. (*Ehrlichia risticii*) Enzootic to certain areas of USA and Canada. Signs include fever, diarrhea, depression, and anorexia. Laminitis is also commonly present.

SALMONELLOSIS. (*Salmonella* spp.) Frequently preceded by stress.

Peracute Form. Septicemia occurs, with death in 6–12 h. Rare.

Acute Form. Signs include fever, anorexia, depression, and mild to moderate abdominal pain. Diarrhea occurs in 1–4 days post infection, is usually profuse and may be fetid. Duration is usually less than 7 days.

Chronic Form. Thought to be a sequel to the acute form, chronic salmonellosis reflects the severe intestinal damage of acute disease.

INTESTINAL CLOSTRIDIOSIS. (*Clostridium perfringens* type A).

Peracute Disease. Signs include severe toxemia, anorexia, and depression. There may also be projectile, watery, dark diarrhea and severe dehydration. Mortality is high. This disease is clinically indistinguishable from other peracute septicemias or toxemias.

PARASITIC COLITIS AND TYPHLITIS. (*Cyathostomum* spp.) Profuse chronic diarrhea. Signs include severe weight loss, muscle atrophy, and occasionally, subcutaneous edema. Occurs in winter to spring in northern hemisphere. Larvae may be identified in scrapings of rectal mucosa.

STACHYBOTRYOTOXICOSIS. (Satratoxins B, H) Hemorrhagic diarrhea. Most frequently reported in Eastern Europe. Signs include thrombocytopenia, and stomatitis. Mortality is high.

COLITIS X. (ill-defined etiology) Peracute toxemia. Death occurs in some cases in 12–18 h. Signs include diarrhea or dysentery, following anorexia, fever, and depression. Clinically indistinguishable from monocytic Ehrlichiosis, salmonellosis, or other acute colitides.

ANTIBIOTIC-INDUCED DIARRHEA. Several cases of equine diarrhea have been linked to prior administration of antibiotics, such as tetracyclines, trimethoprim-sulfa, erythromycin, and lincomycin.

INFILTRATIVE ENTEROCOLITIS. Cellular infiltration of intestinal wall leads to chronic malabsorption or maldigestion, protein loss, chronic weight loss, low grade colic, and occasionally diarrhea. Category of illnesses includes granulomatous enteritis, eosinophilic gastroenteritis, lymphocytic-plasmacytic enteritis, and intestinal lymphosarcoma.

SAND-INDUCED DIARRHEA. Ingestion of large quantities of sand has been associated with weight loss and diarrhea in horses. History of grazing on sandy soils.

Calves (0–4 Weeks Old)

Diarrhea

COLIBACILLOSIS. (*Escherichia coli*)
Septicemic Form
Acute. Affects calves 1–4 days old. Signs include sudden onset of fever, anorexia, and depression, followed by circulatory (septic) shock. Diarrhea is frequently seen, but in peracute cases may not occur. Animals may be found dead.

Chronic. Affects calves older than 4 days. Onset is insidious. Fever and anorexia may wax and wane. Other signs include poor growth and thinness. Infection frequently localizes as arthritis, osteomyelitis, meningitis, omphalophlebitis, panophthalmitis, pneumonia, endocarditis, or pyuria.

Enterotoxigenic Form. Affects calves 0–5 days old. Enterotoxigenic *E. coli* (ETEC) increases secretion of water and electrolytes in small intestine. Commonly associated with Rotavirus. Not a true enteritis, thus absorption of electrolytes is unaffected.

SALMONELLOSIS. (*Salmonella typhimurium, S. dublin*—highly specific for cattle, *S. muenchen, S. copenhagen,* etc.) Affects calves 1–5 weeks of age.

Peracute (Septicemic) Form. Frequent cause of sudden death. Observed calves are depressed: septic shock ensues. Signs include neurologic changes and diarrhea. Colic may be evident. Death occurs in 6–36 h from time of onset.

Acute Form
Enteric. (*S. typhimurium* or *S. dublin*) Signs include fever, inap-

petence, depression, and watery diarrhea, followed by dysentery or frank blood.

Septicemic. (commonly *S. dublin*) Signs include weakness, fever, and depression. Mortality is high. May develop complications, such as meningitis, pneumonia, osteomyelitis, arthritis, or sloughing of extremities.

Chronic Form. Affects calves older than 6 weeks, up to 4 months. Signs include poor growth, loose stool, but no dysentery. Affected calves show poor hair coat and appear thin to emaciated. May have low-grade fever.

CLOSTRIDIAL ENTEROTOXEMIA. (*Clostridium perfringens*) Type C is the cause of hemorrhagic enterotoxemia, usually in calves younger than 10 days old. It causes a severe necrotizing enteritis. May cause sudden death. Types A, B, D, and E have occasionally been associated with neonatal diarrhea.

ROTAVIRUS INFECTION. Affects calves 1–20 days old (average 7 days). Destruction of tips of villi leads to impaired digestive and absorptive functions, resulting in malabsorption and osmotic diarrhea. Severity is influenced by the presence of other enteropathogens, especially ETEC. Uncomplicated infection causes mild to moderate pale yellow diarrhea, lasting 24–36 h.

CORONAVIRUS INFECTION. Usually affects calves 7–10 days old (3–20 days). More severe than rotavirus infection. Sudden onset. Signs include anorexia, depression, and gray mucoid feces, which may contain milk curds or fresh blood. Entire villus and crypt affected, leading to interference with digestion, absorption, and secretion. Severe dehydration and emaciation occur by 48 h. There are no gross lesions at necropsy, but the intestines are fluid-filled.

INFECTIOUS BOVINE RHINOTRACHEITIS. (herpesvirus type 1) Alimentary disease may occur. Mucosal lesions are also present.

OTHER VIRUS INFECTIONS. Parvo-, breda-, calici- and astroviruses have been isolated from calf diarrhea. Their role is uncertain.

CRYPTOSPORIDIOSIS. (*Cryptosporidium* spp.) Usually affects calves 10–12 days old (7–14 days). Signs include diarrhea, anorexia, tenesmus, weight loss, and, occasionally, dehydration. Organism commonly isolated from mixed infections.

COCCIDIOSIS. Usually affects calves older than 17–18 days of age. Most commonly caused by *Eimeria* spp. Signs include diarrhea, frequently with blood and mucus; dehydration; occasionally anemia; and depression. Mortality is generally low. Nervous form seen in older calves, especially in feedlots in early winter.

MYCOTIC INFECTIONS. Usually secondary to oral antibiotic therapy. Genera associated with disease are *Mucor* spp. and *Candida* spp.

ABOMASAL GROOVE DYSFUNCTION. Failure of abomasal groove to close, with subsequent fermentation of milk in the rumen. Can result in chronic diarrhea and mild bloat.

NUTRITIONAL ABNORMALITIES.

Overfeeding. Occurs especially under conditions of artificial rearing.

Milk replacements. Replacements containing starch can cause diarrhea because young calves have low maltase concentrations. Those containing sucrose cannot be digested and lead to osmotic diarrhea. Incorrect dilutions or poor preservation of milk replacer can also cause diarrhea.

DRUG-INDUCED DIARRHEA. Diarrhea in young calves has been associated with certain antibiotics, when administered orally, e.g., chloramphenicol and neomycin.

Weanling and Adult Cattle

Acute Diarrhea

SALMONELLOSIS. (*Salmonella typhimurium, S. dublin*—species-specific, *S. anatum, S. muenster,* and others) Organism shed by stressed latent carriers or active carriers (resides in gallbladder). Pregnancy, parturition, transport, surgery, and feed change are primary stressors. Mortality may be up to 40%, morbidity varies (5–20%).

Peracute Form. Animals may die without developing diarrhea.

Acute Form. Signs include fever, anorexia, depression, and dehydration. Onset of fetid diarrhea may be watery, and contain blood, epithelial casts, fibrin, or mucus. Abortion may accompany acute form, especially with *S. dublin.*

BACTERIAL SEPTICEMIA/ENDOTOXEMIA. Diarrhea may occur in association with septicemia or toxemia due to many conditions, including mastitis, septic metritis, traumatic reticuloperitonitis, and peritonitis.

YERSINIOSIS. (*Yersinia pseudotuberculosis*) Acute watery diarrhea in young cattle (weanlings to yearlings). Recognized in southern hemisphere. Occasionally fatal disease.

BOVINE VIRAL DIARRHEA: BVD. (pestivirus) High morbidity, low mortality. Signs include fever, diarrhea, ocular and nasal discharge, anorexia, and decreased rumen motility. Recovery is rapid (7–10 days). Frequently the infection is inapparent. Oral erosions are mild and transient. There is transient leucopenia.

MUCOSAL DISEASE. (BVD virus) Low morbidity, high mortality. Cattle that develop mucosal disease are thought to have been infected in utero before 125 days of gestation with *noncytopathogenic BVD virus,* and develop tolerance to this form of the virus. Subsequent infection with the *cytopathogenic form* produces clinical disease.

Signs include fever, anorexia, depression, salivation, nasal and ocular discharge, mucocutaneous erosions, blunting of tips of oral papillae, teat ulceration, fetid diarrhea (may have dysentery), tenesmus, dehydration, weight loss, coronitis, and interdigital lesions with lameness. Survivors of acute form may develop chronic disease.

WINTER DYSENTERY. (coronaviral etiology suspected) Occurs in winter months (November–March) in northern hemisphere. High morbidity, low mortality (<1%). Illness is most severe in periparturient animals. Heifers are less severely affected: animals younger than 6 months do not appear to be affected. Tends to be cyclical in occurrence.

Signs include sharp drop in milk output; and fever preceding diarrhea, which is profuse, watery, and variable in color (brown or black, frequently blood-stained). Illness has a short course (1–4 days).

MALIGNANT CATARRHAL FEVER. (herpesvirus) Disease of wild and domestic ruminants: distribution is worldwide. Acute, fatal, generalized disease. Low morbidity, high mortality (100%). Two forms of the disease are recognized.

Wildebeest-Associated Form (Africa). Occurs where cattle and wildebeest share common grazing. Has occurred in zoos in North America.

Sheep-Associated Form. Seen where cattle and sheep intermingle. Sheep show no clinical signs. No virus has been conclusively implicated in this form of the disease. Signs include persistent high fever, profuse diarrhea, tachycardia, nasal discharge, respiratory difficulty due to nasal catarrh, muzzle encrustation. Ocular lesions include corneal opacity, photophobia, and blepharospasm. Lymphadenopathy is generalized. Ulcers occur at mucocutaneous, teat, and skin–horn junctions. Neurologic disease and hematuria may occur. Peracute cases die in 2–3 days; others may survive 7–10 days.

RINDERPEST. (morbillivirus) Acute, highly contagious disease of ruminants. Occurs mainly in Africa. High morbidity and high mortality. Signs include fever and gastrointestinal tract ulceration leading to severe diarrhea or dysentery. Clinically similar to acute mucosal disease.

COCCIDIOSIS. (*Eimeria* spp.) Primarily a disease of young animals (younger than 1 year), especially calves. Infection rates are high; economic losses due mainly to decreased performance. Mortality low. More common in winter months, following close confinement. May occur in summer as a sequel to contamination around watering troughs. Stress may contribute to disease.

Signs include fever and diarrhea with moderate anorexia. May be followed by dysentery, tenesmus, and rectal prolapse. In severe cases anemia and death may occur.

BABESIOSIS. (*Babesia* spp.) "Pipe-stem" diarrhea occurs in the acute febrile stage.

RUMEN FLUKE. (*Paramphistomum* spp.) Fetid diarrhea has acute onset and becomes persistent. May develop submandibular edema (bottle jaw).

ACUTE PYRROLIZIDINE ALKALOID TOXICITY. (*Senecio* spp.—ragwort and *Crotalaria* spp. implicated) Typified by tenesmus and central nervous system involvement.

BRACKEN FERN POISONING. (*Pteridium aquilinum*) Toxin causes severe bone marrow depression, and thrombocytopenia, high fever, diarrhea or dysentery, hematuria, and bleeding from body orifices.

HEAVY-METAL POISONING

Acute Arsenic Poisoning. Signs include ruminal atony and, frequently, regurgitation and fetid diarrhea, followed by convulsions and death in severe cases.

Acute Lead Poisoning. CNS signs are main manifestations; however, gastrointestinal signs, including diarrhea, may occur.

Other Heavy Metals. Acute poisoning with copper, phosphorous, mercury, fluorine, and selenium from environmental or plant sources may cause diarrhea in cattle.

ORGANOPHOSPHATE POISONING. Source is usually topical application or oral administration of organophosphates for parasite control. Signs include salivation, incoordination, excitement, diarrhea, colic, and pupillary constriction.

GRAIN OVERLOAD. History of accidental access to high-energy carbohydrate.

Mild Cases. Signs include mild depression, inappetence, decreased ruminal activity, and mild to moderate diarrhea, often of a pasty consistency.

Severe Cases. Signs include depression, anorexia, agalactia, absence of ruminal motility, fluid-filled rumen, and pasty to watery diarrhea that may contain blood. There may also be bruxism and kicking at abdomen (colic). Later, signs of systemic shock develop, including tachycardia, tachypnea, weakness, recumbency, and coma leading to death.

Sequelae in survivors include peritonitis, liver abscessation, chronic laminitis, fungal rumenitis, ruminal hyperkeratosis, and polioencephalomalacia.

Chronic Diarrhea

SALMONELLOSIS. (*Salmonella* spp.) Relatively uncommon. Usually sequel to acute form. Signs include diarrhea, dysentery, intermittent fever, cachexia, dehydration, and ill-thrift.

PARATUBERCULOSIS: JOHNE'S DISEASE. (*Mycobacterium johnei*) Sporadic occurrence. Afebrile, wasting disease of adult cattle (2 years old or older). Signs include continuous or intermittent diarrhea. Bottle jaw may result from protein-losing enteropathy.

CHRONIC MUCOSAL DISEASE. (BVD virus) Terminal disease; sequel to acute form (see p. 36). Manifested by nasal discharge, recurrent oral ulceration, emaciation, interdigital ulcers, and intermittent or continuous diarrhea.

PARASITIC GASTROENTERITIS. (*Trichostrongylus* spp., *Ostertagia* spp.) Signs include chronic weight loss, diarrhea, and lack of fever.

Usually a herd problem. Mainly affects weanlings and young adults; summer to fall occurrence.

Type 2 Ostertagiasis. Chronic diarrhea in winter and spring.

STOMACH FLUKE. (*Paramphistomum* spp.) Immature flukes may cause acute onset of diarrhea leading to chronic diarrhea, weakness, and depression. Often leads to death. Usually affects yearlings in the late summer.

LIVER FLUKE. (*Fasciola hepatica*) Fluke migrates through the liver, and adults inhabit the bile ducts and gallbladder. Signs include weight loss, submandibular edema, anemia, and diarrhea. Signs are evident in late winter and early spring.

COPPER DEFICIENCY/MOLYBDENUM EXCESS. Signs include chronic diarrhea, anemia, ill-thrift, coat depigmentation, lameness due to bony exostoses, and infertility. Usually a herd problem.

HEAVY-METAL POISONING. Acute arsenic toxicosis (see Acute Diarrhea, p. 38) may be followed by chronic diarrhea, with variable appetite and ill-thrift.

PYRROLIZIDINE ALKALOID TOXICOSIS. Chronic diarrhea may follow the acute syndrome. There may also be tenesmus (frequently accompanied by rectal prolapse) and CNS signs.

AMYLOIDOSIS. Signs include emaciation, profuse diarrhea, polydipsia, and peripheral edema. May lead to death. Renal involvement is main feature. Many cases are presented soon after calving.

BOVINE LYMPHOSARCOMA. Diarrhea may be a feature.

Lambs and Kids (0–4 Weeks Old)

Diarrhea

COLIBACILLOSIS. (*Escherichia coli*) Usually a septicemia, but enteric signs may occur. Affects animals 1–3 days old: may see disease in 1–2-month-olds also. Survivors may develop septic arthritis and lameness. Enterotoxigenic form affects lambs in first 3 days of life, causing severe watery diarrhea and dehydration.

SEPTICEMIA. (*Listeria monocytogenes, Salmonella* spp., and *Erysipelothrix rhusiopathiae*) Diarrhea may be an accompanying sign.

ENTEROTOXEMIA. (*Clostridium perfringens*): Type C, and less commonly type B, occur in lambs younger than 2 weeks old. Kids are mainly affected by type C.

Peracute Form. Animals are found dead or severely depressed, toxemic, colicky, and moribund. Death soon follows.

Acute Form. Usually within a few days of birth, neonates have severe abdominal pain, profuse brown or hemorrhagic diarrhea, and extreme depression. Death usually occurs within 12 h. Maternal vaccination is protective if adequate colostrum is ingested.

ROTAVIRUS INFECTION. Affects lambs younger than 3 weeks old. Signs include mild diarrhea and moderate colic. Recovery is quick in uncomplicated cases. Illness is severe if *Escherichia coli* causes secondary infection.

COCCIDIOSIS. (*Eimeria* spp.) Affects lambs and kids older than 2 weeks of age. Kids appear to be more severely affected. Overcrowding and major stresses induce clinical coccidiosis, typified by acute diarrhea and sometimes dysentery. Severe anemia may accompany dysentery. Occasionally sudden death results. Major problem in housed animals.

CRYPTOSPORIDIOSIS. (*Cryptosporidium* spp.) May cause heavy losses in lambs. Kids are also affected, but usually mortality is low. Animals are commonly infected in first week of life. Diarrhea may persist for several days.

NUTRITIONAL DIARRHEA. Diarrhea caused by excessive intake, especially of milk replacer.

Weanling and Adult Sheep and Goats

PARATUBERCULOSIS: JOHNE'S DISEASE. (*Mycobacterium johnei*) A chronic, wasting disease of adult ruminants. Signs include soft, pasty feces seen late in the course of the disease in sheep, but not usually seen in goats.

YERSINIOSIS. (*Yersinia pseudotuberculosis*) Signs include fetid, green, watery diarrhea in weanling kids especially. Usually precipitated by stress. Closely resembles coccidiosis or a severe helminth infection.

BORDER DISEASE. (pestivirus) Affects weanlings and adults. Spontaneous diarrhea in lambs 2 months old or older. Becomes chronic in the same manner as bovine mucosal disease.

SYNDROME X (AVEYRON) DISEASE. (Probably caused by border disease virus) Reported in France. Signs include leukopenic enterocolitis leading to fever, severe depression, and diarrhea. Lambs and adults are affected.

OSTERTAGIASIS. (*Ostertagia* spp.) Two clinical syndromes.

Type 1. Seen in late summer to fall. Signs include diarrhea and poor growth in lambs. Severity of diarrhea varies. Herd disease.

Type 2. Seen in late winter–early spring in yearlings. Signs include chronic diarrhea, severe weight loss, and bottle jaw. Caused by emergence of hypobiotic larvae from abomasal wall.

NEMATODIASIS. (*Nematodirus* spp.) This disease of lambs occurs in early summer and causes severe black-green diarrhea. Up to 30% mortality. Recovered animals are resistant.

BLACK SCOURS. (*Trichostrongylus* spp.) Occurs in lambs and young goats. Severe cases develop anemia and may die.

COOPERIA INFECTION. (*Cooperia* spp.) Usually subclinical. Severe cases similar to trichostrongylosis.

CHABERTIA INFECTION. (*Chabertia* spp.) Heavy infections lead to diarrhea containing blood and mucus.

HAEMONCHOSIS. (*Haemonchus contortus:* "Barber's pole worm.") Major signs are anemia and hypoproteinemia. Diarrhea or constipation may occur.

STOMACH FLUKE. (*Paramphistomum* spp.) Acute hemorrhagic or catarrhal enteritis in sheep and cattle. May be fatal. Persistent foul smelling diarrhea is characteristic. Seen in fall and early winter.

LIVER FLUKE. (*Fasciola* spp.) Infection with F. *hepatica* or F. *magna*. Acute cases may die suddenly in early fall. Chronic infection with F. *hepatica* is seen in winter and early spring. Signs include anemia, lethargy, bottle jaw, brittle wool, and occasionally, diarrhea.

GRAIN OVERLOAD. History of excessive intake of grain or high-carbohydrate feeds. Signs include severe depression, toxemia, abdominal pain, and soft to pasty feces that may contain grains.

COPPER DEFICIENCY. Usually a herd problem. Most important sign is ataxia in lambs 2–4 months old. Severely deficient adults may have poor quality wool, anemia, ill-thrift, and diarrhea.

COBALT DEFICIENCY. Ill-thrift and anemia are most common signs; diarrhea is less common.

ACUTE HEAVY-METAL POISONING. Acute poisoning with arsenic, lead, copper, or other heavy metals.

Acute Cases. Signs include severe gastroenteritis, depression, and abdominal pain. There may also be regurgitation, and diarrhea may develop. High mortality.

Less Severe Cases. Animal may live for several days. Gastrointestinal disease predominates, manifested by diarrhea, dysentery, and regurgitation.

Chronic Cases. Signs include ill-thrift and depression.

Preweaning Piglets (0–4 Weeks Old)

COLIBACILLOSIS. (enterotoxigenic *Escherichia coli*) Profuse watery diarrhea within the first 5 days of life. High mortality. Signs include severe dehydration; often the whole litter is affected. Chilling and reduced intake of colostrum predispose to illness.

CLOSTRIDIAL ENTEROTOXEMIA. (*Clostridium perfringens*) Type C causes sudden onset of acute, profuse, brown-bloody diarrhea. Usually the best piglets are affected (7–10 days of age). Outbreaks occur on farms, and most of the litter become affected. Severe toxemia occurs, and many die within 12–24 h. Animals are usually afebrile. Type A causes milder disease than type C.

CAMPYLOBACTERIOSIS. (*Campylobacter coli*) Signs include mild fever for 2–3 days and may cause creamy to watery diarrhea, with or without blood, in piglets younger than 3 weeks old. A different form occurs in weaned piglets.

TRANSMISSIBLE GASTROENTERITIS: TGE. (coronavirus) Piglets 6–16 days old are affected. Diarrhea is profuse, watery, and yellowish. There may be milk clots in the stool. Signs include depression and dehydration. Many die if untreated. Sow may show mild fever and anorexia.

HEMAGGLUTINATING ENCEPHALOMYELITIS: VOMITING AND WASTING DISEASE. (coronavirus) Affects suckling pigs 2–20 days old. Signs include transient fever, anorexia, and vomiting. Severe emaciation follows. Some cases, usually in the older piglets, develop diarrhea. Muscle tremors, incoordination, paddling, convulsions, and death are seen as a separate presentation.

ROTAVIRUS INFECTION. Primarily affects piglets 1–4 weeks old. Uncomplicated rotavirus infection produces profuse milky diarrhea and vomiting. Recovery occurs within 1–3 days. Other signs include moderate to severe dehydration. This is a litter problem.

PSEUDORABIES: AUJESZKY'S DISEASE. (porcine herpesvirus) Diarrhea may be part of this disease in piglets. Signs are mainly neurologic and respiratory.

PORCINE EPIDEMIC DIARRHEA. (coronavirus) Occasionally seen in UK and Europe. Clinically similar to TGE. Signs include watery diarrhea lasting 3–4 days and vomiting. Recovery occurs in 1 week. Occasional fatalities.

COCCIDIOSIS. (*Isospora suis*) Affects piglets 5–15 days of age (peak incidence 7–10 days). Signs include mild fever, depression, vomiting, diarrhea, and maybe dysentery. Tenesmus is also a feature. May last several days. Mortality up to 20%.

STRONGYLOIDIASIS. (*Strongyloides ransomi*) Larvae adhere to teats or are transferred in colostrum. Direct penetration of skin by soil-borne larvae also occurs. Signs include anorexia and diarrhea (may progress to dysentery) accompanied by protein-losing enteropathy. Mortality up to 50%.

SALMONELLOSIS. (*Salmonella cholerae suis, S. typhimurium*) Signs include septicemia, neurologic signs, and mucoid dysentery in piglets older than 3 weeks of age.

ERYSIPELAS. (*Erysipelothrix rhusiopathiae*) Septicemia caused by this organism can cause diarrhea in piglets older than 1 week of age.

TOXOPLASMOSIS. (*Toxoplasma gondii*) Diarrhea can be part of this disease, which is primarily a respiratory and nervous system problem.

CRYPTOSPORIDIOSIS. (*Cryptosporidium* spp.) May cause watery, brown diarrhea.

IRON DEFICIENCY. Signs include anemia, ill-thrift, and diarrhea. Signs develop after 2–3 weeks of age.

Postweaning and Adult Pigs

SALMONELLOSIS. (*Salmonella cholerae suis* and sometimes *S. typhimurium*) Formerly occurred in outbreaks, similar to hog cholera (swine fever). Disease varies widely in presentation.

Septicemic Form. Signs include purple discoloration of skin and general signs of septicemia. There may be CNS signs. Commonly fatal.

Acute Enteric Form. Signs include enteritis or dysentery and, occasionally, pneumonia and/or meningoencephalitis. Animals that die may have "turkey egg kidney" (also seen with hog cholera and African swine fever).

Chronic Form. May follow acute form or can be primary. Signs include fever, persistent watery diarrhea, and anorexia. Rectal stricture may develop.

SWINE DYSENTERY. (*Treponema hyodysenteriae*) Affects large numbers in a group. Most prevalent in postweaning and fattening pigs (7–15 weeks old). May be precipitated by stress. Signs include insidious onset, mild fever, depression, and moderate inappetence. Characteristic feces are partially formed, grey to black, and contain mucus, blood, and perhaps epithelial casts. Occasional deaths. Severe weight loss is typical in chronic cases (razorback). Lesions limited to colon.

COLIBACILLOSIS. (*Escherichia coli*) Differs from the neonatal form and from edema disease. There may be sudden deaths later in outbreaks. Signs include moderate pyrexia followed by yellow, watery diarrhea. Animals tend to be poor doers.

PORCINE INTESTINAL ADENOMATOSIS. (*Campylobacter sputorum* subsp. *mucosalis, C. hyointestinalis*) Usually affects pigs 6–20 weeks old. Often causes retarded growth. Diarrhea is often accompanied by wasting. Anemia, peritonitis, melena, and diarrhea may also occur. Recovery is common in uncomplicated cases.

EDEMA DISEASE. (*Escherichia coli*) Seen in postweaning pigs (6–14 weeks old). Often follows dietary changes or other stresses. Primarily a neurologic disease, with ataxia and palpebral edema. Diarrhea may be seen.

CAMPYLOBACTERIOSIS. (*Campylobacter coli*) Chronic mucoid diarrhea in postweaning pigs.

LEPTOSPIROSIS. (*Leptospira* spp.)

Acute Form. Signs include anorexia, fever, depression, diarrhea, and, occasionally, hemoglobinuria.

Chronic Form. Manifested by abortion.

TRANSMISSIBLE GASTROENTERITIS: TGE. (coronavirus) Mild disease in adult pigs. Most severe in young pigs. Characterized by mild fever, anorexia, and agalactia in sows. There may be diarrhea. May be subclinical.

ROTAVIRUS INFECTION. May cause diarrhea in piglets soon after weaning. Milky scours are prominent sign.

PORCINE EPIDEMIC DIARRHEA. (coronavirus) Similar to TGE. Limited to Europe and China. Many animals affected in epizootics, but severity varies greatly. Diarrhea is the major presentation.

HOG CHOLERA: SWINE FEVER. (pestivirus)

Peracute Form. Viral septicemia in young pigs. Sudden death.

Acute Form. Signs include fever, anorexia, depression, and consti-pation followed by diarrhea and vomiting. Severe conjunctivitis is a feature. Occasionally there are neurologic signs.

Chronic Form. Signs include ill-thrift and inappetence. Other man-ifestations of hog cholera infection in a herd include reproductive failure and congenital defects in piglets.

AFRICAN SWINE FEVER. (Iridovirus) Clinically similar to hog chol-era, but more severe. Mortality very high. Outbreaks occur, seen in Africa, Cuba, and South America.

INTESTINAL PARASITISM. (*Oesophagostomum* spp., *Trichuris suis, Ascaris suum*) Mild diarrhea is sometimes seen with *Oesophagosto-mum* infection; inappetence, mild dysentery, and anemia may also occur. Occasionally infection with *A. suum* causes mild diarrhea.

TOXOPLASMOSIS. (*Toxoplasma gondii*) Usually subclinical. Clini-cal signs include respiratory disease and abortion in sows (diarrhea occasionally).

TRICOTHECENE TOXICITY. (*Fusarium* spp.) Fungal toxin in feed causes stomatitis, vomiting, inappetence, and intestinal disease leading to diarrhea. Recovery is quick once toxin is eliminated from the diet.

OCHRATOXICOSIS. (*Aspergillus* spp.) The presence of fungal toxin in feed may cause diarrhea.

ANTIBIOTIC-INDUCED DIARRHEA. Several antibiotics can precipitate diarrhea, although such illness is not common. Tylosin and lincomycin have been implicated.

GASTRIC ULCERS. Signs include anemia, melena, and diarrhea. Animals may be found dead from acute peritonitis, due to gastric erosion or internal hemorrhage.

New World Camelids

The diarrheal diseases of New World camelids (NWCs) are poorly documented. In general, the parasitic and infectious diseases of NWCs are similar to those of ruminants, and they are likely to be susceptible to similar plant poisonings and other toxicoses as are the domestic ruminants.

PATIENT EVALUATION AND DIAGNOSTIC PLAN

1. History: ages affected, vaccination status, colostrum intake, recent introductions to herd, environmental or management changes, ac-cess to toxins, and parasite control.
2. Physical findings.
3. Hematologic and biochemical evaluation: serum chemistry, acid–base status, immunoglobulin determination (neonates), hematocrit, and total serum protein.

4. Collection of material for diagnostic procedures.

   Specimens must be fresh and properly preserved. Postmortem autolysis can destroy lesions within 1 h of death, and bacterial overgrowth can mask true pathogens.

   a. Loops of fresh intestine are needed for bacterial cultures and virus and ETEC identification using fluorescent-antibody tests. These specimens should be refrigerated (but *not* frozen) for transport. Other tissues should also be examined as part of the complete postmortem examination.

   b. Intestine preserved in formalin is required for histopathologic examination and virus identification using electron microscopy.

   c. Feces from litter mates should be examined if fresh necropsy material is not available.

   d. Enzyme-linked immunosorbent assay (ELISA) kits are available for the detection of rotavirus in fresh fecal samples.

   e. Impression smears of the ileal wall may be Gram stained.

   f. Fecal flotation is used for detection of cryptosporidial and coccidial oocysts and worm eggs.

   g. In herd outbreaks, euthanasia and immediate postmortem examination of an affected animal may facilitate diagnosis.

PATIENT MANAGEMENT

1. Maintain electrolyte, water, and acid–base status. In mild dehydration, oral fluids may be suitable. In severe dehydration, parenteral fluids are indicated. (See section on fluid therapy in Chapter 12, pp. 247–250.)

2. Parenteral antibiotics are indicated when septicemia is suspected. Tetracyclines are recommended for treatment of Potomac horse fever.

3. Antisecretory drugs (such as bismuth subsalicylate, flunixin meglumine) may be used if secretory diarrhea is suspected. Other agents with demonstrated antisecretory properties include calcium channel blockers (e.g., iodochlorhydroxyquin), alpha$_2$-adrenergic agonists (e.g., clonidine), alpha$_1$-adrenergic antagonists (e.g., chlorpromazine). Sedation is an unwanted side effect of alpha-adrenergic agents.

4. When parasitism is suspected, anthelmintics are indicated. Coccidiosis is best treated with sulfonamides or amprolium orally, and improvement of management is recommended to prevent reinfection.

5. Isolate affected animals, and avoid cross-contamination of feeding utensils and stall cleaning equipment. Where feasible, separate disposable clothing, gloves, and boots should be used when entering an infected area and removed when leaving it. An effective disinfectant foot bath should be available immediately outside the affected stall. Infected bedding should be disposed of appropriately.

EXCESSIVE SALIVATION AND DROOLING, VOMITING, AND REGURGITATION

EXCESSIVE SALIVATION AND DROOLING

Horses

FOREIGN BODIES
Oropharyngeal. Pieces of wood, wire, or needles may become lodged in the tongue, in the gums, or between the dental arcades.

Esophageal. Impaction of food material may result secondary to poor quality feed or poor dentition.

DENTAL PROBLEMS. Dental points may traumatize oral or lingual mucosa.

VESICULAR STOMATITIS. (viral disease) Signs include oral vesicles, ulceration, and fever. Seasonal on North American continent.

CLOSTRIDIAL MYOSITIS. (*Clostridium* spp.) Lingual or cervical involvement with secondary lowering of the head may lead to dependent edema and salivary losses.

TRAUMA. Fractures of the bones of the facial area or trauma to the soft tissues may lead to salivary loss. There is usually physical evidence of injury.

IRRITANTS. Irritants include oral phenylbutazone, licking at blistered sites, cantharidin (blister beetle toxin).

NEUROLOGIC DISEASES
Central Diseases. Rabies, encephalitis (e.g., viral), and yellow star thistle toxicity may lead to failure of deglutition and/or dependent drainage of saliva during lowering of the head.

Peripheral Nerve Disease. Disease of cranial nerves 5, 7, 9, 10, and 12, including botulism, tetanus; may also lead to salivary loss.

ORGANOPHOSPHATE POISONING. Overdose of organophosphate anthelmintics may cause salivation, colic or diarrhea, and miosis.

SLAFRAMINE: SUMMER SLOBBERS. (mycotoxin) Causes excessive salivation and lacrimation. Seasonal incidence, late summer, early fall in North America.

STACHYBOTRYOTOXICOSIS. (satratoxins B, H; fungal toxin) Causes stomatitis, hemorrhagic diarrhea, and death.

Cattle

FOREIGN BODIES
Oropharyngeal. Pieces of wood, wire, or needles, lodged between the dental arcades, in the cheeks, or in the pharyngeal region may cause drooling.

Esophageal. Food (e.g., tuber) may lodge in the esophagus, leading to impaired swallowing.

FOOT AND MOUTH DISEASE. (picornavirus) Endemic to certain areas of the world. Herd outbreaks. Signs include fever; anorexia; salivation; and buccal, coronary, and interdigital ulceration. High morbidity: mortality about 2% in adults.

BOVINE VIRAL DIARRHEA: BVD. (pestivirus) Signs include mild fever, mild nasal discharge, and diarrhea. Abortions occur in some cows. There is hyperemia of oral mucosa and some drooling.

MUCOSAL DISEASE. (pestivirus) Signs include severe diarrhea, fever, depression, inappetence, and nasal and ocular discharge. Oral erosions occur, frequently involving much of oral cavity. Papillae are blunted. Erosions are also seen at the interdigital spaces, coronary band, and teats.

MALIGNANT CATARRHAL FEVER. (herpesvirus) Signs include fever, anorexia, depression, increased heart and respiratory rate, and severe nasal congestion with encrustations on the muzzle. Corneal opacity, hypopyon, blepharospasm, photophobia also occur. Peripheral lymphadenopathy and, occasionally, neurologic signs occur. Hematuria occurs infrequently. Outbreaks in cattle are associated with close contact with sheep or wildebeest.

RABIES. (rhabdovirus) May present with great variety of signs, including drooling.

INFECTIOUS BOVINE RHINOTRACHEITIS. (bovine herpesvirus type 1) Signs include cough, fever, and nasal discharge with muzzle encrustation. Outbreaks occur in herd. There may be a history of abortions in herd.

BLUETONGUE. (orbivirus) Arthropod-borne. Occurs in west coast and midwest of USA and in South Africa. May be subclinical. Signs include fever, hyperemia of mucous membranes, oral mucosal ulcerations, necrosis of dental pad, hyperemia and encrustations on the muzzle, swollen tongue, and nasal discharge. Coronary band may be affected. Lameness results. Decreased reproductive efficiency may occur.

VESICULAR STOMATITIS. (rhabdovirus) Enzootic in USA and Central America. Resembles other stomatitides, such as foot and mouth disease. Younger cattle are more severely affected, but adults also show signs. Mild fever gives way to vesicle formation in the mouth, leading to ulceration. There may be teat lesions and coronary band lesions on occasion. Recovery is quick.

RINDERPEST. (morbillivirus) Occurs in Africa and the Middle East. Major signs are fever and gastroenteritis with dysentery. Salivation may be excessive due to necrotic stomatitis. May be purulent. Acute form may be fatal.

TIMBER TONGUE: WOODEN TONGUE. (*Actinobacillus lignieresii*) The base of the tongue is swollen initially: later the tongue protrudes.

Animal chews as if foreign body were present. Local lymph nodes may enlarge and drain pus.

LUMPY JAW. (*Actinomyces bovis*) Mandible slowly enlarges, destroying the bone. Misalignment of dentition may lead to drooling.

BOVINE PAPULAR STOMATITIS. (parapoxvirus) Not a systemic disease. Younger animals generally are affected, with outbreaks occurring. Signs include raised papular lesions on muzzle and lips. Papule becomes gray in center and sloughs, leaving erosion. Teat lesions also occur.

CALF DIPHTHERIA. (*Fusobacterium necrophorum*)

Oral Form: Necrotic Stomatitis. Signs include fever, depression, anorexia, salivation, and buccal ulcers. There is occasional fatal pneumonia. Mainly affects calves.

Laryngeal Form. Affects older calves and yearlings (feedlots). Signs include fever, pain on swallowing, foul breath, and snoring. May be possible to palpate swollen laryngeal area.

CLOSTRIDIAL MYOSITIS. (*Clostridium chauvoei, C. septicum, C. novyi*) May affect the tongue causing necrotizing myositis. Signs include acute depression and signs of toxemia. High mortality.

SARCOCYSTOSIS. (*Sarcocystis* spp.) Nonspecific signs include fever, mild depression, anemia, cachexia, oral ulcers, and salivation.

TRAUMA. Fracture of the mandible or maxilla, trauma to soft tissues (e.g., balling gun), or malocclusion of or injury to teeth may cause salivation.

CHEMICAL STOMATITIS. Caustic substances, such as acids or alkalis, may damage mucosa and cause stomatitis.

CHRONIC MERCURY POISONING. Stomatitis may be evident.

ORGANOPHOSPHATE POISONING. History of exposure to organophosphates. Signs include salivation, diarrhea, moderate abdominal pain, and pupillary miosis.

SLAFRAMINE. (mycotoxin) Salivation and lacrimation are major signs. Bloat may also be evident.

NEUROLOGIC DISEASE. Central or peripheral lesions of cranial nerves 5, 7, 9, 10, and 12 may lead to saliva loss.

MISCELLANEOUS CAUSES. Tumors, tooth root abscess, and uremia may result in excessive salivation.

Sheep and Goats

FOOT AND MOUTH DISEASE. (picornavirus) Buccal vesicular lesions are less pronounced than in cattle.

BLUETONGUE. (reovirus) Arthropod-borne. Signs include fever, depression, coronitis, salivation, edema of the head, and impaired wool growth. Morbidity 80–100%.

VESICULAR STOMATITIS. (rhabdovirus) Signs include fever; depression; anorexia; teat and coronary band vesicles; and vesicles on tongue, lips, and gums. Zoonotic.

MUCOCUTANEOUS ULCERATION. Diseases such as orf (contagious echthyma) may secondarily cause excessive salivary losses.

RINDERPEST. (morbillivirus) Occurs in Africa and Middle East. Signs include fever, necrotic stomatitis, and gastroenteritis. Less common in small ruminants than in cattle.

PESTE DES PETITS RUMINANTS. Occurs in Africa and Middle East. Infectious agent is antigenically related to the morbillivirus that causes rinderpest. Spreads very rapidly in goat population. Sheep rarely get clinical disease. Signs include fever, oral mucosal lesions, diarrhea, pneumonia, and preputial/vulvar erosions.

Miscellaneous Causes

Choking (Esophageal choke)
Organophosphate Poisoning
Trauma
Chemical Stomatitis

Pigs

Causes include foreign body in oropharynx (uncommon); chemical/irritant stomatitis; pharyngeal form of anthrax; vesicular stomatitis (vesicles on snout and feet; lameness is common); foot and mouth disease; organophosphate poisoning; and trauma to oropharynx.

VOMITING

Piglets

TRANSMISSIBLE GASTROENTERITIS: TGE. (coronavirus) Signs include vomiting and severe watery to yellow diarrhea. Usually affects pigs 6–16 days old. Other signs include dehydration and depression. Sows may show mild signs of disease.

HEMAGGLUTINATING ENCEPHALOMYELITIS: VOMITING AND WASTING DISEASE. (coronavirus) Affects piglets 2–20 days old. Signs include transient fever, anorexia, depression, rapid emaciation, vomiting (yellow to green in color), and difficulty in drinking. Feces are hard and dry. Dehydration develops. Encephalitic form also occurs.

COCCIDIOSIS. (*Isospora suis*) Affects piglets 5–15 days old (peak incidence 7–10 days). Diarrhea/dysentery and tenesmus are typical. Vomiting may also occur. May last several days. Up to 20% mortality.

PORCINE EPIDEMIC DIARRHEA. (coronavirus) Occurs in Europe,

U.K., and Taiwan. TGE-like syndrome in piglets. Watery diarrhea and vomiting is typical.

ROTAVIRUS INFECTION. Signs include diarrhea, depression, and sporadic vomiting, in piglets under 4 weeks of age.

PSEUDORABIES. (porcine herpesvirus) May cause vomiting in neonatal to 4-week-old pigs. Diarrhea and neurologic signs follow.

HOG CHOLERA: SWINE FEVER. (pestivirus) Vomiting may accompany the acute form of the disease (see pp. 43–44).

AFRICAN SWINE FEVER. (iridovirus) Signs are similar to hog cholera. Exotic disease.

Weaned and Adult Pigs

MOLDY CORN. (mycotoxins, especially vomitoxin and trichothecenes) Signs include vomiting and inappetence.

EPIDEMIC DIARRHEA. (coronavirus) Occurs in Europe, U.K., and Taiwan. Signs include vomiting and diarrhea in pigs of all ages. Occurs in outbreaks.

PSEUDORABIES. (porcine herpesvirus) Occasionally vomiting is seen in growing pigs (3–6 months of age). Neurologic or respiratory signs predominate.

SWINE FEVER. (pestivirus) Vomiting is a less important sign; diarrhea, respiratory distress, and neurologic signs predominate.

AFRICAN SWINE FEVER. (iridovirus) In acute form, diarrhea, depression, fever, and neurologic signs occur. Vomiting is occasionally seen.

PORCINE INTESTINAL ADENOMATOSIS COMPLEX. (*Campylobacter mucosalis*) Occurs in growing pigs and young adults. Anemia, melena, depression, and weight loss also seen. Animals may be found dead.

ANTHRAX. (*Bacillus anthracis*) Three forms occur: septicemic, pharyngeal, and intestinal. Signs include vomiting, depression, anorexia, and blackening and necrosis of the cervical skin.

FURAZOLIDONE TOXICITY. High concentrations of furazolidone in the feed may induce vomiting and anorexia.

REGURGITATION

Ruminants

True vomiting does not occur in ruminants. Causes of regurgitation include ingestion of caustic substances, e.g., arsenic; plant poisoning—mountain laurel, rhododendron (especially in small ruminants); frothy bloat; ruminal acidosis; passive regurgitation in recumbent animals, e.g., milk fever; and diaphragmatic hernia.

COLIC, ABDOMINAL DISTENTION, AND TENESMUS

COLIC

Horses

Adult Horses

Colic is a nonspecific term used to describe the clinical manifestation of abdominal pain. Early signs of colic include behavioral changes, such as pawing, inappetence, looking at the flanks, recumbency and rolling. In serious cases these signs progress, sometimes rapidly, to severe abdominal pain with constant rolling, depression, and signs of circulatory shock.

SPASMODIC AND GAS COLIC. These are the most common causes of acute colic. They result from the accumulation of gas in the stomach or intestine and have an acute onset. Cribbing may predispose the animal to this form of colic. Signs include normal to mildly increased heart rate, increased gut sounds, and normal to mildly distended loops of bowel that are palpable per rectum. Usually responds to analgesics.

IMPACTION COLIC. Impaction can occur in the stomach, small intestine, or large intestine. Large-colon impactions are the more common. Impactions of fecal material at the pelvic flexure, cecum, and small colon are usually palpable per rectum. Poor dentition, poor quality hay, and dehydration may be predisposing causes. These impactions are usually of insidious onset, with an initial mild colic, which may worsen. Obstruction at the transverse colon with fecoliths or enteroliths may cause partial or total obstruction (ball-valve effect) to outflow into the small colon. These are generally not palpable per rectum. Chronic low-grade or acute colic may accompany these obstructions.

STRANGULATING OBSTRUCTIONS. Partial or complete vascular occlusion.

Small Intestine. Small intestinal strangulating obstruction is accompanied by ileus, with resultant gastric distention. There is rapid onset of cardiovascular collapse. Strangulating obstructions are of the following types:

1. Volvulus—often at mesenteric root
2. Lipoma—affects older horses
3. Mesenteric rent
4. Epiploic foramen entrapment—usually in horses older than 7 years
5. Fibrous adhesions (may be sequelae of peritonitis)
6. Inguinal hernia

7. Intussusception.
8. Diaphragmatic hernia.

Large Intestine. Torsion occurring along the long axis of the large colon may cause acute onset of severe colic, with subsequent abdominal distention, and rapidly ensuing cardiovascular collapse.

INCARCERATIONS. Incarceration is an entrapment of bowel without vascular compromise.

Small Intestine. Incarceration of the small bowel occurs in the following ways:

1. Inguinal hernia—especially in foals and stallions
2. Epiploic foramen entrapment—early stages
3. Diaphragmatic hernia.

Large Intestine. Incarceration of the large bowel may result from the following problems:

1. Large colon displacement
2. Nephrosplenic entrapment
3. Diaphragmatic hernia.

ENTEROCOLITIS. Diseases such as salmonellosis, Potomac horse fever, or ingestion of irritant substances, such as heavy metals or cantharidin, may cause acute colic in association with intestinal inflammation. Fever may be part of the syndrome, with depression and sometimes laminitis.

PARASITISM. Migrating strongyle larvae in the cranial mesenteric artery may cause ischemic colic. Other verminous infections may lead to poor growth, weight loss, and intermittent colic.

PERITONITIS. Associated with intestinal perforations, cholangitis, mesenteric abscesses, and breeding, or foaling injuries in mares.

GASTROINTESTINAL ULCERATION. Gastric ulcers due to chronic administration of nonsteroidal antiinflammatory drugs (NSAIDs). Bot larvae or very fibrous feed may induce colic; bouts are particularly associated with feeding. Ulcers throughout intestinal tract may also induce colic. Causes include NSAIDs, irritants, and infectious agents.

INFILTRATIVE ENTEROPATHY. Lymphosarcoma, granulomatous enteritis, and lymphocytic-plasmacytic enteritis may give rise to low-grade colic; fever, anorexia, and weight loss may also be seen. Per-rectum exam indicates thickened bowel or masses in the mesentery or intestinal wall.

BILIARY COLIC. Occasionally, choleliths may occur in the common bile duct, causing colic. Jaundice and fever are usually clinical features.

Conditions That May Be Confused with True Colic

Differential diagnosis for nonenteric colic includes the following conditions when accompanied by normal findings per-rectum and absence of nasogastric reflux.

MYOSITIS

Exertional: Tying-Up. History of exercise. Signs include acute onset of stiff gait, generalized or localized muscle swelling, and coffee-colored urine.

Infectious. (*Clostridium* spp.) Often results from intramuscular injection. Severe localized swelling and signs of toxemia or shock are common.

LAMINITIS. Abnormal stance, reluctance to move, positive response to toe pressure (hoof tester), and abnormal digital pulses support the diagnosis.

PLEURITIS. Fever, increased respiratory rate, decreased lung sounds (or friction rubs), and cough may be noted.

UROGENITAL. Urinary tract obstruction from calculi may cause colic signs, as may hemorrhage into broad ligament postfoaling or estrus cycle activity.

METABOLIC. Lactation tetany in the mare may present as colic.

NEUROLOGIC. Rabies has many clinical presentations, including colic. Stiff gait in cases of tetanus may be misinterpreted as reflecting abdominal pain.

Patient Evaluation

HISTORY AND SIGNALMENT. Obtain detailed information about the following areas of the horse's medical history:

Age of animal: Older horses are more prone to tumors than younger horses.
Sex: Mares—record their history of breeding and any resultant injury to the reproductive tract.
    Stallions—inquire about inguinal hernia acquired during mating.
Diet: Record any recent changes and investigate the possibility of grain overload.
Deworming history: Determine the probability of thromboembolic lesions. Establish if tapeworm medications or organophosphates have been recently administered.
Vaccinations: Establish dates for most recent rabies and Potomac horse fever vaccinations.
Environment: Ask about the presence of sandy pastures.
Medical history: Determine if there has been previous abdominal surgery (possibly adhesions) or exposure to strangles.

PRESENTATION. Observe the following presenting features of the illness:

Duration of colic: Large-bowel impactions may be manifested by low-grade colic of a few days' duration.
Progression of signs: Small-intestine lesions usually deteriorate rapidly.

Volume, nature, and frequency of feces over previous 12 h: In large-bowel displacement or torsion fecal output is reduced or absent.

Response to medication: Spasmodic and gas colics usually respond well to analgesics.

PHYSICAL EXAMINATION. Thoroughly examine the animal, recording the following data:

Pulse rate and quality: Increased heart rate (greater than 60 in adult) and weak pulse suggest surgical lesion.

Temperature: Many colic cases may show mild pyrexia (up to 39°C) due to pain and increased muscle activity. Fever >39°C (102°F) suggests enteritis or peritonitis.

Abdominal tympany: Indicative of large-colon torsion or displacement.

Per-rectum examination: Large or small bowel distended from gas, with tachycardia and cardiovascular compromise, suggests surgical lesion.

Nasogastric intubation: Copious gastric reflux suggests small-intestine obstruction or anterior enteritis.

Abdominocentesis: Examination of peritoneal fluid can determine the existence of cytological abnormalities, and changes in protein and specific gravity.

DECISION MAKING. In the interpretation of physical findings, generally speaking, no one sign is diagnostic. Decisions should be based on history and clinical signs; for example, an adult horse with a heart rate greater than 60 and a weak pulse could have severe enteritis or an obstructive small-bowel lesion. The findings per-rectum and the presence or absence of diarrhea will aid in the diagnosis.

Surgery may be indicated when:

1. Analgesic therapy has failed to control pain.

2. Gastric reflux is present in association with small- or large-bowel dilation and deteriorating cardiovascular status.

3. Medical therapy has failed to relieve impactions or tympany.

4. Per rectum findings indicate large- or small-bowel dilation, displacement, or torsion.

5. Abdominocentesis indicates an increase in erythrocytes, leucocytes, or the specific gravity of the peritoneal fluid.

FINDINGS ON PALPATION PER RECTUM

Small Intestine. The duodenum is not palpable per rectum. The jejunoileum may be distended with gas, fluid, or ingesta. In severe cases, loops of small intestine may be palpable throughout the caudal abdomen, extending even into the pelvic inlet. A sausage-shaped mass may be palpable in cases of intussusception. Thickening of the small intestinal wall may be due to edema or inflammation (including infiltrative disease).

Colon. When large colon or cecum is distended with gas, fluid or ingesta, taut colonic band(s) are palpable. In colonic torsion the pelvic cavity may be filled with distended colon, making the palpation of abdominal contents difficult or impossible. The small colon may be identified by its mesenteric and antimesenteric bands—fecoliths or impactions occasionally occur here.

Medical Management of Equine Colic

PAIN CONTROL. The following drugs should be used with caution and dosages tailored to the animal's needs and physical status.

Nonsteroidal Antiinflammatory Drugs. A variety of agents are used, the most frequently used of which include dipyrone (20–22 mg/kg, i.v. or i.m.), flunixin meglumine (1.0 mg/kg, i.v. or i.m.), and phenylbutazone (2.2–8.8 mg/kg, i.v. only; irritant if given i.m.).

Opioids. Butorphanol (0.05–0.1 mg/kg), pentazocine (0.5–1.0 mg/kg), and buprenorphine (0.006 mg/kg), i.v. or i.m.

Alpha$_2$ Agonists. Xylazine (0.2–0.5 mg/kg, or to effect, i.v. [i.m. dose rate is two to three times that required for i.v.]) is highly effective but of short duration; detomidine (0.005–0.015 mg/kg, i.v. or i.m.).

LAXATIVES

Mineral Oil. Administer 4–6 L orally to adult horses to help soften impactions. May be repeated daily if necessary.

Dioctyl Sodium Succinate: DSS. May be given for relief of impactions. Acts as a wetting agent. Administer 10–20 mg/kg as 5% solution in warm water.

FLUIDS. Oral electrolyte solutions or water may be given by nasogastric tube for large-bowel impactions. Two to three gallons (8–12 L) may be administered every 6–8 h. Saves time and money over intravenous method.

Intravenous Fluids. Indicated when oral intake is contraindicated, as in ileus, and when circulatory compromise is present.

GASTRIC DECOMPRESSION. As needed to relieve gastric distention secondary to ileus.

ANTIBIOTICS. Indicated where bowel compromise, peritonitis, or septicemia is suspected.

HEPARIN. The clinical use of heparin remains controversial. It has been recommended for prevention of laminitis and for its antiendotoxemic effects.

Neonatal Foals

MECONIUM RETENTION. Failure to pass meconium, more common in colts. Signs include tenesmus and recumbency or rolling. Animals usually respond satisfactorily to enemas.

ILEUS. Caused by lack of exercise, inadequate colostrum, or peritonitis.

ENTERITIS. Acute enteritis may be accompanied by colic. Signs include fever, toxemia, hypoglycemia, and weakness.

RUPTURED BLADDER. Colts are more commonly affected. Usually occurs at parturition. Signs manifest at 2–5 days of age. Signs include tenesmus and small quantities of urine voided. Depression, abdominal enlargement, and weakness follow.

GASTRIC ULCERS. Signs include salivation, rolling (often assume dorsal recumbency), and inappetence.

INTESTINAL ACCIDENTS. Less common in foals than in adults. Intussusception may be a sequel to enteritis.

Patient Evaluation

In general, the principles outlined for evaluation of the adult equine apply to the neonate. One obvious difference is the inability to perform per-rectum examination.

Cattle

Adult Cattle

Signs of abdominal pain in cattle include depression, anorexia, kicking at the abdomen, and grunting. Some may adopt a "saw-horse" stance, others may shift weight from one rear foot to the other. Some may be recumbent.

TRAUMATIC RETICULOPERITONITIS. (hardware, foreign body) Mainly seen in adult dairy cattle. Signs are compatible with acute peritonitis and include depression, anorexia, fever, scant feces, hunched back, abducted elbows and reduction of ruminal motility, with shallow respiration and grunting. Mild tachycardia may be seen. Palpation of abdomen elicits a painful response on probing or pressurizing the paracostal or xiphoid regions.

RUMINAL ACIDOSIS. (grain overload) Excessive intake of grain or fermentable feed. Signs include depression, anorexia, "full rumen," abdominal pain, tachycardia, lack of fever, diarrhea, and groaning. Laminitis may develop. Examination of rumen fluid may verify the diagnosis.

PERITONITIS. Causes include

1. Traumatic reticuloperitonitis
2. Perforated abomasal ulcer (local/diffuse)
3. Septic metritis
4. Rumenitis (sequel to acidosis)
5. Penetrating wounds.

ABOMASAL ULCERATION. Nonperforated ulcers are generally sub-clinical. Associated with concurrent diseases and stress (e.g., heavy grain diet postcalving).

Signs include melena, anemia, and abdominal pain. Sudden death may occur. Pain exacerbated by deep palpation behind right costal arch.

TORSION OF ABOMASUM. Torsion may result from abomasal dilation and right-sided displacement. Usually seen in adult dairy cows soon after parturition. Torsion leads to rapid onset of circulatory shock. Signs include scant, soft feces, depression, anorexia, decreased ruminal activity, distension on right side of abdomen, and colic in advanced stages. Auscultation reveals high-pitched ping over right paracostal region and a splashiness on deep palpation of this area. Viscus in right cranial abdomen may be palpated per rectum.

OMASAL OR ABOMASAL IMPACTION. Poor quality forage or high sand content in diet (sandy pasture, contaminated feed). Nonspecific signs include abdominal pain, scant feces, depression, and poor appetite. Pain over abomasal area may be detected by deep palpation.

RUMINAL TYMPANY. May be primary or secondary.

Primary. Lush leguminous feed causes frothy bloat. Highly fermentable feed causes gas bloat.

Secondary. Functional obstruction (e.g., tetanus) from vagal indigestion, reticulitis, or actinobacillosis. Mechanical (e.g., esophageal) obstruction, reticular foreign body, abscess, enlarged lymph node (e.g., lymphosarcoma).

Signs include distention of left paralumbar fossa (may be bilateral in severe cases), increased respiratory rate, recumbency, regurgitation, and signs of systemic shock.

INTUSSUSCEPTION. Signs include scant feces, which may be mucoid or tarry, and kicking at abdomen. Examination per rectum indicates sausage-shaped mass and distended small intestine. Upon auscultation of the right flank, small discrete pings may be heard. Acute onset of pain. Late in the course of the illness, signs of shock may be evident.

INTESTINAL VOLVULUS. Often occurs at mesenteric root or may be segmental. Sporadic occurrence. Signs include acute onset of severe abdominal pain and bilateral distention. Examination per rectum indicates many distended loops of small intestine. Pings may be auscultated on right side. Rapid progression.

CECAL DILATION: CECAL TORSION/VOLVULUS. Signs include abdominal pain and small volume of dark feces. Gas pings may be heard on right side in dorsal paralumbar fossa. Distended cecum is palpable per rectum and may occupy pelvic cavity.

INGUINAL HERNIA. Occurs in mature bulls. Signs similar to other causes of intestinal obstruction. Scrotal swelling may be evident.

ABDOMINAL FAT NECROSIS. Affects Channel Island breeds. Signs include small amounts of feces passed. Often a chronic condition.

ENTERITIS. Salmonellosis, acute mucosal disease, and other causes of enteritis may cause colic signs. Animal may be febrile, and more than one animal may be affected.

HEAVY-METAL POISONING. Acute arsenic intoxication may cause severe gastrointestinal discomfort.

RENAL DISEASE. (*Escherichia coli* or *Actinomyces pyogenes*) Pyelonephritis. May present with colic signs, as may urolithiasis.

MISCELLANEOUS CONDITIONS. Rabies, calving/abortion, and laminitis.

Calves

ENTERITIS. Abdominal discomfort and depression may precede the development of diarrhea.

ABOMASAL DISEASES

Ulceration. May perforate.

Dilatation and Torsion. Most common between 6–12 weeks of life.

INTESTINAL VOLVULUS/STRANGULATION. Uncommon.

PERITONITIS. Can occur as a sequel to perforating ulcer.

TRICHOBEZOARS. Hairballs may obstruct the pylorus or intestinal tract.

HEAVY-METAL POISONING. Subacute lead poisoning may have colic as a presenting sign.

ABDOMINAL DISTENTION IN CATTLE

Location of Distention

LEFT-SIDED DISTENTION. The left side can be distended as a result of the following:

Free gas bloat (impaired gas removal or increased production)
Frothy bloat
Vagal indigestion. Progressive anorexia leading to abdominal enlargement, especially on the left side (involves lower right side also)
Ruminal impaction
Left displaced abomasum
Pneumoperitoneum.

RIGHT-SIDED DISTENTION. The right side can be distended because of the following:

Severe ruminal bloat (involves left side also)
Abomasal dilatation and volvulus/torsion

Cecal dilatation/volvulus
Pneumoperitoneum.

BILATERAL ABDOMINAL DISTENTION. Both sides of the abdomen are distended with these conditions:

Ruminal bloat
Rapid abdominal distention in hydrops allantois (late pregnancy)
Ascites, e.g. cardiac failure
Pregnancy (advanced)
Mesenteric volvulus
Uroperitoneum; usually affects steers under feedlot conditions
Peritonitis
Vagal indigestion—Progressive anorexia leading to abdominal enlargement, primarily on left side.

Other Causes of Misshapen Abdomen

RUPTURE OF PREPUBIC TENDON. Most commonly associated with advanced pregnancy.
VENTRAL ABDOMINAL HERNIA. Results from trauma.
UMBILICAL HERNIA. Usually congenital.
HEMATOMA. May be due to trauma to milk vein, or other superficial abdominal vessels.
UDDER EDEMA. May be normal prior to calving. Condition should resolve in 10–14 days postpartum.

TENESMUS

Adult Horses

1. Parturition/abortion
2. Colitis
3. Cystitis, urinary outflow obstruction
4. Proctitis, e.g., from rectal neoplasia.

Foals

1. Retention of meconium
2. Ruptured bladder (90% are colts)
3. Severe enteritis
4. Atresia ani.

Adult Cattle

1. Second-stage parturition in cows, abortion
2. Vaginitis/metritis/retained placenta

3. Coccidiosis
4. Salmonellosis
5. Mucosal disease
6. Rabies
7. Chronic pyrrolizidine alkaloid toxicity
8. Rinderpest (acute form)—exotic disease
9. Proctitis (traumatic, inflammatory)
10. Pyelonephritis—cystitis, urinary tract obstruction
11. Estrogen toxicity in steers
12. Fusarium toxicity
13. Lower spinal cord disease.

Calves

1. Coccidiosis
2. Salmonellosis
3. Other infectious diarrheas
4. Atresia ani
5. Ruptured bladder/urinary obstruction.

Pigs

1. Coccidiosis
2. Salmonellosis
3. Constipation (in pregnant sows)
4. Dystocia
5. Vaginitis/metritis

Small Ruminants

Many of the conditions described for adult cattle and calves may cause tenesmus in small ruminants.

Respiratory System

EXAMINATION OF THE RESPIRATORY SYSTEM

The case history should include information about the presence of nasal discharge, coughing, abnormal sounds associated with breathing, and increased respiratory rate and effort. Normal respiratory rates are shown in Table 3–1. The duration of the illness should be noted. Where applicable, the type of housing and the health of animals with whom the patient has contact should be determined. Information on vaccination and deworming programs is especially pertinent in herd situations.

Initially, the animal should be observed at rest and from a distance, to determine the rate, character, rhythm, and depth of respiration. The observation should take place from both sides and from behind the animal, to assess bilateral symmetry and the thoracic and abdominal components of respiration. In the horse, reduced thoracic movement is a feature of acute pleuritis, and an increase in the abdominal component is a feature of advanced small airway disease (heaves).

In the resting state, no audible sound is produced during respiration, and abnormalities should be classified according to their origin, character, and timing in relation to the respiratory cycle. Examples of abnormal sounds include the "snoring" sounds associated with pharyngeal obstruction and the "roaring" sounds associated with laryngeal stenosis.

The patency of the nasal passages is checked by placing a hand close to the nostrils in order to assess air flow. The presence of obstruction can be verified by occluding each nostril in turn. The breath odor can be determined at this time. Abnormal odors include those associated with ketosis (in cattle) and infection, such as tooth infection, stomatitis, laryngitis, and pneumonia (particularly anaerobic infections). Normally cattle's breath has a characteristic sweet odor. The muzzle and nares are examined for abnormalities such as discharge, and the volume, color, consistency, and odor of such discharges are noted.

TABLE 3–1. NORMAL RESPIRATORY RATES*

Species	Age	Rate
Horses	Adult	10–15
	Foal	15–20
Cattle	Adult	10–30
	Yearling	15–40
Sheep and goats	Adult	20–30
Pigs	Adult	10–20
New World Camelids	Adult	20–30

*The respiratory rate will vary with excitement, environmental temperature, and exercise.

Examination of the paranasal sinuses includes inspection for swelling and external injuries. Percussion may be performed on the nasal cavities and the paranasal sinuses. The normal hollow sound heard during percussion can be amplified by holding the mouth open during the procedure.

The pharynx and larynx are palpated externally for gross abnormalities. Direct visualization of these structures can be achieved in horses and ruminants using a flexible endoscope and in ruminants using a tubular speculum and light source. The throat latch of the horse should be checked for scars that would indicate a previous ventriculectomy. The cervical trachea is palpated to determine its shape and sensitivity to pressure. Endoscopic examination of the trachea is easily performed in awake animals large enough to accommodate the endoscope.

Auscultation of the lungs and trachea is the principal means of clinically examining the lung fields. The lung fields must be auscultated in their entirety. Their extent varies with the species and may be determined using percussion (Table 3–2).

The character of abnormal lung sounds and their timing in the respiratory cycle should be recorded. In the larger species, it is frequently necessary to amplify the lung sounds by forcing the animal to rebreathe for 1 to 2 minutes prior to auscultation. This can be achieved by placing a suitably sized plastic bag over the nostrils while the animal breathes or by occluding the nostrils for a brief period.

Diagnostic imaging, including plain radiography and ultrasonography, are used in differentiating diseases of the upper and lower airways. Ultrasonography is especially useful in the diagnosis of pleural effusion and lung tissue consolidation.

If infection is suspected, swabs of the upper and lower airways may be cultured. Thoracic fluid may be cultured and examined cytologically in cases of pleural effusion.

Bronchoalveolar lavage is a method of collecting lower airway cells for examination.

TABLE 3–2. CAUDAL BORDER OF PERCUSSION IN DOMESTIC ANIMALS

	Intercostal Space		
	Dorsal Border of Scapula	*Shoulder Joint*	*Elbow*
Horse	16	11–12	6
Cattle	11	9	5
Sheep, goats	11	7	6

DISORDERS OF THE RESPIRATORY SYSTEM

HORSES

Epistaxis (Bleeding from the Nose)

TRAUMA. May follow nasogastric intubation or endoscopy.
T R E A T M E N T: Not generally necessary for mild cases.

EXERCISE-INDUCED PULMONARY HEMORRHAGE. Common. Usually the nasal bleeding is bilateral. Subclinical form is associated with reduced exercise tolerance.
T R E A T M E N T: Since specific etiology is not understood, treatment is palliative. Furosemide appears to help in some cases.

GUTTURAL POUCH MYCOSIS. (fungal) Uncommon. Fungal infection of one or both guttural pouches. Associated arterial damage leads to unilateral or bilateral hemorrhage. Often preceded by foul-smelling mucopurulent nasal discharge.
T R E A T M E N T: Requires (internal carotid) arterial ligation, in addition to topical antifungal therapy.

ETHMOID HEMATOMA. Uncommon. Intermittent nasal hemorrhage. The lesion may occlude one nostril and deviate nasal septum.
T R E A T M E N T: Surgical removal is successful in some cases.

NEOPLASIA. Uncommon. Usually associated with chronic mucopurulent (sometimes foul-smelling) nasal discharge.

Nasal Discharge

EQUINE VIRAL RHINOPNEUMONITIS. (equine herpes virus type 4) Mainly affects young horses. Signs include fever, anorexia, depression, and enlarged submandibular lymph nodes. Animal may have cough. Neurologic disease and abortion are mostly caused by EHV-1.
EQUINE INFLUENZA. (myxovirus) Major sign is coughing. There may also be slight nasal discharge and fever.
EQUINE RHINOVIRUS. Signs include profuse watery nasal discharge, fever, lymphadenitis, and coughing.
EQUINE ADENOVIRUS. Nasal discharge may be present.

T R E A T M E N T: See under Coughing, p. 67.

EQUINE VIRAL ARTERITIS. (togavirus) Signs include fever; serous, later mucopurulent nasal discharge; conjunctivitis; and limb and palpebral edema. May produce abortions.
T R E A T M E N T: None specific. Administer supportive care.

AFRICAN HORSE SICKNESS. (orbivirus) Occurs in Southern Europe and Africa. Epizootics occur. Signs include fever, paroxysmal coughing, profuse nasal discharge, ataxia, recumbency, and death.
 T R E A T M E N T: None specific.

STRANGLES. (*Streptococcus equi*) Early signs include serous nasal discharge, pharyngeal discomfort, fever, and anorexia. Subsequent signs include lymphadenopathy, mucopurulent nasal discharge, lymph node rupture, and drainage.
 T R E A T M E N T: See under Strangles, p. 68.

PARASCARIASIS. (*Parascaris equorum*) Affects foals. Signs include nasal discharge, cough, ill-thrift, and pot-bellied appearance.
 T R E A T M E N T: Administer a broad spectrum anthelmintic.

ALLERGIC RHINITIS. (environmental allergens) Signs include serous nasal discharge. There are usually no systemic signs.
 T R E A T M E N T: Remove from source of allergen. Administer corticosteroids in severe cases.

SINUSITIS. Relatively uncommon. Usually a sequel to upper respiratory tract infection. May result from tooth root infection. Nature of discharge varies from serous to mucopurulent and tenacious depending on stage of disease.
 T R E A T M E N T: Antibiotics are effective in some cases. Surgical drainage and/or tooth removal in other cases.

GUTTURAL POUCH DISEASE. Mycosis or inflammation of guttural pouch may produce bilateral or mostly unilateral nasal discharge.
 T R E A T M E N T: Antifungal agents and aeration of pouch using an indwelling catheter; arterial ligation if epistaxis is present.

CHRONIC OBSTRUCTIVE PULMONARY DISEASE: HEAVES. See under Coughing, below.

MISCELLANEOUS CONDITIONS. Ethmoidal hematoma, tumors, and fungal plaque on the ethmoids are potential causes of nasal discharge.

Coughing

CHRONIC OBSTRUCTIVE PULMONARY DISEASE: HEAVES. (environmental allergens) Nasal discharge may be slight or profuse, mucopurulent or serous. Usually affects older animals, and is associated with poorly ventilated barns. In advanced cases, respiratory distress can be severe, with an obvious expiratory phase.

T R E A T M E N T: Improve environment through ventilation and removing obvious source of allergens (e.g., moldy hay). Atropine (0.02–0.04 mg/kg, i.v., i.m.) will relieve respiratory distress in severe cases. Bronchodilators suitable for longer term administration include beta$_2$ agonists (e.g., clenbuterol) and xanthines, (e.g., aminophylline). Corticosteroids (e.g., prednisolone) will reduce airway inflammation.

Viral

EQUINE VIRAL RHINOPNEUMONITIS. (equine herpes virus 4) Common. Young, previously unexposed animals are most often affected. Signs include fever, anorexia, depression, nasal discharge, and lymphadenopathy. Coughing is common. Adults may also present with ataxia and posterior paralysis, and mares may abort (although it is uncommon for respiratory disease to develop in association with these latter diseases, which are due to EHV-1).

EQUINE INFLUENZA. (myxovirus common) Outbreaks occur. Cough is usually dry and hacking. Signs include fever, anorexia, and small amount of nasal discharge. Course is 1–2 weeks.

EQUINE RHINOVIRUS. Signs include mild cough, nasal discharge, lymphadenitis, and moderate fever.

EQUINE ADENOVIRUS. (equine adenovirus) Disease is mild in adults. Causes pneumonia, fever, nasal discharge, and coughing in foals. Immunodeficient Arabian foals often suffer a fatal pneumonia.

T R E A T M E N T: Isolation of infected animals. Rest and supportive care. Antibiotics and antiinflammatories, e.g., phenylbutazone, if secondary bacterial infection is suspected and if the disease process is prolonged.

Bacterial

BACTERIAL PLEUROPNEUMONIA. (*Streptococcus zooepidemicus* and gram-negative bacteria frequently involved) Commonly occurs after long-distance transport or other stresses. Signs include nasal discharge, coughing, fever, depression, and occasionally colicky signs. There may also be foul-smelling breath, indicating anaerobic involvement.

T R E A T M E N T: Antibiotic therapy should be based on culture and sensitivity of pleural or tracheal fluid. Nonsteroidal antiinflammatory drugs are indicated in severe cases. Drainage of pleural cavity is indicated if pleural effusion is copious.

SEPTICEMIA. Affects neonates primarily. Gram-negative septicemia (e.g., *Escherichia coli, Klebsiella*) may lead to pneumonia of hematogenous origin. Signs include fever, weakness, and depression; signs of septic arthritis or meningitis may also be present. Coughing is not a common sign in these animals.

T R E A T M E N T: Provide supportive care; administer broad-spectrum antibiotics.

RHODOCOCCUS EQUI INFECTION. Affects foals 1–6 months old. Common. Outbreaks may occur. Associated with poor hygiene. Signs include fever, tachypnea, coughing, and joint effusion.

T R E A T M E N T: Early cases respond well to combined treatment with erythromycin and rifampicin.

STRANGLES. (*Streptococcus equi*) Common. Outbreaks may occur. Signs include suppuration of enlarged submandibular or parotid lymph nodes, coughing, and fever.

T R E A T M E N T: Hotpacking to encourage drainage of abscesses. Penicillin administration in the acute phase may halt the disease. A tracheostomy is indicated for respiratory tract obstruction.

BACTERIAL PNEUMONIA. (*Streptococcus zooepidemicus*) Signs include coughing, nasal discharge, and fever.

T R E A T M E N T: Penicillin is usually effective.

Parasitic

PARASCARIASIS. (*Parascaris equorum*) Common. Affects foals 6–9 months old. Signs include coughing, nasal discharge, and ill-thrift.

DICTYOCAULUS INFECTION. (*Dictyocaulus arnfieldi*) Uncommon. Horses are rarely a source of infection, donkeys more commonly so. Chronic cough is the major sign.

T R E A T M E N T: Administer broad-spectrum anthelmintic (e.g., ivermectin).

CATTLE

Epistaxis and Hemoptysis

BRACKEN FERN POISONING. (*Pteridium aquilinum*) Signs include fever, melena or dysentery, and excessive salivation. Bleeding occurs from body orifices including nostrils. Petechial and ecchymotic hemorrhages on mucosal surfaces are common. Hemorrhage into anterior chamber of eye can result from thrombocytopenia.

T R E A T M E N T: None specific. Supportive care including fluids and blood transfusions in severe cases.

VENA CAVAL THROMBOSIS. Affects young to adult cattle on high-grain diets. Occurs as a sequel to rumenitis or hepatic abscessation. Signs associated with septic embolism in lung, and subsequent pulmonary arterial aneurysm and rupture. Signs include fever, moist lung sounds, hemoptysis, and potentially fatal pulmonary hemorrhage.

T R E A T M E N T: None successful.

MOLDY SWEET CLOVER POISONING. Dicoumarol produced by action of molds on sweet clover. Interferes with coagulation. Epistaxis is an occasional finding. Subcutaneous hemorrhage is common.
   ANTHRAX. (*Bacillus anthracis*) Usually a fatal septicemia. Epistaxis, a feature in more prolonged cases, is especially evident after death sometimes.
   TRAUMA. External (e.g., fractured nasal or maxillary bones) or internal injury (e.g., nasogastric tube) may cause epistaxis.
   TUMORS. Rare.

Nasal Discharge

The following illnesses can cause nasal discharge: infectious bovine rhinotracheitis; malignant catarrhal fever; mucosal disease; sinusitis (usually after dehorning); bovine ephemeral fever (occurs in Australia, Asia, and Africa); bovine respiratory disease complex; summer snuffles (rhinosporidiosis—mucopurulent to caseous discharge); pasteurellosis; rinderpest (Initially serous, later mucopurulent. Occurs in Africa and Middle East); and respiratory syncytial virus.

Coughing and Respiratory Difficulty

CALF DIPHTHERIA. (*Fusobacterium necrophorum*) Stomatitis is occasionally followed by laryngitis. Cases with laryngeal involvement have fever, depression, and inspiratory stridor. May spread to lungs, causing suppurative pneumonia.
   T R E A T M E N T: Responds well to penicillin, sulfonamides, or oxytetracycline in early stages; a temporary tracheotomy is indicated in severe cases.

HAEMOPHILUS SOMNUS INFECTION. Most frequently seen in young animals in the fall and winter, following entry into a feedlot. Forms of the disease include an acute neurologic form, with lameness and respiratory tract involvement in some cases. The animals are febrile and have rapid, shallow respirations. Outbreaks of disease may occur.
   T R E A T M E N T: If treated early, most animals respond well to antibiotic therapy, e.g., penicillin or oxytetracycline. In-contact animals should be monitored closely.

PASTEURELLOSIS. (*Pasteurella haemolytica*) Common. Follows episode of stress or viral infection. Signs include fever, anorexia, depression, coughing, and respiratory difficulty. Sudden death may occur at commencement of outbreak. Course is short and mortality high if untreated. Typically occurs in feedlots within 2–3 weeks of arrival.

T R E A T M E N T: Reduce stress and administer broad-spectrum antibiotics.

TUBERCULOSIS. (*Mycobacterium bovis*) Signs include soft, moist cough; crackles and wheezes develop terminally. Reportable disease.

ENZOOTIC PNEUMONIA. (viruses [parainfluenza virus, respiratory syncytial virus, bovine viral diarrhea virus]), *Mycoplasma* spp., *Ureaplasma* spp., and secondary bacterial pneumonia are implicated) Common. Associated with waning colostral immunity. Usually affects housed calves, occasionally beef calves on pasture. Signs include chronic coughing, ill-thrift, and intermittent fever.
T R E A T M E N T: Improve management and administer broad-spectrum antibiotics.

RESPIRATORY SYNCYTIAL VIRUS INFECTION. (paramyxovirus) Variety of presentations range from subclinical to severe pneumonia. Signs include fever, cough, and nasal discharge. Herd outbreaks occur. Secondary bacterial pneumonia may ensue. Disease may be fatal.
T R E A T M E N T: Reduce stress and administer broad-spectrum antibiotics if secondary infection suspected.

INFECTIOUS BOVINE RHINOTRACHEITIS. (bovine herpesvirus type 1) Occurs in weanlings and young feedlot cattle; complicated by secondary bacterial pneumonia. Signs include fever, nasal discharge, coughing, salivation, lacrimation, and tachypnea. Low mortality. Occasionally diarrhea occurs. Rarely, neurologic signs occur in neonates.
T R E A T M E N T: Antibiotics are indicated in severe cases to control secondary bacterial infection.

HUSK/HOOSE. (*Dictyocaulus viviparus*) Common in temperate climates. Affects calves late in first season at pasture. Signs include respiratory distress, moist cough, and mild fever. Severe cases have respiratory distress, cyanosis, and subcutaneous emphysema.
T R E A T M E N T: Administer anthelmintics (e.g., fenbendazole, levamisole, ivermectin). Severe cases may benefit from corticosteroids.

EXTRINSIC ALLERGIC ALVEOLITIS: BOVINE FARMER'S LUNG. (*Micropolyspora faeni*) Caused by exposure to fungal spores. Affects housed adult cattle. Acute onset of coughing and tachypnea may occur. Chronic form includes history of chronic cough and weight loss with audible crackles and wheezes on auscultation. Fever is rarely a feature. Mainly an environmental problem.
T R E A T M E N T: Improve ventilation and decrease exposure to molds. Corticosteroids may be useful to stabilize severe cases.

ASPIRATION PNEUMONIA. May be a sequel to drenching of medication or an improper tube feeding technique in calves. Signs include fever, anorexia, depression, and coughing. May have nasal discharge. Fatalities are common.

T R E A T M E N T: Administer broad-spectrum antibiotics.

RETROPHARYNGEAL MASSES. Abscessation most common. Associated with foreign bodies, drenching, or balling-gun injuries. Signs may include stridor, swelling in parotid region, fever, and inappetance.

T R E A T M E N T: Removal of foreign body where possible. Abscesses may be amenable to drainage.

OCCLUSIVE LESIONS

Fractured Ribs. Occurs in calves as a sequel to dystocia. May cause lung damage or compression of trachea (first rib). Respiratory distress may be a feature.

Thymic or Multicentric Juvenile Lymphosarcoma. May compress trachea, leading to inspiratory and/or expiratory noise in young cattle.

ACUTE BOVINE PULMONARY EMPHYSEMA: FOG FEVER. (3-methyl indole) Disease of adult cattle, mainly beef cows. Usually occurs following transfer from poor quality to lush pasture. Caused by ingestion of L-tryptophan in grass, metabolized to 3-methyl indole in rumen. Respiratory difficulty occurs, but coughing is not a feature. Lung sounds are variable. Fever and tachypnea are common.

T R E A T M E N T: Corticosteroids or nonsteroidal antiinflammatories may be beneficial.

CHRONIC INTERSTITIAL PNEUMONIA

Fibrosing Alveolitis. Cause unknown. May be a form of chronic exposure to 3-methyl indole (see Fog Fever above). Signs include chronic cough, tachypnea, difficulty in breathing, and weight loss.

T R E A T M E N T: None effective.

Bronchiolitis Obliterans. Chronic disease of young cattle, of unknown etiology. Signs include coughing, tachypnea, difficulty in breathing, and lack of fever. Postmortem diagnosis.

T R E A T M E N T: None effective.

PLEURAL EFFUSION. Rarely primary. May cause respiratory embarrassment.

T R E A T M E N T: Address underlying cause.

SHEEP AND GOATS

Nasal Discharge

SHEEP NASAL BOTFLY INFESTATION. (*Oestrus ovis*) Larvae parasitize nasal cavity and frontal sinus. Adult fly deposits larvae on nostril.

Signs include head-shaking, nasal irritation with discharge, and anorexia. Invasion of CNS occurs in rare cases.
T R E A T M E N T: Administer rafoxanide (7.5 mg/kg, p.o.), or
ivermectin (0.2 mg/kg).

ENZOOTIC NASAL ADENOCARCINOMA. (Viral etiology suspected)
Sheep are affected. Occurs sporadically in North America. Nasal
discharge is serous, mucous, or mucopurulent. Signs also include
progressive anorexia and respiratory difficulty leading to open-mouth
breathing. Usually fatal within 3 months.
T R E A T M E N T: None successful.

MISCELLANEOUS CONDITIONS

Neoplasms
Foreign bodies
Mycotic nasal granuloma
Nasal schistosomiasis (blood fluke)
Trauma (e.g., from fighting)

Coughing and Respiratory Distress

ENZOOTIC PNEUMONIA. (many agents, including viruses [PI$_3$, RSV,
reovirus], *Mycoplasma* spp., *Chlamydia* spp., and bacteria [e.g., *Pasteurella haemolytica*] implicated) Signs include poor performance,
nasal discharge, and coughing. Mainly occurs in housed animals.
Deaths may occur with secondary bacterial infection.
T R E A T M E N T: Improve management, especially ventilation.
Antibiotics are indicated for secondary bacterial infection.

PNEUMONIC PASTEURELLOSIS. (*Pasteurella haemolytica* type A, less
commonly type T, also *P. multocida*) Common. Outbreaks occur;
sudden deaths are seen early in outbreak. Signs include cough, fever,
nasal discharge, and respiratory distress. Deaths may occur in 12 h,
but the course of the illness usually lasts several days. Mortality is
high in young animals. Stress or environmental changes may precipitate outbreaks.
T R E A T M E N T: Administer broad-spectrum antibiotics, e.g.,
oxytetracycline (10 mg/kg, i.v. or i.m. b.i.d.). Nonsteroidal antiinflammatory drugs or corticosteroids may be helpful in early stages of the
disease.

CASEOUS LYMPHADENITIS. (*Corynebacterium pseudotuberculosis*) Commonly associated with abscess formation and chronic weight loss. May cause acute, fatal bronchopneumonia in sheep.

T R E A T M E N T: None effective.

OVINE PROGRESSIVE PNEUMONIA (sheep)/CAPRINE ARTHRITIS EN-CEPHALITIS (goats). (lentivirus) Long incubation; onset of disease is heralded by weight loss. Signs include lack of fever, exercise intolerance, and respiratory embarrassment. Respiratory signs are rare in goats. May also cause chronic mastitis. Neurologic disease is seen in sheep with some virus strains, but only rarely accompanies respiratory form.

T R E A T M E N T: None effective.

PULMONARY ADENOMATOSIS. (retroviral etiology suspected) Affects sheep. Uncommon in USA. Mainly seen in Europe. Fatal disease. Signs include lack of fever, slow onset, exercise intolerance, weight loss, respiratory distress, and copious, watery nasal discharge.

T R E A T M E N T: None effective.

HOOSE. (*Dictyocaulus filaria*) Worldwide. Sheep and goats affected; usually young animals, chronic coughing, weight loss, nasal discharge.

T R E A T M E N T: Administer broad-spectrum anthelmintics, e.g., levamisole, ivermectin, and newer benzimidazoles at standard dosages.

MUELLERIUS CAPILLARIS INFECTION. Occurs worldwide. Usually subclinical; occasionally, severe infection may cause coughing and respiratory distress. May be complicated by secondary pneumonia.

T R E A T M E N T: Administer fenbendazole (15 mg/kg, p.o.).

PROTOSTRONGYLUS RUFESCENS INFECTION. Affects only kids and lambs. Signs are similar to those for infection by *Dictyocaulus filaria*.

T R E A T M E N T: Administer broad-spectrum anthelmintics.

PIGS

Epistaxis and Nasal Discharge

ATROPHIC RHINITIS. Common. Complex disease associated with concurrent *Bordetella bronchiseptica* and *Pasteurella multocida* infection. Signs include sneezing and nasal discharge in pigs up to 6–8 weeks of age. There is often subsequent turbinate atrophy with deviation of snout. Epistaxis occurs occasionally.

T R E A T M E N T: None specific.

INCLUSION BODY RHINITIS. (cytomegalovirus) Signs usually include subclinical or mild fever in pigs over 3 weeks old. Neonatal piglets may develop sneezing and nasal discharge. Occasionally viral septicemia occurs and results in death.

T R E A T M E N T: None specific.

NECROTIC RHINITIS. (*Fusobacterium necrophorum*) Disease usually spread by fighting. Affects young pigs. Signs include cellulitis of soft tissues of face (may also involve bone), respiratory embarrassment, anorexia, and nasal discharge.

T R E A T M E N T: Penicillin, sulfonamides, or tetracyclines are effective.

Coughing and Respiratory Distress

ENZOOTIC PNEUMONIA. (*Mycoplasma hyopneumoniae*) Common.

Acute Form. Rare. Signs include fever, coughing, and inappetance. Usually affects specific pathogen free (SPF) herds.

Chronic Form. Common in postweaning piglets. Signs include moderate fever, hacking cough, and weight loss. Occasionally animals may develop secondary bacterial pneumonia.

T R E A T M E N T: Medication of water with tetracycline prevents disease. Other drugs found to be effective include tylosin, tiamulin, and lincomycin. Improve ventilation.

MYCOPLASMA HYORHINIS INFECTION. Signs include fever, decreased growth rate, and polyserositis. Occasionally respiratory signs result from pleuritis.

T R E A T M E N T: Same as for enzootic pneumonia.

PASTEURELLOSIS. (*Pasteurella multocida*) Generally a secondary invader in enzootic pneumonia. Acute form, with fever, coughing, and respiratory distress, may be fatal. Frequently the chronic form develops with fever, coughing, and ill-thrift.

T R E A T M E N T: Administer broad-spectrum antibiotics.

PLEUROPNEUMONIA. (*Actinobacillus pleuropneumoniae*) May occur in outbreak form with sudden deaths. Signs include fever, anorexia, and increased work of breathing. Bloody froth may be evident at nostrils or mouth terminally. A chronic or subacute form occurs with chronic coughing, ill-thrift, and respiratory difficulty.

T R E A T M E N T: Improve management, e.g., all-in, all-out system. Remove carriers (serologic testing). Affected animals may be treated with antibiotics, including penicillin, potentiated sulphonamides, and tetracyclines.

GLASSER'S DISEASE. (*Haemophilus parasuis*) All ages are affected, but young pigs especially. Signs include acute polyserositis with fever, anorexia, and respiratory distress. Many die; others may develop meningitis or chronic arthritis.

T R E A T M E N T: Administer penicillin or potentiated sulphonamide.

PSEUDORABIES. (herpesvirus) Neurologic disease in young pigs. Infection in adults may cause mild cough, fever, and nasal discharge of short duration. Reproductive efficiency is affected, with increased stillbirths and increased returns to service.

SWINE INFLUENZA. (orthomyxovirus, type A influenza virus) Occurs in North America, Europe, and Asia. High morbidity, low mortality. Outbreaks occur. Signs include coughing, respiratory distress, lacrimation, and prostration, with fever and inappetence. Animals recover in 7–10 days.

T R E A T M E N T: None specific. Vaccine available.

PARASITISM. (*Metastrongylus apri, Ascaris suum*) Infection with large number of *M. apri* or *A. suum* in young pigs may cause coughing, nasal discharge, and respiratory difficulty.

T R E A T M E N T: Administer broad-spectrum anthelmintic.

ANTHRAX. (*Bacillus anthracis*) Uncommon. Pharyngeal, intestinal, and septicemic forms occur. Pharyngeal form may manifest as swelling of throat area, with fever and respiratory distress.

MISCELLANEOUS CONDITIONS

1. **Cardiac failure** due to mulberry heart disease or monensin poisoning
2. **Nitrate ingestion** leads to nitrite formation in gut; nitrite causes methemoglobinemia, muddy mucous membranes, and increased respiratory effort due to hypoxia
3. **Other poisons** including carbon monoxide
4. **Dusty environment** associated with dry feeding

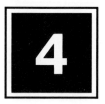

Cardiovascular System

CONGENITAL CARDIAC DISEASES

Congenital cardiac diseases are uncommon in ruminants, pigs, and horses, but appear to be quite common in New World camelids in North America. Some of the more commonly diagnosed conditions in horses and ruminants include:

1. interventricular septal defect
2. ectopia cordis
3. ventricular hypoplasia
4. valvular hematomas (bovine)
5. patent foramen ovale
6. tetralogy of Fallot
7. patent ductus arteriosus.

EXAMINATION OF CARDIOVASCULAR SYSTEM

Examining the cardiovascular system involves inspection, palpation, percussion, and auscultation. If disease is suspected or if the examination is part of a soundness examination, the procedures should be conducted at rest and following exercise. Needless to say, the decision to exercise the animal depends on its physical state.

Inspection

The animal should be inspected for gross signs of cardiac disease, including the presence of edema, distention of jugular veins, and abnormal jugular pulses. The mucous membranes should be pink, and the capillary refill time should be less than 2 s.

Palpation

The peripheral arterial pulse can be palpated in a number of locations, such as facial, transverse facial, auricular, coccygeal (bovine especially), brachial, femoral (neonates), and metatarsal arteries. The rate, strength, and regularity of the pulse should be noted.

The cardiac impulse should be palpated using the flat of the hand. In the horse, the cardiac impulse is palpable between the third and fifth intercostal space on the left side, about the middle or lower third of the thorax. It is strongest at the fifth intercostal space. On the right side, the impulse is detected between the third and fourth intercostal space above the sternal border.

Percussion

The boundaries of percussion vary with the animal's conformation and body condition. The area of dullness on percussion is increased in the presence of extensive cardiomegaly and pericardial effusion.

Auscultation

Although heart sounds may radiate over a wide area, there are specific areas or points of maximal intensity (PMI) where the heart sounds are loudest. These specific points are the areas where the heart sounds reach the surface first.

In the horse, the specific locations on the chest wall associated with PMI for each heart valve are:

1. **Mitral:** The fifth intercostal space on the left side, halfway between the point of the shoulder and sternum.

2. **Aortic:** The fourth intercostal space on the left side, approximately 1 in. below the point of the shoulder.

3. **Pulmonic:** The third or fourth intercostal space on the left side, approximately in the middle of the lower third of the chest wall.

4. **Tricuspid:** The third or fourth intercostal space on the right side.

Table 4–1 lists normal heart rates.

Heart Sounds

"There are strings," said Mr Tappertit, . . . in the human heart that had better not be vibrated."

Charles Dickens (*Barnaby Rudge*)

The mechanical activity of the myocardium propagates transverse vibrational waves that traverse the surfaces of the ventricles, great vessels, and thorax. These transverse vibrations cause the column of air in the stethoscope to vibrate in a longitudinal fashion, and the resultant waveform is received by the listener as a true sound wave.

Heart sounds vary in loudness among animals. Of importance in individual cases is the relative loudness of the heart sounds. Factors such as the force of ventricular contraction and the degree of valve opening prior to the closure affect the loudness of the corresponding heart sound.

The timing of heart sounds follows the pattern described below and illustrated in Figure 4–1.

First Heart Sound (S₁)

The S_1, or first heart sound, is primarily caused by closure of the atrioventricular (AV) valves. A minor contribution is due to movement in the ventricular wall at the start of ventricular systole.

A split S_1 is the result of many factors, including the length of the sound, ventricular motion prior to AV valve closure, and the rapid ejection phase. S_1 follows the QRS complex of the electrocardiogram (ECG).

Second Heart Sound (S₂)

The S_2, or second heart sound, is caused by closure of the aortic and pulmonic valves and occurs following the T wave of the ECG.

TABLE 4–1. NORMAL HEART RATES

Species	Age of Animal	Range of Normal Heart Rates
Horses	Adults	28–42
	Foals <1 mo	70–80
	Older foals	50–60
Cattle	Adults	50–80
	Calves	90–110
Sheep and Goats	Adults	70–90
	Lambs and kids	100–180
Pigs	Adults	70–80
	Piglets	150–200
Llamas	Adults	60–70
	Crias	140–180

Splitting of the S_2 occurs owing to asynchrony of pulmonic and aortic valve closure. The degree of asynchrony is dependent on the respiratory cycle. During inspiration, S_2 is split into an aortic and pulmonic component, whereas in expiration the sounds merge.

Third Heart Sound (S₃)

The S_3, or third heart sound, occurs almost immediately after S_2, between the T and P waves of the ECG. It is caused by vibration of the ventricular myocardium and closure of the atrioventricular valves subsequent to vortex formation during the period of rapid ventricular filling.

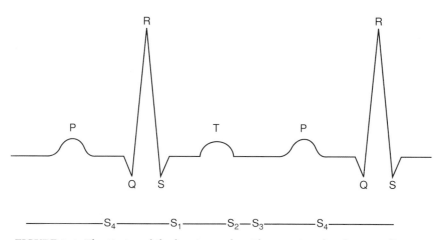

FIGURE 4–1. The timing of the heart sounds with respect to the electrocardiogram.

Fourth Heart Sound (S₄)

The S_4, or fourth heart sound, is caused by contraction of the atrium and occurs between the P wave and QRS complex of the ECG. It occurs close to S_1, and its presence may give the impression of a split S_1. S_4 is absent in certain diseases of the conduction pathways, such as atrial fibrillation. S_4 is particularly audible in the llama on the left side of the thorax.

Murmurs

Murmurs are sounds produced by turbulent flow. Generally, blood flow in vessels is silent because the flow profile is laminar. The laminar stream is smooth and lacks vibrations, as the laminae (layers) move silently over each other.

The point at which laminar flow becomes turbulent—the critical velocity (Vc)—is dependent on the viscosity (η) and density (ρ) of the fluid and the radius of the tube (r), according to the formula

$$Vc = \frac{R\eta}{\rho r}$$

where R is Reynold's number, a dimensionless number described by the formula

$$R = \frac{v\rho r}{\eta}$$

Here *v* is the velocity of flow.

In long straight tubes, an R value ≥ 2000 signifies turbulent flow; however, values <200 have been calculated in experimental models of stenosis.

Murmurs are always associated with an abnormally high flow velocity through vessels or valves, but innocent or functional systolic murmurs occur with intensive exercise (increased velocity), increased fluid density (ρ), increased vessel radius (r), or decreased blood viscosity (η). The formula above explains why murmurs are more likely to occur in large animals (increased r).

Murmurs are classified according to the following criteria.

Location in the Cardiac Cycle

SYSTOLIC MURMURS. These occur between S_1 and S_2. Proto-, meso- and telesystolic murmurs occur in early, middle, or late systole, respectively. Holosystolic murmurs occupy the time between S_1 and S_2, and pansystolic murmurs span systole and encompass S_1 and S_2.

DIASTOLIC MURMURS. Holodiastolic murmurs occur between S_2 and S_1. Protodiastolic murmurs occur early in diastole (between S_2 and S_3), and mesodiastolic murmurs (between S_3 and S_4) occur in mid-diastole. Presystolic (i.e., late diastolic) murmurs occur between S_4 and S_1.

CONTINUOUS MURMURS. These encompass systole and diastole.

Intensity of Murmurs

The following grading system may be used for describing the intensity of murmurs.

GRADE 1. Faintest murmur auscultated.

GRADE 2. Faint murmur that can be heard readily after a few seconds of auscultation.

GRADE 3. Immediately audible over a wide area. A loud grade 3 murmur has an associated thrill.

GRADE 4. Loudest murmur that is inaudible after removal of stethoscope. Always has an associated thrill.

GRADE 5. Audible even without auscultation. Always has an associated thrill.

CARDIAC DISEASE IN HORSES

Cardiac Murmurs

A large percentage of horses (up to 50% in some surveys) have systolic murmurs, and approximately 25% have diastolic murmurs. It appears that the anatomy of the equine cardiovascular system and the characteristics of blood flow in the horse predispose to the development of murmurs. Thus, there occur functional murmurs that are frequently present at rest and that are not associated with pathologic states.

Significant Murmurs*

The following murmurs probably constitute an unsoundness.

SYSTOLIC MURMURS. Systolic murmurs that are grade 3 or higher, or that persist throughout systole, e.g., tricuspid valve incompetence, pulmonic stenosis, mitral valve incompetence, aortic stenosis, or ruptured chordae tendineae of the mitral valve.

---

*It should be noted that valvular endocarditis may cause a wide variety of murmurs and therefore warrants inclusion in the differential diagnosis of murmurs associated with poor form, fever, or inappetance.

DIASTOLIC MURMURS

1. Diastolic murmurs of grade 3 intensity or higher and those that persist for half or more of the diastolic period, e.g., aortic insufficiency (common) typified by a whistling or musical sound.

2. Murmurs accompanied by a thrill.

3. Decrescendo diastolic murmurs with a grade 2 intensity or higher, associated with a presystolic murmur, e.g., atrioventricular valve stenosis.

4. Machinery murmurs due to patent ductus arteriosus in adults.

Functional Murmurs

SYSTOLIC MURMURS. Early systolic, stopping by midcycle and grade 3 or less. They result from turbulent flow in the aortic and pulmonary outflow tracts in early systole when flow velocity is high.

DIASTOLIC MURMURS. Less than grade 3 and occurring in early diastole.

Arrhythmias

Heart Block

SINOATRIAL (SA) BLOCK. The basic rhythm is preserved, but an occasional beat is absent. A junctional escape beat may occur if the P-P interval is prolonged. SA block is less common than atrioventricular block.

There are two forms of SA block.

Sinus Block. The pauses are less than or equal to two of the previous P-P intervals.

Sinus Arrest. The pauses are greater than twice the P-P interval.

Junctional escape beats occur occasionally during these prolonged intervals.

ATRIOVENTRICULAR (AV) BLOCK

First-Degree AV Block. Heart rate is normal and P wave and QRS complex are normal. An ECG is required for diagnosis. The P-R interval is consistently increased, and its duration is greater than 0.44 s.

Second-Degree AV Block

Mobitz Type 1 (Wenckebach). The P wave and QRS complexes are within normal limits. The P-R interval increases progressively until eventually a P wave occurs that fails to be conducted.

Mobitz Type 2. This type is much less common than type 1. It is detected as an absent QRS complex following a P wave, without any premonitory ECG signs.

It appears that sinoatrial block, first-degree AV block, and second-degree Mobitz type 1 AV block are common at rest and can be attributed to the predominance of vagal tone.

In a horse, single dropped beats at rest that disappear after exercise can be regarded as normal if no other abnormalities are present.

Third-Degree AV Block. This condition is pathologic. The P-P interval is normal. The P waves are of normal configuration, but they are not conducted through the AV node. Ventricular rate is often very slow but regular, and the QRS complex and T wave may be of normal configuration (as in an AV nodal pacemaker) or widened (reflecting a ventricular pacemaker).

Atrial Fibrillation (AF)

Atrial fibrillation appears to be relatively common in horses. AF affects large horses, commonly draught breeds. It is more common in older draught animals; however, it is commonest in racing animals between 3 and 4 years old. Signs may develop suddenly if the animal is at work and may include incoordination, respiratory distress, and collapse. Poor performance is the most common finding in competitive horses. In other cases, AF may be an incidental finding and these animals function adequately unless stressed. If myocardial failure is clinically evident (jugular pulsation and peripheral edema) or detected echocardiographically, prognosis is guarded and treatment may not be justified. In general, a heart rate in excess of 60 beats per minute indicates significant cardiac disease (Table 4–2).

T R E A T M E N T: The prognosis is better if treatment is instituted soon after the condition is detected, and reversion to sinus rhythm is less likely if the condition has been present for longer than 3 months. In some cases sinus rhythm cannot be regained, and in other cases AF may recur.

1. Animals such as brood mares with a stable ventricular rate and no signs of distress may not require treatment.

2. Animals with signs of cardiac failure generally respond poorly to treatment, and treatment may not be justified in such cases.

3. Quinidine sulphate (administered orally) or quinidine gluconate (administered intravenously) are the drugs of choice at present.

TABLE 4–2. DATA SUPPORTING DIAGNOSIS OF ATRIAL FIBRILLATION

Clinical Findings
Irregular cardiac rhythm
Absence of S_4
Variable pulse strength
Variation in loudness of heart sounds reflecting changing end-diastolic volumes

ECG Changes
Absence of P waves
Presence of fibrillation or flutter waves
Irregular R-R interval
T wave changes, reflecting myocardial hypoxia

Since quinidine is a negative inotrope and positive chronotrope, digoxin should be administered initially to animals with a rapid ventricular rate and those with signs of cardiac failure. Digoxin may be given (0.001 mg/kg, i.v. or 0.005 mg/kg) orally.

Quinidine Sulphate (oral). Due to the frequency of toxicity, which includes edema of the nasal passages, gastrointestinal upset (diarrhea, colic), urticaria, and laminitis, a test dose of 5.0 g quinidine sulphate, is commonly given orally on the day prior to treatment. Quinidine sulphate (10.0 g/450 kg) is given orally every 2 h until sinus rhythm returns, signs of toxicity develop, or a total dose of 60–80 g has been given in 24 h. Treatment may be repeated on the following day(s) and the frequency of administration reduced if signs of toxicity become evident. Frequent monitoring of the ECG is recommended during treatment.

Quinidine Gluconate (intravenous). Intravenous quinidine is a more convenient method of therapy. The dosage is approximately 1.1 mg/kg (over 3–4 min) given every 15 min for a total of 10 doses or until normal sinus rhythm returns or signs of toxicity occur. There appears to be wide individual variation in the amount of quinidine required for conversion. Likewise, the serum quinidine concentration associated with toxicity seems to vary. On this basis, the commonly recommended maximum daily dosage could be exceeded if toxicity is not evident. Once again, ECG monitoring is recommended throughout the treatment period. Prolongation of QRS complex is the primary sign of toxicity.

PAROXYSMAL ATRIAL FIBRILLATION. Whereas the majority of cases of AF are persistent, paroxysmal AF has been recorded in horses following severe exercise. Most cases appear to regain a normal sinus rhythm within a 24-h period and go on to race again uneventfully. This type of arrhythmia may be responsible for some cases of unexplained poor racing performance.

Premature Ventricular Contractions (PVCs)

An ectopic focus may arise anywhere in the ventricles. The degree of aberrancy depends on the site of the ectopic focus (foci) and its distance from the Purkinje system. Activation of the atria rarely occurs, so that the SA node is not reset. Auscultation of a single PVC is probably insignificant; however, it must be appreciated that PVCs may occur intermittently and unpredictably if an irritable focus is present in the ventricular myocardium. Multifocal PVCs are indicative of myocardial disease and carry a poor prognosis. If they occur with a greater frequency, a closer evaluation of the cardiovascular system is warranted.

The first heart sound is louder than normal as the AV valves are open when the ventricular contraction begins. Since the atria are not contracting in sequence with the ventricles, no S_4 precedes the ventricular contraction.

T R E A T M E N T: Administer intravenous lidocaine (1.0–1.5 mg/kg) as a bolus and repeat if necessary. It is generally safe to administer 4.0 mg/kg, i.v., over a 5-min period. Low doses of lidocaine have a sedative effect; however, high doses (≥ 10.0 mg/kg) over a short period may cause excitation and convulsions. To control persistent ectopic beats, a continuous i.v. infusion (0.02–0.04 mg/kg/min) may be given following a bolus injection.

Causes of Inflammatory and Degenerative Cardiac Disease

Viral

Viral diseases that have been implicated in myocarditis include:

AFRICAN HORSE SICKNESS. Signs in the subacute (cardiac) form include edema of the head region, eyelids, lips and limbs; fever; and petechiae of the mucous membranes. Hydropericardium is a common postmortem finding.

EQUINE INFECTIOUS ANEMIA
EQUINE VIRAL ARTERITIS
EQUINE INFLUENZA

Bacterial

Streptococcus equi infection
Septicemia in neonates

Parasite Migration

Aberrant migration of *Strongylus vulgaris* larvae.

Toxins

IONOPHORES (LASALOCID, MONENSIN): Used as feed additive for cattle. Accidental feeding to horses may cause toxic myocardial degeneration. Signs include colic, diarrhea, and cardiac failure.

VITAMIN D TOXICITY. Inappropriate administration of vitamin D or ingestion of plants containing high concentrations of vitamin D–like steroids, e.g., *Cestrum diurnum* (wild jasmine) may cause calcification of myocardium and endocardium.

CANTHARIDIN POISONING: BLISTER BEETLE POISONING. Southern USA. Signs include colic, frequent urination, hematuria.

T R E A T M E N T: Administer supportive care.

Miscellaneous Conditions

SELENIUM DEFICIENCY. Linked to myocardial degeneration.

EXERTIONAL RHABDOMYOLYSIS. Degeneration of the cardiac muscle has been reported in the horse.

COR PULMONALE. Hypertrophy of the right ventricle secondary to chronic pulmonary disease develops in horses suffering from chronic small-airway disease (heaves). It is a consequence of long-standing increases of pulmonary arterial pressure.

RUPTURE OF BASE OF AORTA. Uncommon cause of sudden death. Stallions more often affected.

Diseases in Which Edema Is a Prominent Sign

EQUINE VIRAL ARTERITIS. (togavirus) Worldwide disease. Signs include fever, depression, serous nasal discharge (which may become purulent), conjunctivitis, palpebral edema, nasal mucosal petechiation, keratitis, and lacrimation. Uveitis occurs with cloudiness of aqueous humor. Respiratory distress and coughing are secondary to pulmonary congestion. Limb edema and edema of prepuce and scrotum are common. Abortion frequently occurs in infected pregnant mares. Arteritis is prominent.

T R E A T M E N T: None specific. Institute supportive care.

GETAH VIRUS INFECTION. Present in Japan. Signs include fever, limb edema, and mucosal exanthema, but no respiratory signs are evident. Recovery without complications in most cases.

AFRICAN HORSE SICKNESS. (orbivirus) Occurs in North Africa, Mediterranean, and Southwest Asia. Edema of the head, eyes, and lips is a prominent feature of the subacute form. High mortality rate.

EHRLICHIOSIS. (*Ehrlichia equi*) Occurs in western USA. Clinical signs include fever, anorexia, edema of limbs, stiffness, jaundice, and mucosal petechiation. Signs persist for 10–14 days.

T R E A T M E N T: Responds to tetracyclines.

PURPURA HEMORRHAGICA. Uncommon. Usually a sequel to streptococcal respiratory disease. Signs include widespread subcutaneous edematous swellings, particularly in head and neck areas.

T R E A T M E N T: Administer corticosteroids, e.g., dexamethasone (0.05 mg/kg, i.v. or i.m.), once or twice daily initially; reduce frequency of treatment according to response. Treatment may have to be continued for 4–6 weeks. Antibiotics, e.g., penicillin, may be indicated initially. Supportive care includes leg bandaging and cold-water hosing of affected areas.

DOURINE. (*Trypanosoma equiperdum*) Occurs in Africa, Asia, southeastern Europe, and parts of southern USA. Spread by coitus, lesions start on external genitalia and spread to surrounding areas. In both sexes edema of the genitalia is prominent. A mucopurulent urethral discharge is seen in stallions. Perineum, udder, and vulva are affected in mares, with copious watery discharge. Reddening and ulceration of vaginal mucosa may be evident.

T R E A T M E N T: Poor response to treatment with diminazene or suramin.

IMMUNE-MEDIATED THROMBOCYTOPENIA. Affects any age and either sex. May be primary (idiopathic) or secondary due to certain therapeutic agents. Clinical signs include petechiae on mucous membranes and subcutaneous swellings. Hemorrhage from body orifices may occur in severe cases.

T R E A T M E N T: Administer corticosteroids and provide supportive care. Blood transfusions are needed in severe cases.

SPORADIC LYMPHANGITIS. Uncommon. Thought to develop secondary to skin wounds. Signs include acute onset of fever and swelling of one or both hindlimbs, pain and heat in the affected limbs, and cording of the lymphatics. Signs persist for 7–10 days. Occasionally abscesses may develop in the lymphatics and rupture to the exterior.

T R E A T M E N T: Administer antibiotics (e.g., penicillin), antiinflammatories, hot packing, and support bandages.

ANGIONEUROTIC EDEMA. (plant allergens) Signs include localized areas of painless edematous swellings commonly around eyes, muzzle, and, occasionally, in the perineal area. Usually seen in animals at pasture, suggesting a plant allergen as a cause.

T R E A T M E N T: Administer corticosteroids when indicated.

BLACK WALNUT POISONING. (*Juglans nigra*) Wood shavings have caused the following clinical signs within 18 h of exposure: mild to marked edema of the limbs and signs of laminitis, especially an unwillingness to move. Illness may result from ingestion or skin exposure.

T R E A T M E N T: Administer nonsteroidal antiinflammatories, provide supportive care.

EQUINE INFECTIOUS ANEMIA. (lentivirus) Edema may be a feature of the recurrent episodes of EIA. Other signs include anemia, fever, jaundice, inappetence, and weight loss.

T R E A T M E N T: None specific.

BABESIOSIS. (*Babesia caballi, B. equi*) Infection with *B. caballi* occurs in USA, Canada, and Central America. Infection with *B. equi* occurs in Europe, Asia, and India. Signs include fever; jaundice; and edema of the legs, head, and ventral abdomen. Hemoglobinuria is uncommon.

TREATMENT: See Chapter 16.

HYPOPROTEINEMIA. Usually occurs subsequent to the failure of absorption (e.g., infiltrative bowel disease) or as a result of excessive loss of protein in the intestine, (e.g., parasitism), kidney, or skin (rare). Edema is a prominent sign, usually involving the lower limbs, ventral abdomen, and the prepuce. Poor prognosis in infiltrative bowel disease.

TREATMENT: Depends on cause.

CARDIAC FAILURE. Rare. May be accompanied by edema of limbs, ventral aspect of thorax and abdomen, and the prepuce. Other signs may include distended jugular veins, respiratory distress, cardiac arrhythmias, murmurs, or thrills.

TREATMENT: Generally unsuccessful.

Lymphangitis

EPIZOOTIC LYMPHANGITIS. Exotic disease. Occurs in Africa, Asia, and the Mediterranean area. Chronic disease, manifested by suppurative lymphangitis, lymphadenopathy, and ulceration of skin. Lesions generally restricted to legs, especially the hock region, but may occur on other parts of the integument. Other signs may include keratitis, conjunctivitis, and pneumonia. Contagious.

TREATMENT: Generally unsuccessful.

SPOROTRICHOSIS. (*Sporotrichum schenkii*) Characterized by cutaneous nodules and ulcers on the limbs, sometimes accompanied by lymphangitis. Skin nodules occur on the lower limbs, especially around the fetlocks. No pain is associated with the lesions. Scab forms on the surface of the nodule following rupture and purulent discharge. Cording of lymphatics may be a feature.

TREATMENT: Antifungal agents, e.g., natamycin, or iodides.

GLANDERS. (*Actinobacillus mallei*)
Acute Form. Signs include fever, cough, and skin ulceration on lower limbs and abdomen. Ulcers may be present on nasal mucosa. High mortality rate.

Chronic Form. A pulmonary form is seen. Alternatively, the skin may be affected, with the development of subcutaneous nodules, which ulcerate to release a syrup-like discharge and later heal with a characteristic scar.

TREATMENT: Prolonged treatment with sulfadiazine may be effective.

ULCERATIVE LYMPHANGITIS. (*Corynebacterium pseudotuberculosis*) Nodules develop on the skin. Lower limbs are usually affected but can spread to any part of the body. The nodules rupture to discharge a thick, creamy pus. Thickening of lymphatics may occur and the disease may continue to recur for several months.

T R E A T M E N T: Provide wound care and systemic penicillin.

SPORADIC LYMPHANGITIS. Develops secondary to skin wounds. May involve one or both hindlimbs. Signs include pain, fever, swelling and lameness of the affected leg, cording of lymphatics, and enlargement of lymph nodes (which may rupture to the exterior). Chronic thickening of the affected limb occurs.

T R E A T M E N T: Systemic antibiotics, e.g., penicillin; administer antiinflammatories and provide wound care.

CARDIAC DISEASE IN RUMINANTS

Arrhythmias

Atrial Fibrillation (AF)

Auscultatory findings include a rhythm irregularity, variation in the heart sound intensity, and an absence of S_4.

Fibrillation may be primary or secondary. The primary form is associated with myocardial diseases or bacterial endocarditis. Cardiac lesions are absent. The secondary form is associated with gastrointestinal disease and electrolyte or acid–base abnormalities.

In cows with a rapid heart rate (>100 beats/min) a pulse deficit is generally present. Signs of heart failure are usually absent. Some cows will convert to a normal sinus rhythm, but therapeutic intervention should occur if AF persists for longer than 7 days.

T R E A T M E N T:

1. Correct underlying disease (e.g., abomasal torsion) and correct associated dehydration, acid–base imbalances, and electrolyte imbalances.

2. If the heart rate is >120 beats/min, digoxin (0.001 mg/kg, i.v.) should be administered prior to quinidine therapy.

3. Administer quinidine sulphate (20.0 mg/kg in 4 L of saline, orally). Repeat in 1 h.

4. Alternatively, administer quinidine sulphate (50.0 mg/kg in 4 L of saline, i.v.) at a rate of 1 L/h (0.20 mg/kg/min), until conversion to normal rhythm.

5. Alternatively, administer quinidine gluconate (12.0 mg/kg, i.v.) in 1 L of saline over 2 h. Repeat if necessary.

Premature Atrial Contractions

This type of arrhythmia is commonly encountered in some types of gastrointestinal disease, especially left-sided abomasal displacement. They usually respond to rest and antiinflammatory drugs.

Premature Ventricular Contractions

This type of arrhythmia is uncommon and may be associated with irritable foci in the ventricular myocardium, resulting from degenerative disease (cardiomyopathy) or from myocarditis of infectious or toxic origin. For treatment, see p. 85.

Causes of Inflammatory and Degenerative Cardiac Disease

Viral

FOOT AND MOUTH DISEASE. (picornavirus) In the acute form myocarditis may occur.

BLUETONGUE. (orbivirus) May cause myocardial necrosis in sheep.

Bacterial

ENDOCARDITIS. (*Streptococcus* spp., *Actinomyces pyogenes*, and coliforms) Relatively uncommon in cattle. The right AV valve is the most frequently affected. Murmurs are common, reflecting valvular insufficiency or stenosis. Infection usually spreads to the heart valve from a septic focus, e.g., liver abscess, mastitis, or metritis. Fever, tachycardia, cardiac thrill, jugular venous distension, and brisket edema are common signs. Sudden death can occur.

T R E A T M E N T: Administer antibiotics and antiinflammatories; provide supportive care. Poor response in many cases.

PERICARDITIS. Relatively uncommon. Usually results from penetration of diaphragm and pericardial sac by foreign body in reticulum. Signs include fever, depression, and anorexia. Pericardial friction rubs occur in early stages, later there are signs of cardiac failure with muffled heart sounds, distended jugular veins, and brisket edema.

T R E A T M E N T: Medical treatment as for endocarditis. Generally a poor response to surgical intervention.

BLACKLEG. (*Clostridium chauvoei*) Cardiac myositis has been observed in cattle.

T R E A T M E N T: Animals are likely to die before treatment is instituted.

TICK PYEMIA. (*Staphylococcus aureus*) May cause cardiac lesions in lambs.

T R E A T M E N T: Early cases may respond to penicillin.

HEARTWATER. (*Cowdria ruminantium*) Occurs in Africa and West Indies. Heart lesions occur.

T R E A T M E N T: Early cases respond to tetracyclines.

Parasitic Infections

CYSTICERCOSIS. (*Cysticercus bovis*) Metacestode of *Taenia saginata*. Commonly found as a small white nodule in myocardium.

SARCOCYSTOSIS. (*Sarcocystis* spp.) Myocarditis is present in acute and chronic infections. May be fatal.

T R E A T M E N T: None specific.

Toxins

IONOPHORES (MONENSIN, LASALOCID)

Cattle. Signs include weakness, ataxia, and tachycardia. Death in acute disease is due to cardiac failure. Signs in subacute form include congestive heart failure, with distension of jugular veins, and respiratory distress. Myoglobinuria may be evident.

Sheep. Skeletal muscle involvement is more common, although heart muscle may be involved.

T R E A T M E N T: Supportive care.

Nutritional Deficiencies

COPPER DEFICIENCY. In Australia, a form of copper deficiency termed "falling disease," causes cardiac muscle degeneration. May be due to anemic anoxia or disturbances of tissue oxidation. Sudden death is usually the only sign, although pivoting on the forelimbs is regarded as a premonitory sign.

IRON OR COBALT DEFICIENCY. May lead to anemia and hypoxic myocardial degeneration.

VITAMIN E/SELENIUM DEFICIENCY. May be a cause of sudden death associated with myocardial degeneration and white muscle disease.

Miscellaneous Conditions

MYOCARDIAL LIPOFUSCINOSIS. Occurs in older or cachexic cattle, especially in Ayrshire breeds.

HIGH-ALTITUDE DISEASE: BRISKET DISEASE. Signs include edema of brisket, distension of jugular veins, increased respiratory rate, cyanosis, and ill-thrift. Common in young animals soon after introduction to high altitudes.

CONGENITAL CARDIOMYOPATHY

Polled Hereford Calves. Tight, woolly haircoat; rapid growth rate;

and protruding eyes are a feature. Signs appear by 3–6 months of age and include respiratory distress, later followed by bloody froth at nostrils and death.

Japanese Black Cattle. Affects calves 1–3 months old. Death is preceded by respiratory distress.

Holstein-Friesian Cattle. Occurs in this breed in Japan and Canada and in red Holstein-Simmental crosses and black-spotted Friesians in Switzerland. Most common in 3- to 4-year-olds. Appears to be precipitated by stress, e.g., lactation. Sudden onset of signs of right heart failure, including jugular distension, brisket edema, ascites, and muffled heart sounds.

Diseases in Which Edema Is a Prominent Sign

Lymphangitis

ULCERATIVE LYMPHANGITIS. (*Corynebacterium pseudotuberculosis*) Uncommon. Characterized by enlargement of lymph nodes with lymphatic cording, especially in lower limbs. Abscesses may form in lymph nodes and rupture to exterior. Infection enters through wounds on lower part of limb.

T R E A T M E N T: Provide wound care and systemic penicillin.

BOVINE FARCY. (*Nocardia farcinica, Mycobacterium farcinogenes*) Tropical disease. Signs include lymphatic thickening and lymph node enlargement. Vessels may rupture and discharge or ulcerate. Lesions may affect limbs or head region.

T R E A T M E N T: Provide wound care, administer sodium iodide parenterally.

LUMPY SKIN DISEASE. In UK, a severe form is caused by the Neethling poxvirus; a mild form is caused by Allerton herpesvirus. In USA, the mild form is caused by dermatotrophic bovine herpesvirus. Highly infectious. Generally restricted to African continent. Cutaneous nodules develop over the entire body; many are shed, leaving craters that scar over. Limb, udder, or scrotal edema may occur as a result of lymphatic inflammation. Thickening of lymphatics and enlargement of lymph nodes is evident.

T R E A T M E N T: None specific.

CARDIAC DISEASE IN NEW WORLD CAMELIDS

Examination

There is little difference between New World camelids and the other large animal species in terms of cardiovascular examination.

Close auscultation often reveals the presence of S_4. Murmurs at rest are unusual, although in neonates closure of the ductus arteriosus may be delayed, evidenced by a machinery murmur that usually disappears by 6 weeks of age.

Arrhythmias

Although apparently uncommon, when present arrhythmias are associated with underlying diseases, such as septicemia or toxemia, or plant poisoning from species such as oleander, which causes bradycardia and heart block.

Congenital Diseases

Congenital diseases appear to be common in this species and include

1. atrial septal defect
2. ventricular septal defect
3. patent ductus arteriosus
4. persistent right aortic arch
5. tetralogy of Fallot
6. transposition of the great vessels.

5

Urogenital System, Abortion, and Mastitis

"Only when we know little do we know anything; doubt grows with knowledge."

Goethe

UROGENITAL SYSTEM

CAUSES OF RED OR DARK URINE

HORSES

Hematuria

BACTERIAL CYSTITIS. Rare. Occasionally a sequel to neurologic impairment of normal voiding, resulting from sorghum poisoning, neuritis of cauda equina, or equine herpes myelitis.
T R E A T M E N T: Administer broad-spectrum antibiotics.

BLISTER BEETLE POISONING: CANTHARIDIN TOXICITY. Occurs in southern USA. Hematuria accompanied by stomatitis, sweating, colic, history of exposure to contaminated hay. High mortality rate.
T R E A T M E N T: None specific.

URINARY TRACT CALCULI. Rare. May be located anywhere in urinary tract.
T R E A T M E N T: Surgical removal is possible in some cases.

MEDULLARY CREST NECROSIS. Uncommon. Has been associated with phenylbutazone administration.
T R E A T M E N T: Cease phenylbutazone administration. Provide supportive care.

URINARY TRACT NEOPLASIA. Uncommon.
T R E A T M E N T: Usually not attempted.

CLOTTING ABNORMALITY. Warfarin toxicity causes clotting abnormalities. Inherited clotting factor deficiencies occur rarely.
T R E A T M E N T: Administer vitamin K_1, 50 mg/kg, i.v., in warfarin toxicity.

Hemoglobinuria

BABESIOSIS. (*Babesia equi, B. caballi*) Occurs in Asia and USA. Tick-borne. Signs include fever, anorexia, depression, and recumbency. Intravascular hemolysis leads to hemoglobinuria.
T R E A T M E N T: Administer amicarbalide, diminazene aceturate, or imidocarb.

PHENOTHIAZINE POISONING. Rare. Formerly seen when phenothiazine was used as an anthelmintic.

T R E A T M E N T: Usually not necessary.

ISOIMMUNE HEMOLYTIC ANEMIA. Antibody to foal's red cells in dam's colostrum. Onset of signs follows colostrum ingestion and includes depression, anemia, jaundice, weakness, hemoglobinuria, and death in severe cases.

T R E A T M E N T: Prevent access to dam's colostrum for 2–3 days (antibodies are then no longer absorbed across gut). Provide supportive care. Red cell transfusions are necessary in severe cases.

AUTOIMMUNE HEMOLYTIC ANEMIA. Rare.

T R E A T M E N T: Administer steroids and provide supportive care.

RED MAPLE POISONING. Ingestion of wilted leaves or branches may cause methemoglobinemia, exhibited as a brown discoloration of mucous membranes.

T R E A T M E N T: Administer new methylene blue (5.0 mg/kg, i.v.); repeat every 12 h. Provide supportive care and blood transfusion in severe cases. Prognosis is poor if the mucous membranes are severely discolored. *Caution* is advised when treating with methylene blue, as the drug may produce methemoglobin. This drug is not as beneficial in the horse as it is in other species.

TRANSFUSION REACTION. Not common.

T R E A T M E N T: Stop the transfusion and administer corticosteroids, such as dexamethasone (0.1–1.0 mg/kg, i.v.).

Myoglobinuria

EXERTIONAL RHABDOMYOLYSIS: MONDAY MORNING DISEASE. Usually follows intense or prolonged exercise, especially after a period of inactivity.

POSTANESTHETIC MYOSITIS. Prolonged recumbency with resultant ischemic damage to muscle leads to myoglobin release.

T R E A T M E N T: Mild cases of muscle injury resolve with rest, followed by a gradual reintroduction of exercise. More severely affected animals may require the administration of antiinflammatory drugs and supportive care (i.e., fluids). Mild exercise (walking) should be started on the second day after injury. Mannitol (0.25g/kg, i.v.) is recommended to reduce muscle edema and prevent renal damage in severe cases. Treatment may be repeated two to three times in the first day. Maintain hydration.

CATTLE

Hematuria

ENZOOTIC HEMATURIA. Caused by bracken fern poisoning. Usually affects animals older than 1 year. Enzootic to certain areas. Signs include persistent intermittent hematuria.

T R E A T M E N T: None specific. Provide supportive care. Blood transfusions may be indicated.

PYELONEPHRITIS. (*Corynebacterium renale, Escherichia coli,* other bacteria) More common in female (associated with breeding and parturition). Signs include fever, colic, hematuria, loss of condition, pollakiuria, and stranguria.

T R E A T M E N T: Administer antibiotics. If the organism is *C. renale*, response to penicillin is good; if *E. coli*, an aminoglycoside antibiotic is indicated.

MALIGNANT CATARRHAL FEVER. (herpesvirus type 1) Signs include fever, nasal discharge, respiratory distress, ocular discharge, scleral injection, oral ulceration, lymphadenopathy, dysentery, and hematuria.

T R E A T M E N T: None effective.

GOSSYPOL POISONING. A toxic substance present in cottonseed cake. Long-term feeding may result in toxicity. Signs include weakness, anorexia, and occasionally hematuria.

T R E A T M E N T: None specific.

MISCELLANEOUS CONDITIONS. Cystitis due to infection, trauma (calculi), or infarction.

T R E A T M E N T: Remove inciting factor if possible (e.g., calculus), and administer broad-spectrum antibiotics.

Hemoglobinuria

BABESIOSIS. (*Babesia bigemina, B. bovis, B. divergens*) Tick-borne. Rare in animals younger than 6 months. Signs include acute hemolytic crisis with fever, jaundice, depression, hemoglobinuria. Diarrhea is an early sign, followed by constipation.

T R E A T M E N T: Administer amicarbalide, diminazene acetutrate, or imidocarb. Provide supportive care with fluids. Blood transfusion is necessary in severe cases.

POSTPARTURIENT HEMOGLOBINURIA. Occurs 2–6 weeks postpartum. Affects high-producing dairy cows. Signs include sudden onset of weakness, anorexia, hemoglobinuria, and tachycardia. Animals are generally afebrile. High mortality. Associated with low serum phosphorus and possibly low copper and selenium.

T R E A T M E N T: Administer sodium acid phosphate (60 g, i.v., diluted), twice daily for 2 days. Provide supportive care with fluids. Blood transfusions are necessary in severe cases.

BRASSICA POISONING. Overfeeding of rape, kale, turnips, and swedes. Toxic principle is converted to dimethyl disulfide. Signs include extravascular and intravascular hemolysis, hemoglobinuria, general weakness, and sudden death.

T R E A T M E N T: None specific. Provide supportive care. Blood transfusion is necessary in severe cases.

COPPER POISONING. Chronic poisoning. High copper concentration in feed may lead eventually to an acute hemolytic crisis. Signs include anorexia, hemoglobinuria, icterus, and pink/red serum. Death occurs in 24–48 h.

T R E A T M E N T: Provide supportive care. Administer (i) penicillamine to promote urinary exertion of copper (very expensive), (ii) ammonium molybdate (1.6 mg/kg, i.v.) on alternate days, for a total of four to six treatments, or (iii) daily dosing with sodium molybdate (3.0 g), and sodium thiosulphate (5.0 g).

BACILLARY HEMOGLOBINURIA. (*Clostridium novyi* type D) Occurs mainly in western USA. May cause sudden death. Liver damage precedes clinical signs, which include abdominal pain, fever, tachypnea, and hemoglobinuria. High mortality rate.

T R E A T M E N T: Administer penicillin and provide supportive care.

LEPTOSPIROSIS. (*Leptospira pomona*) Young animals are more susceptible. Signs include fever, anorexia, petechiae, jaundice, and hemoglobinuria.

T R E A T M E N T: Administer penicillin or tetracyclines.

CLOSTRIDIUM PERFRINGENS TYPE A. Occurs in Australia. Cattle and sheep are affected. Signs include acute onset of depression, anemia, jaundice, respiratory distress, and hemoglobinuria. High mortality rate.

T R E A T M E N T: Unlikely to succeed. Hyperimmune serum is the only agent that may effect a cure.

WATER INTOXICATION. Usually affects calves. Sudden ingestion of a large volume of water may lead to hemoglobinuria and CNS signs. Animals are afebrile. Usually several animals in group are affected.

T R E A T M E N T: Often resolves spontaneously. Diuretics have been recommended. Hypertonic saline (5.0%), 4–6 mL/kg may be helpful in severe cases.

ISOIMMUNE HEMOLYTIC ANEMIA. Newborns are affected. Hemolysis is due to reaction of maternal colostral antibody with fetal red blood cells. Depression, pale mucous membranes, jaundice, and anemia occur.
T R E A T M E N T: Same as for horses (see p. 98).

AUTOIMMUNE HEMOLYTIC ANEMIA. Rare.
T R E A T M E N T: Administer steroids and provide supportive care.

TRANSFUSION REACTION. Uncommon.
T R E A T M E N T: Stop transfusion. Maintain hydration and administer corticosteroids, e.g., dexamethasone (0.1–1.0 mg/kg, i.v.).

PROPYLENE GLYCOL POISONING. May cause hemolysis when administered intravenously as a base for drugs such as tetracyclines. Usually mild effects.
T R E A T M E N T: Usually not necessary. Administer oral or intravenous fluids in severe cases.

Myoglobinuria

EXERTIONAL MYOPATHY. Usually follows intense exercise, such as turnout after prolonged confinement. Inflammation of muscle leads to release of myoglobin. May be a consequence of low serum vitamin E or selenium concentrations.
T R E A T M E N T: Maintain hydration. Administer antiinflammatories if condition is severe. Provide vitamin E/selenium supplement.

SHEEP AND GOATS

Hematuria

Uncommon in small ruminants. Some of the diseases described for cattle might occur.

Hemoglobinuria

CHRONIC COPPER POISONING. Signs include acute hemolytic crisis, jaundice, and hemoglobinuria. High mortality. Goats are more resistant than sheep.
T R E A T M E N T: Same as for cattle (see p. 100).

BABESIOSIS. *(Babesia motasi, B. ovis)* Occurs in southeastern Europe, Africa, and South America. Signs include fever, depression, anorexia, weakness, tachycardia, pallor of mucous membranes, and hemoglobinuria. Animals may develop jaundice if they survive earlier stages.

T R E A T M E N T: Administer antiprotozoal, such as amicarbalide, diminazene aceturate, or imidocarb. Provide supportive care.

BRASSICA/ONION POISONING. History of intake. Toxic principle is S-methyl cysteine sulfoxide, which is converted in the rumen to dimethyl disulfide, the active toxin. Heinz-Ehrlich bodies in erythrocytes are due to hemoglobin precipitation. May be a cause of sudden death. Signs include fever, blindness, hemoglobinuria, weakness, and pallor.

T R E A T M E N T: Provide supportive care.

BACILLARY HEMOGLOBINURIA. *(Clostridium novyi* type D) Worldwide distribution. Signs include short duration of illness, colic, fever, jaundice, hemoglobinuria, and shallow rapid respiration. Relatively rare in sheep.

T R E A T M E N T: Administer penicillin and provide supportive care.

Myoglobinuria

Can result from muscle trauma, such as sheep traumatized by dogs.

T R E A T M E N T: Provide supportive care. Administer antiinflammatories and analgesics.

PIGS

Hematuria

CYSTITIS AND PYELONEPHRITIS. *(Eubacterium* (formerly *Corynebacterium) suis)* Signs include fever; depression; purulent, bloody urine; and abdominal discomfort in gilts and sows. May be fatal. Several animals in group affected. Bacteria other than *E. suis* may cause sporadic disease with similar signs.

T R E A T M E N T: Administer antibiotics, e.g., high doses of penicillin.

WARFARIN POISONING. Uncommon. Access to warfarin rat bait. Signs include hemorrhage from nose and mouth. May cause hematuria.

T R E A T M E N T: Administer vitamin K and provide supportive care.

Hemoglobinuria

ACUTE LEPTOSPIROSIS. (*Leptospira canicola, L. pomona, L. ictero-haemorrhagiae*) Signs include fever, icterus, depression, and occasionally diarrhea. Hemoglobinuria accompanies these signs. Neurologic signs are rare.

T R E A T M E N T: Administer streptomycin, dihydrostreptomycin, or other broad-spectrum antibiotics.

BABESIOSIS. (*Babesia trautmanni, B. perroncitoi*) Rare. Occurs in southeastern Europe and Africa. Tick-borne. Signs include fever, icterus, hemoglobinuria, and anemia.

T R E A T M E N T: Not well described.

HEMOLYTIC DISEASE OF NEWBORN. Occurs in first 2–3 days of life. Signs include jaundice, anemia, and death in many cases. Antibodies to piglet red cells are ingested in the colostrum and intravascular hemolysis results.

T R E A T M E N T: Provide supportive care.

Myoglobinuria

Uncommon in pigs.

RENAL DISEASES

HORSES

Toxicities

Antibiotics

AMINOGLYCOSIDES. Concentrate in renal tubular epithelium. Toxicity is associated with volume depletion or with long-term high dosages. Foals are especially susceptible.

T R E A T M E N T: Provide supportive care.

SULFONAMIDES. Toxicity favored by volume depletion and acidic urine. Crystal formation in tubules leads to renal disease.

T R E A T M E N T: Provide supportive care.

TETRACYCLINES. Potentially nephrotoxic. Inhibition of oxidative metabolism impairs ability of kidney to concentrate urine.

T R E A T M E N T: Provide supportive care.

Other Toxic Agents

NONSTEROIDAL ANTIINFLAMMATORY DRUGS. NSAIDs may cause renal medullary crest necrosis, with focal necrosis in the medulla. Inhibition of prostaglandin-mediated renal autoregulation may lead to kidney failure, especially in dehydrated states and when other nephrotoxic drugs are administered concurrently.

T R E A T M E N T: Discontinue drug therapy. Administer parenteral fluids and provide supportive care.

HEAVY METALS. Arsenic and, especially, mercury (from blistering agents) may cause renal failure.

T R E A T M E N T: None specific. Provide supportive care.

VITAMIN D. Overdosage of vitamin D_3 (cholecalciferol) or D_2 (ergocalciferol) may lead to renal calcification and damage to tubular function. Other systemic signs are usually present, e.g., lameness due to bony changes or ossification of ligaments or tendons.

T R E A T M E N T: None specific.

VITAMIN K_3. Menadione sodium bisulfite has been associated with renal failure. Tubular nephrosis is the primary lesion.

T R E A T M E N T: None specific.

OXALATES. Ingestion of plants containing high concentrations of oxalates may cause renal failure.

T R E A T M E N T: None specific.

HEMOGLOBIN, MYOGLOBIN. Hemoglobinuria or myoglobinuria may cause renal failure. Tubular damage occurs owing to the formation of free radicals. Examples include oak poisoning (rare) with hemoglobinuria, and exertional rhabdomyolysis leading to myoglobinuria.

T R E A T M E N T: Provide supportive care. Maintain hydration. Administer mannitol (0.25 g/kg, i.v.); may be repeated two or three times in the first day, in severe cases.

BLISTER BEETLE POISONING: CANTHARIDIN TOXICITY. Potent irritant, may cause severe gastrointestinal irritation, myocardial and renal insufficiency, hematuria due to bladder mucosa ulceration. High mortality rate.

T R E A T M E N T: None specific.

Infectious Diseases

SEPTICEMIA, ENDOTOXEMIA. Septicemia is more common in foals, usually due to gram-negative organisms, such as *Escherichia coli*,

Actinobacillus equuli. Renal failure may be a sequel. Endotoxemia is common in gastrointestinal crises, such as colitis and strangulation, and in septic metritis.

T R E A T M E N T: Provide supportive care. Maintain hydration. Administer antibiotics.

PYELONEPHRITIS. Rare. Ascending bacterial infection may result from trauma to urinary tract; for example, during parturition in mares or from retention cystitis caused by neurologic damage. Renal abscessation with pyuria, hematuria, fever, and abdominal pain are common signs.

T R E A T M E N T: Administer broad-spectrum antibiotics, especially those that are excreted by the urinary tract, e.g., penicillins.

Miscellaneous Conditions

GLOMERULONEPHRITIS. Deposition of immune complexes in glomerular wall or production of antiglomerular basement membrane antibody may cause protein loss. Equine infectious anemia, equine viral arteritis, and purpura hemorrhagica have been associated with the disease. Signs include anorexia, weight loss, ventral edema, and isosthenuria.

T R E A T M E N T: Administer corticosteroids and provide supportive care.

AMYLOIDOSIS. Uncommon. Amyloid production occurs due to chronic antigenic stimulation. Deposition in kidney leads ultimately to renal failure with polyuria and polydipsia, proteinuria, weight loss, and ventral edema.

T R E A T M E N T: None effective.

NEPHROLITHS. Uncommon. May be associated with chronic renal failure. Thought to be a sequel to pyelonephritis or mineralization of fibrotic tissue. Usually made up of calcium salts.

T R E A T M E N T: None specific.

RUMINANTS

Congenital Abnormalities

RENAL CYSTS. May be single or multiple. Other congenital abnormalities may coexist in the same animal.

RENAL OXALOSIS. Recorded in aborted fetuses in conjunction with other congenital defects. Postulated to be associated with abnormal glycine metabolism.

Toxicities

Antibiotics

AMINOGLYCOSIDES. Accumulates in proximal tubular epithelium. May reach toxic concentration with prolonged administration at high doses, especially in dehydrated animals.
T R E A T M E N T: Provide supportive care.

SULFONAMIDES. Toxicity favored by volume depletion and acidic urine. Crystal formation in tubules leads to renal disease.
T R E A T M E N T: Provide supportive care.

TETRACYCLINES. May cause renal failure. Affects oxidative metabolism in renal tubular cells, leading to inability to concentrate urine.
T R E A T M E N T: Provide supportive care.

Other Toxic Agents

NONSTEROIDAL ANTIINFLAMMATORY DRUGS. By inhibition of prostaglandin-dependent renal autoregulation, NSAIDs may lead to kidney failure, especially in volume-depleted states. Toxicity is more probable when other nephrotoxic drugs are administered concurrently.
T R E A T M E N T: Provide fluid therapy and supportive care. Discontinue inciting drug.

HEAVY METALS. Arsenic, mercury, and some other heavy metals have been implicated in kidney failure. Toxicity may follow accidental ingestion.
T R E A T M E N T: None specific.

PLANT TOXINS. Ingestion of oak (contains tannins) may cause acute tubular necrosis.
T R E A T M E N T: None specific.

MYCOTOXINS. Ochratoxin A and citrinin may cause toxic nephrosis in cattle. Source is moldy feed.
T R E A T M E N T: None specific.

HEMOGLOBIN, MYOGLOBIN. Hemoglobinuria and myoglobinuria may cause tubular damage, with resultant renal failure.
T R E A T M E N T: Provide supportive care. Maintain hydration. Administer mannitol (0.25 g/kg, i.v.); may be repeated two or three times in the first day, in severe cases.

Infectious Diseases

LEPTOSPIROSIS. *(Leptospira interrogans* var. *hardjo, L. interrogans* var. *pomona)* Affects cattle mainly. Acute, subacute, and chronic forms occur. Acute endothelial damage to the renal blood vessels can cause permanent kidney damage. Leptospirae may be deposited in interstitium, leading to chronic interstitial nephritis and shedding of organisms.

T R E A T M E N T: Poor response to treatment.

PYELONEPHRITIS. *(Corynebacterium renale,* coliforms) Affects cattle, sheep, and goats. Sporadic occurrence. Signs include fever, abdominal pain, anorexia, depression, pyuria, and hematuria. Renal failure may occur as parenchyma becomes abscessed and scarring progresses. May be a sequel to ascending infection from bladder or, rarely, a sequel to septicemia.

T R E A T M E N T: Administer a long course (7–14 days) of appropriate antibiotic.

PULPY KIDNEY. *(Clostridium perfringens,* type D) "Overeating" disease. Affects rapidly growing lambs and kids. May also affect adults. Postulated that overgrowth of organism occurs in intestinal tract with subsequent absorption of toxin. Severe vascular endothelial damage ensues. Death results from toxemia. Rapid autolysis occurs, hence the name "pulpy" kidney. Characterized by sudden death, or sudden onset of neurologic signs followed by death.

T R E A T M E N T: Ineffective.

Miscellaneous Conditions

GLOMERULONEPHRITIS. Very uncommon. Rarely associated with persistent BVD virus infection. Proteinuria with hypoproteinemia and peripheral edema result from glomerular membrane damage. Finnish Landrace lambs under 4 months old develop mesangiocapillary glomerulonephritis. Disease is probably inherited.

T R E A T M E N T: Usually impractical. Where practical, administer corticosteroids and provide supportive care.

AMYLOIDOSIS. Rare. Associated with chronic antigenic stimulation such as occurs in chronic suppurative disease. Deposition of amyloid in renal medulla and glomeruli eventually compromises glomerular filtration. Enlarged pale kidneys are a feature.

T R E A T M E N T: None effective.

RENAL ISCHEMIA. Usually a sequel to shock (septic, endotoxic, or hemorrhagic, most commonly). Hypoxic damage to tubules leads to renal failure.

T R E A T M E N T: Provide fluids and supportive care. Response is poor if there is large-scale involvement of renal tissue.

PIGS

Toxicities

Antibiotics

SULFONAMIDES. Toxicity favored by volume depletion.
T R E A T M E N T: Provide supportive care.

TETRACYCLINES. Affects oxidative metabolism in renal tubular cells, leading to inability to concentrate urine.
T R E A T M E N T: Provide supportive care.

AMINOGLYCOSIDES. Toxicity favored by volume depletion and prolonged administration.
T R E A T M E N T: Provide supportive care.

Mycotoxins

OCHRATOXIN A. May cause renal disease. Present in moldy feed. Signs include reduced appetite, polydipsia, polyuria, and poor growth rate. Tubular degeneration and interstitial fibrosis are features. Less commonly, weaned piglets may develop incoordination and die suddenly. Perirenal edema is evident post mortem. Mortality rates are up to 80%.
T R E A T M E N T: None specific.

Miscellaneous Conditions

PYELONEPHRITIS. *(Eubacterium suis)* May occur in outbreak form in sows. Associated with an infected boar. Some animals die suddenly; others are found with fever, arched backs, painful urination, hematuria, and pyuria. Vaginal and vulval discharge may occur; in mild cases it is the only clinical sign.
T R E A T M E N T: Administer a long course (7–14 days) of the appropriate antibiotic.

PIGMENT NEPHROSIS. Rare. Myoglobinuria or hemoglobinuria may cause renal failure.
T R E A T M E N T: Provide supportive care.

Parasitism

STEPHANURIASIS. *(Stephanurus dentatus)* Tropical disease. Adult worms inhabit cysts in the renal pelvis and the wall of the ureter. Eggs are passed in the urine. Results in fibrosis, abscessation, and scarring in kidney and perirenal tissue.

T R E A T M E N T: Prevention by regular anthelmintic use. Poor response to anthelmintics in advanced cases.

DISEASES OF THE LOWER URINARY TRACT

HORSES

Urinary Bladder Problems

RUPTURE. Common in foals, particularly colts (1%). Occurs during foaling, probably due to pressure on abdomen. Signs occur within 24–36 h after birth and include depression, loss of suck reflex, and frequent attempts to urinate. Foal may pass small amounts of urine or sometimes fail to urinate. Progressive distension of abdomen, increased respiratory rate, abdominal discomfort, and shock may develop later. Tachycardia and arrhythmias may accompany electrolyte and acid–base abnormalities. Early stages of disease mimic meconium retention.

Occurs infrequently in adults. Is associated with foaling (mare) or may happen spontaneously.

T R E A T M E N T: Repair surgically, following stabilization of cardiovascular system.

CYSTITIS. Uncommon. Infection may follow foaling trauma or neurologic damage to bladder, from such causes as equine herpesvirus, cauda equina syndrome, or sorghum toxicity. Signs include frequent urination, pyuria, foul-smelling urine in some cases, or hematuria. Appears to be more common in mares. (See Bladder Paralysis, below.) Blister beetle poisoning may cause cystitis due to the irritant effects of cantharidin.

T R E A T M E N T: Administer antibiotics such as penicillin for 7–10 days.

BLADDER PARALYSIS. Uncommon. Signs include urinary incontinence, with staining of hindlimbs. May be associated with ataxia of hindlimbs or other neurologic signs. Bacterial cystitis may develop secondarily.

Causes include equine herpesvirus myelitis, sorghum toxicity, neuritis of cauda equina, and, occasionally, rabies.

T R E A T M E N T: No specific treatment. Provide supportive care and catheterize the bladder.

BLADDER DISPLACEMENT. Affects mares. Rare. Eversion through urethral sphincter is most common and seems to be related to abdominal straining. Prolapse of bladder also occurs, where it accompanies vaginal prolapse. Prolapse of bladder can also occur through a tear in the floor of vagina, anterior to the urethral orifice.

T R E A T M E N T: Administer epidural anesthesia; then replace manually or repair surgically.

CYSTIC CALCULI. Usually affects older horses, and more commonly males. Signs include straining, dribbling of urine, hematuria, and frequent posturing to urinate. Urine scalding of legs may occur. May be an incidental finding on examination per rectum. Commonly caused by calcium carbonate crystals.

T R E A T M E N T: Remove surgically.

NEOPLASIA. Uncommon.

Diseases of the Urethra

URETHRAL CALCULI. Uncommon. Occur in males. May occur anywhere in urethra, but frequently at the ischial arch. Signs include dribbling of urine (amount passed depends on degree of obstruction), frequent posturing and straining to urinate, extrusion of penis, and, occasionally, hematuria.

T R E A T M E N T: Remove surgically.

URETHRITIS. May be sequel to cystitis or a urethral calculus. Signs are consistent with the presence of pain on urination.

T R E A T M E N T: Administer antibiotics and remove calculus.

Lesions of the External Genitalia

TRAUMA. Damage to penis may occur at mating or from attempts to clear high fences. Contusions or lacerations may be present. Outcome depends on amount of tissue damage.

T R E A T M E N T: Depends on lesions. Maintain patency of urethra.

Infectious Disease

COITAL EXANTHEMA. (equine herpesvirus type 3) Venereal disease characterized by small papules or vesicles in vagina, which may spread to vulva, later ulcerate, and may coalesce. Disease has a short course if no secondary bacterial infection occurs.

Stallions may develop similar lesions on penis and prepuce.

T R E A T M E N T: Apply topical antibiotic cream; sexual rest.

DOURINE. (*Trypanosoma equiperdum*) Occurs in parts of southern USA, Africa, southeastern Europe, and Asia. Venereal disease.

Male. Signs include edema of prepuce, scrotum, and ventral abdomen, with mucopurulent urethral discharge.

Female. Signs include edema of perineal region and ventral and mammary gland edema. Occasionally ulcerations of vaginal mucosa may develop. Neurologic signs occur later, consisting of ataxia and paralysis.

TREATMENT: Reportable disease. Usually not treated. Administer diminazene aceturate in early cases.

CUTANEOUS HABRONEMIASIS. (*Habronema* spp.) Occurs worldwide, but is more important in warmer climates. Also known as summer sore and swamp cancer. Lesions often occur on face and from midline of abdomen extending to penis and prepuce in some cases. Lesions may become large, with depressed center and raised fibrotic edges. Center consists of gray necrotic material covering a granulation bed. Inciting cause is deposition of larvae by stable flies and domestic flies.

TREATMENT: Usually excise surgically.

Neoplasia

SQUAMOUS CELL CARCINOMA. Affects penis and prepuce and may extend to urethra. Diffuse involvement of area carries grave prognosis.

TREATMENT: Surgically excise and/or administer cryotherapy.

OTHER NEOPLASMS. Melanomas, sarcoids, and papillomas.

RUMINANTS

Urinary Bladder Problems

RUPTURE. Common sequel to urinary tract obstruction. Usually occurs in castrated males. Usual cause is urethral calculi. Especially common in feedlots. Signs include depression and anorexia, due to uremia and abdominal discomfort.

TREATMENT: Repair surgically, following correction of underlying cause.

CYSTIC CALCULI. Common in animals under feedlot conditions. Often subclinical. Clinical importance is in castrated males on high-concentrate diets, and where estrogens are administered (growth promoters) or occur in feed, e.g., clover hay, mycotoxins. Decreased water intake, low vitamin A status, and high vitamin D intake have been implicated.

T R E A T M E N T: Ensure adequate calcium and phosphorus ratio. Provide adequate access to water. Add sodium chloride to feed to increase water intake. Adding ammonium chloride to feed will help prevent the formation of phosphate calculi.

ENZOOTIC HEMATURIA. Occurs in cattle older than 1 year following chronic ingestion of bracken fern. Neoplasia of bladder wall transitional cells occurs, with ulceration leading to bleeding. Signs include poor condition and weight loss, with hematuria.

T R E A T M E N T: None successful.

CYSTITIS. May be sequel to ascending bacterial infection or bladder calculi, trauma at parturition, iatrogenic manipulation, or, less commonly, bladder paralysis. Signs include frequent urination, accompanied by grunting and prolonged posturing, and discoloration of urine (cloudy and/or bloody).

T R E A T M E N T: Address inciting cause. Administer prolonged course of antibiotics in bacterial cystitis.

NEOPLASIA. Rare, with the exception of enzootic hematuria.

T R E A T M E N T: Not undertaken.

Diseases of the Urethra

URETHRAL OBSTRUCTION. Common in castrated males, especially in those on high-grain diets. Usually caused by urolithiasis. Calculi commonly lodge at the sigmoid flexure or at the vermiform appendage in sheep and goats. May resolve with passage of calculus, or may proceed to the rupture of the bladder or urethra. Signs include constant shifting of weight on hindlimbs, straining to urinate with frequent posturing, pulsations of urethra on palpation of ischial arch region, and dribbling of urine.

T R E A T M E N T: Perform subischial urethrostomy if calculus is not passed.

"WATERBELLY." Castrated males are affected most often. Urethral rupture, most commonly caused by urolithiasis. Signs include swelling of scrotal area and ventrum, which may extend back to perineal region. Affected animals are depressed owing to uremia and abdominal discomfort. Sloughing of skin of affected area may occur.

Urethral damage may also occur owing to improper technique when using the Burdizzo method of castration.

T R E A T M E N T: Poor response to treatment. Subischial urethrostomy may be tried as salvage procedure.

Lesions of the External Genitalia

INFECTIOUS PUSTULAR VULVOVAGINITIS: INFECTIOUS BALANOPOS-THITIS. Caused by infectious bovine rhinotracheitis (IBR) virus. Affects cattle.

IPV. The disease occurs within days of mating. May be mild or severe. Signs include dysuria, frequent urination, tail-swishing, edema of vulva, and formation of small pustules on vaginal mucosa, which later ulcerate. A mucopurulent discharge is present. Signs abate in 10–14 days.

IBP. Similar vesicles and ulcers develop on preputial mucosa and penis. A discharge from the prepuce is present, especially with secondary bacterial infection.

TREATMENT: None specific. Administer broad-spectrum antibiotics to obviate secondary bacterial disease.

ENZOOTIC POSTHITIS: PIZZLE ROT. (*Corynebacterium renale*) Occurs mainly in castrated sheep. Bulls may be affected. A scab forms on exterior of prepuce and may extend to inside of prepuce, leading to ulceration. Signs include discomfort, with kicking at the belly, and dribbling of urine. In some infected herds, a vaginitis in ewes, with ulcers at the vulvar lips, has been ascribed to this organism.

TREATMENT: Reduce plane of nutrition and put animal(s) on a dry pasture. Irrigate lesion with copper sulfate or antiseptic solution. Debride surgically in severe cases.

PENILE FIBROPAPILLOMA. (bovine papillomavirus) Worldwide disease. Lesions have a cauliflowerlike appearance. May grow to considerable size, causing inability to retract the penis into the sheath.

TREATMENT: May resolve spontaneously. Surgical excision is also practiced.

TRAUMA. An example is penile hematoma. Usually occurs during breeding.

TREATMENT: Surgical drainage of hematoma 10–12 days after the injury may be beneficial. Other forms of trauma are treated as appropriate.

ULCERATIVE DERMATOSIS. (an unclassified virus, antigenically unrelated to orf virus) Lips, nares, feet, and the external genitalia may be affected. The glans, prepuce, and vulva of ewes are affected. Resembles contagious ecthyma but lesions are ulcerative rather than proliferative.

TREATMENT: None specific.

CONTAGIOUS ECTHYMA: SORE MOUTH, ORF. (parapoxvirus, related to pseudocowpox) Common in sheep and goats. Papules develop into ulcers covered by scabs and then granulate. Oral commissures usually are affected first, followed by proliferative lesions, which extend to lips, gums, muzzle, and face. In localized form, reduced food intake, especially among lambs and kids, is the main problem. A systemic form occurs rarely. Lesions may involve facial area, vulva or prepuce, and anus, and may spread to the gastrointestinal tract or cause bronchopneumonia.
T R E A T M E N T: None specific.

CHRONIC MUCOSAL DISEASE. Affects cattle. Chronic cases may develop scab-covered ulcers on vulva or prepuce, accompanied by oral and digital ulceration, wasting, and diarrhea.
T R E A T M E N T: None effective.

GRANULAR VULVOVAGINITIS. (*Ureaplasma* spp.) Affects cattle. May lead to infertility.
T R E A T M E N T: None specific. Tylosin or lincomycin might be effective.

PIGS

Lesions of the External Genitalia

Uncommon in pigs.

ZEARALENONE. Ingestion of zearalenone (mycotoxin produced by *Fusarium* spp.) may cause edematous enlargement of the vulva, which may prolapse in severe cases. Sows may deliver piglets early or run milk prior to parturition. Piglets may be small and weak. Preputial edema may occur in males.
T R E A T M E N T: None.

SCROTAL ENLARGEMENT

The following conditions may be associated with scrotal enlargement in all species.

Scrotal/inguinal hernia
Testicular torsion
Hydrocele
Varicocele
Urethral rupture

Lymphatic obstruction
Testicular tumors
Orchitis
Trauma with associated edema or hematoma.

ABORTION

HORSES

Viral Diseases

EQUINE HERPESVIRUS INFECTION. (equine herpesvirus type 1) Abortion associated with episode of stress. May become widespread. Ten per cent of diagnosed abortions are due to EHV. Onset is sudden. Fetus is fresh and may be contained in membranes. Placental retention is relatively rare. Focal hepatic necrosis in fetus is pathognomonic.

EQUINE VIRAL ARTERITIS. (togavirus) Signs include moderate depression, fever, edema of the extremities, and keratoconjunctivitis. Abortion usually follows 7–10 days after initial illness. Severe autolysis is due to fetal retention.

EQUINE INFECTIOUS ANEMIA. (lentivirus) Very rare cause of abortion.

Bacterial Diseases

STREPTOCOCCAL INFECTION. (*Streptococcus zooepidemicus*) Multifocal inflammation of the chorionic surface may be evident.

MISCELLANEOUS BACTERIAL CAUSES. Bacteria isolated include *Streptococcus* spp., *Escherichia coli*, *Klebsiella* spp., *Salmonella abortus equi*, and *Pseudomonas* spp.

Miscellaneous Causes

FUNGAL. (*Aspergillus fumigatus*, *Mucor* spp.) The placenta has a thickened, dry, and leathery appearance. Not pathognomonic.

PLACENTAL INSUFFICIENCY. Results from loss of functional endometrial surface area from conditions such as endometrial fibrosis.

ABORTIONS DUE TO TWINNING. Accounts for up to 30% of all diagnosed abortions.

UTERINE BODY PREGNANCIES. Rare. May lead to abortion.

UMBILICAL CORD ABNORMALITIES. Twisting of cord and other aberrations.

MISCELLANEOUS CAUSES. Sorghum toxicity, iodine or selenium deficiency, and organophosphate toxicity.

CATTLE

Viral Diseases

INFECTIOUS BOVINE RHINOTRACHEITIS. (IBR virus or IPV—infectious pustular vulvovaginitis virus) Abortions usually occur between fourth and seventh month, often independent of respiratory disease, and may be only signs of IBR infection. Expulsion of fresh or mummified fetus. No pathognomonic lesions of fetus or placenta.

BOVINE VIRAL DIARRHEA: BVD. (pestivirus) Potentially a cause of abortion, more likely in first half of gestation. May cause other fetal abnormalities including cerebellar hypoplasia, cavitation of brain, and skeletal abnormalities.

AKABANE VIRUS INFECTION. Occurs in Australia, Japan, Israel, and Turkey. Hydranencephaly and arthrogryposis are seen in calves that survive virus infection in utero.

AINO VIRUS INFECTION. Occurs in Australia and Japan. Occasionally affects pregnant cows. Survivors of in utero infection may have arthrogryposis.

RIFT VALLEY FEVER. (bunyavirus). Occurs on African continent. Arthropod-borne. Fever, diarrhea, salivation, and abortion are features of this disease. High mortality in calves.

Bacterial Diseases

SALMONELLOSIS. *(Salmonella dublin, S. typhimurium)* Sporadic occurrence. Fever, depression, and dysentery may be accompanied by abortion, or abortion may be the only sign. Fetus shows no lesions. Placenta is usually retained and is edematous and yellow with adherent purulent exudate. Positive culture from fetal stomach supports diagnosis.

LEPTOSPIROSIS. *(Leptospira hebdomadis* serogroup *hardjo)* Abortions occur in last trimester. Primarily a winter disease associated with confinement. Frequently subclinical; abortion may be the only clinical feature but is not a consistent finding. Mastitis, agalactia, and induration of udder may be seen. No characteristic lesions.

ACTINOMYCOSIS. *(Actinomyces pyogenes)* Sporadic. Rare outbreaks. Fetus is usually autolyzed. Signs include purulent placentitis.

LISTERIOSIS. *(Listeria monocytogenes)* Sporadic abortions. Yellow necrotic foci appear in fetal liver. Silage feeding is implicated.

CAMPYLOBACTERIOSIS. *(Campylobacter fetus* var *veneralis)* Occurs at 5–7 months of gestation. Thick, dark brown material apparent in intercotyledonary areas. Fetal stomach contents are thick and yellow.

LICHENIFORMIS INFECTION. *(Bacillus licheniformis)* Associated with conditions of poor hygiene.

BRUCELLOSIS. *(Brucella abortus)* Abortion occurs from 6 months of gestation onward. Herd outbreaks occur. Signs include edema of placenta and necrosis of cotyledons. Major zoonosis.

Miscellaneous Causes

MYCOTIC ABORTION. *(Aspergillus, Absidia, Mucor* spp.) Up to 5% incidence on some farms. Occurs in cows 3–7 months pregnant. Lesion is a mycotic placentitis with leathery appearance. Retention of placenta is common. Fetus may have gray mycotic patches on skin.

BOVINE TRICHOMONIASIS. *(Trichomonas foetus)* Abortion occurs at 2–4 months' gestation. Signs include fetal maceration, possibly with associated pyometra. Flocculent uterine exudate is also a sign.

PONDEROSA PINE POISONING. May cause abortion in cattle. Occurs in western USA and Canada. Dried, wilted, or green pine needles are toxic. Placental retention and septic metritis may follow.

BOVINE SARCOCYSTOSIS. *(Sarcocystis cruzi, S. hirsuta)* Signs include salivation, stiffness due to myositis, fever, and weight loss. Abortion may occur in acute disease.

OTHER. Nutritional and hormonal abnormalities must always be considered in cases of abortion. In many cases of abortion there is no etiologic diagnosis.

SHEEP

More than half of the abortions seen in sheep remain undiagnosed etiologically. Both infectious and noninfectious causes have been identified. If more than 2% of flock are affected, an infectious agent is likely.

Viral Diseases

AKABANE VIRUS INFECTION. Occurs in Australia, Japan, and Israel. May cause abortions. Lambs that survive in utero infection may be born with hydranencephaly, microencephaly, and other defects.

BORDER DISEASE. (pestivirus) May cause embryonic and fetal death with or without abortion.

WESSELBRON DISEASE. (mosquito-borne flavivirus) Occurs in Africa. Humans, sheep, and other species are affected. Abortion occurs in ewes, and congenital hydranencephaly and arthrogryposis occur in lambs infected in utero. High mortality in newborn lambs.

Bacterial Diseases

CAMPYLOBACTERIOSIS. *(Campylobacter fetus var intestinalis)* Initial outbreaks have a high herd incidence; incidence decreases as flock immunity develops. Abortions occur in last 6 weeks of gestation. Placentitis is evident.

SALMONELLOSIS. *(Salmonella spp., several serotypes; important ones include S. dublin, S. typhimurium, S. abortus ovis, S. montevideo)* Less than 2% of ovine abortions in UK are caused by the disease. Clinical signs include pyrexia, depression, and diarrhea. More severe signs occur with *S. dublin* and *S. typhimurium*.

BRUCELLOSIS. *(Brucella melitensis)* A potential cause of abortion, usually in late pregnancy. Abortion storms may be seen. Can cause systemic involvement.

LEPTOSPIROSIS. *(Leptospira pomona)* Abortion may be the only sign or animal may also have systemic illness.

LISTERIOSIS. *(Listeria monocytogenes)* Causes abortion in late pregnancy.

Miscellaneous Causes

MYCOTIC ABORTION. *(Aspergillus fumigatus, Claviceps purpurea)* See entry for cattle, pp. 117–118.

Q FEVER. *(Coxiella burnetti)* Zoonosis. Potentially a cause of abortion. Causes influenza-like symptoms and occasionally meningitis in man.

PREGNANCY TOXEMIA: TWIN LAMB DISEASE. Common. Seen in last 6 weeks of gestation. Associated with multiple fetuses and inadequate nutrition. Signs include depression, somnolence, blindness, hypoglycemia, and abortion (late gestation).

TICK-BORNE FEVER. *(Ehrlichia phagocytophilia)* Occurs in UK, Europe, and Africa. Signs include fever, anorexia, depression, and lameness. Abortion occurs in up to 30% of affected animals. Some ewes may die.

CHLAMYDIAL/ENZOOTIC ABORTION. *(Chlamydia psittaci)* Abortion occurs in last half of gestation, often near term. Aborted lambs are clean and well preserved; some are born weak. Characteristic necrotic cotyledons. Flaky yellow exudate covers intercotyledonary areas. May recur year after year. Killed vaccine is available for prevention.

TOXOPLASMOSIS. *(Toxoplasma gondii)* Worldwide disease. Stillbirths and abortions occur; fetus is occasionally mummified. Infection before 40 days leads to fetal resorption; infection between 40 and 100 days' gestation results in fetal death and abortion. Cotyledons have white nodules.

OTHER. Stresses, such as transport or handling; Brucellosis *(Brucella abortus ovis)*.

GOATS

Viral Diseases

PESTE DES PETITS RUMINANTS. (paramyxovirus) Occurs mainly on African continent. Generalized signs include fever, depression, stomatitis, erosions of the vulva, and abortions.

Bacterial Diseases

MYCOPLASMOSIS. (*Mycoplasma agalactia*) Uncommon.

CAMPYLOBACTERIOSIS. (*Campylobacter* spp.) Uncommon.

PARATUBERCULOSIS. (*Mycobacterium johnei*) Uncommon.

LISTERIOSIS. (*Listeria monocytogenes*) Abortion occurs in late pregnancy.

BRUCELLOSIS. (*Brucella melitensis*) May cause abortion, usually in late pregnancy. Abortion storms can occur. Animal can have systemic involvement.

SALMONELLOSIS. See entry for sheep, p. 118.

LEPTOSPIROSIS. (*Leptospira* spp.) Abortion may be associated with systemic disease (*L. pomona*) or independent of other signs (*L. hardjo*).

Miscellaneous Causes

ENZOOTIC ABORTION. (*Chlamydia* spp.) Abortion occurs in last trimester of pregnancy. Placentitis is evident.

TOXOPLASMOSIS. (*Toxoplasma gondii*) Causes abortion and perinatal deaths in kids.

Q FEVER. (*Coxiella burnetti*) Causes placentitis and abortion.

PREGNANCY TOXEMIA. See entry for sheep, p. 119.

PIGS

Viral Diseases

PSEUDORABIES. (porcine herpesvirus) Up to 50% of pregnant sows may abort or deliver macerated or mummified fetuses. Infertility and respiratory signs may also be evident.

HOG CHOLERA: SWINE FEVER. (pestivirus) Pregnant sows may abort during acute disease. Other clinical signs are fever, lethargy, conjunctivitis, diarrhea, or constipation.

PARVOVIRUS INFECTION. (parvovirus) Can cause infertility, fetal mummification, decreased litter size, stillbirths, and, rarely, abortion.

SMEDI. The acronym SMEDI refers to stillbirths, mummification, embryonic death, and infertility. Originally it was thought to be a specific disease, but it is now considered to represent a syndrome.

SWINE INFLUENZA. (orthomyxovirus) Signs include respiratory signs, weakness, and fever. May be followed within 3 weeks by abortion in sows in latter half of gestation.

AFRICAN SWINE FEVER. (iridovirus) Signs are similar to those of swine fever: hog cholera. Sows may abort.

JAPANESE ENCEPHALITIS. (flavivirus) Occurs in Asia. Abortion or stillbirth occurs. Encephalitis occurs in young pigs.

MYSTERY SWINE DISEASE: BLUE EAR DISEASE. A recently described disease in Europe and North America. Possibly of viral etiology (lelystad virus). Causes abortion, stillbirth, and mummification.

Bacterial Diseases

LEPTOSPIROSIS. *(Leptospira pomona, L. canicola)* Abortion may follow infection with *Leptospira* spp. Other signs include fever, depression, icterus, especially in young pigs, and agalactia in sows. Neonatal losses also occur.

BRUCELLOSIS. *(Brucella suis)* Usually introduced by carrier boar. Abortion occurs in sows in early gestation (mummified fetuses), or piglets are weak or stillborn.

ERYSIPELAS. *(Erysipelothrix rhusiopathiae)* Acute form may be accompanied by abortion.

ACTINOBACILLOSIS. *(Actinobacillus [Haemophilus] pleuropneumoniae)* May occasionally cause abortions following pleuropneumonia.

NEW WORLD CAMELIDS

Causes are poorly documented. Infectious causes include toxoplasmosis, leptospirosis, and chlamydiosis. Ingestion of needles or bark of Ponderosa pine has been implicated in abortion cases.

MASTITIS

Mastitis is defined as inflammation of the mammary gland. In clinical medicine, infectious agents are the only important cause of the disease. Bacteria are the most important group of pathogens, with fungi and viruses being of lesser importance.

CLASSIFICATION

Mastitis may be broadly classified as being either clinical or subclinical.

Clinical Mastitis

Clinical mastitis is classified in four categories:

1. *Peracute* mastitis is present when there is sudden onset of severe inflammation of one or more quarters, in association with severe systemic illness.

2. *Acute* mastitis is present when there is sudden onset of inflammation of one or more quarters, which may be accompanied by signs of mild systemic illness.

3. *Subacute* mastitis is present when there is continued inflammation of one or more quarters with persistent changes in milk quality.

4. *Chronic* mastitis is present when repeated episodes of inflammation occur with moderate changes in the milk.

Subclinical Mastitis

Subclinical mastitis is present when there are no clinically detectable changes in the mammary gland or the milk, but the white cell count in the milk is increased.

EVALUATION OF THE MAMMARY GLAND AND MILK

The mammary gland should be observed for symmetry and palpated for evidence of heat, swelling, pain, lymph node enlargement, or changes associated with chronic disease, such as fibrosis or atrophy.

The milk should be examined for the presence of clots or discoloration due to blood or serous effusion. Tests that may be used to evaluate the milk include:

1. Visual assessment, e.g., strip cup

2. Indirect assessment
    a. California Mastitis Test (CMT)
    b. total nucleated cell count (which may be carried out either on a bulk milk sample for screening of herd status or on an individual sample)
3. Culture and sensitivity.

Subclinical mastitis is a major cause of economic loss to dairy farmers. The indirect tests for subclinical mastitis are designed to detect subclinical infection of quarters.

California Mastitis Test

The CMT is based on detecting the presence of DNA in the milk sample; thus, it detects somatic cells—both leukocytes and epithelial cells. The CMT accurately reflects the leukocyte count in milk, with the exception of early lactation and toward the end of lactation, when high epithelial cell counts may give false positive reactions.

Nucleated Cell Count

The total nucleated cell count (NCC) measures the number of leukocytes and epithelial cells in the individual quarter. It can also be used to screen bulk milk to determine the existence of mastitis in the herd. It does not detect the number of affected quarters, rather the presence of a problem.

Although accepted limits for somatic (nucleated) cell counts vary internationally, a count of more than 300,000 cells/mL in a bulk sample indicates the presence of mastitis in the herd, and requires examination of individual animals.

Culture and Sensitivity

Initial screening for affected quarters with an indirect test such as CMT may be followed by bacteriologic culture and sensitivity.

FACTORS INFLUENCING OCCURRENCE OF MASTITIS

Susceptibility of Animal

1. Stage of lactation—mastitis is more likely early in lactation
2. Pendulous udder—more likely to be traumatized
3. Incompetence of teat sphincter—direct trauma or viral infections of the teat may predispose to mastitis.

Virulence of Agent

The ability of the agent to survive in the animal's environment and the agent's invasiveness are important factors.

Environment

Contamination of the environment with fecal material promotes the build-up of coliform organisms. Sawdust bedding is associated with an increased incidence of mastitis due to *Klebsiella* spp. Malfunction of milking equipment or poor milking technique may predispose to mastitis.

Other animals or other quarters of the same animal act as the source of new infections where streptococci and staphylococci are the causative agents.

HORSES

Clinical Mastitis

Uncommon disease in the mare. Mastitis may occur at any stage of lactation, but most cases occur in the postweaning period. Organisms isolated include *Streptococcus* spp., *Staphylococcus* spp., *Pasteurella* spp., and *Klebsiella pneumoniae*.

T R E A T M E N T: Administer broad-spectrum antibiotic and antiinflammatory agents. Stripping and hot-packing are also advisable.

CATTLE

Peracute Mastitis

STAPHYLOCOCCUS INFECTION. (*Staphylococcus aureus*) Signs include fever, anorexia, severe depression, and firm swelling of the udder, which is often cold to the touch, with bluish discoloration and gangrene developing as the infection progresses. Usually seen within a few days of calving. Signs of circulatory shock develop later. A serous or blood-stained mammary secretion is evident, with or without clots.

INFECTION WITH COLIFORMS. (*Escherichia coli, Klebsiella* spp., *Enterobacter aerogenes*) Signs of mastitis are similar to those for *Staphylococcus aureus*, with the exception of the gangrenous changes in the udder. The mammary secretion may be normal initially, but later becomes serous. Occurs most frequently in the periparturient period. Sawdust bedding and a high degree of fecal contamination of the environment are predisposing factors.

T R E A T M E N T: Cardiovascular support with intravenous fluids is essential. Antibiotic therapy should be instituted. Staphylococci are often resistant to penicillin and most penicillin derivatives; thus, oxytetracycline, macrolides, cephalosporins, or cloxacillin is useful in therapy of staphylococcal mastitis. The benefit of antibiotics is not established for coliform mastitis; the problem is related to the toxemia. Nonsteroidal antiinflammatory agents may be beneficial.

Frequent stripping of the affected quarter is essential to remove bacterial toxins and inflammatory debris.

Acute and Subacute Mastitis

The important causative agents of acute and subacute mastitis include *Staphylococcus aureus* and *Streptococcus* spp. *(S. agalactiae, S. uberis, S. dysgalactiae)*. Systemic illness is usually mild or inapparent. *Mycoplasma* spp. typically involves all four quarters, and there is marked swelling of the udder with an acute decrease in milk production and marked changes in milk quality.

T R E A T M E N T: Antibiotic therapy may be administered by the intramammary or parenteral routes. Procaine penicillin is very effective against streptococci, but considerable resistance is encountered among staphylococcal isolates. Other antibiotics that may be efficacious for staphylococcal mastitis include novobiocin, cloxacillin, and tetracyclines. Mycoplasmal mastitis does not respond well to therapy, but in very early cases parenteral erythromycin, tylosin, or oxytetracycline should be considered.

Chronic Mastitis

Ineffective treatment of acute or subacute cases may result in a chronic recurrent mastitis. These cases are best treated, after drying off the gland, with intramammary infusions of the appropriate antibiotic.

Miscellaneous Conditions

SUMMER MASTITIS. *(Actinomyces [Corynebacterium] pyogenes)* Onset of mastitis is acute and usually occurs in dry cows or heifers. Signs include profound toxemia, fever, and firm, painful swelling of the affected quarter. The secretion is characteristically foul-smelling, purulent, and creamy. The function of the affected quarter is usually lost. Abortion may be a sequel to the toxemia.

Amputation of the teat from the affected quarter may assist drainage.

Other Causes

Pseudomonas aeruginosa
Mycobacterium spp.
Serratia marcescens
Bacillus cereus
Clostridium perfringens

Subclinical Mastitis

Quarter cell-counts are increased in subclinical mastitis, although there is no clinical evidence of quarter infection. It is recognized that there is an inverse relationship between nucleated cell counts and the milk yield from a quarter. The organism most commonly involved is Staphylococcus aureus.

Quarters with positive CMTs are usually treated with long-acting intramammary antibiotics at the end of lactation. This selective approach is used where quarter infection rates in the herd are less than 15%. In situations where quarter infection rates are greater, dry-cow therapy is usually administered to all cows at the end of lactation.

SHEEP AND GOATS

Peracute Mastitis

Signs are similar to those in cows with peracute mastitis and include fever, anorexia, and depression. Usually only one half of the udder is affected. Later the affected gland may turn cold, blue, and eventually gangrenous. Profound toxemia may precipitate cardiovascular collapse and death.

The two agents commonly associated with this syndrome are Staphylococcus aureus and Pasteurella haemolytica.

Acute Mastitis

Signs include sudden onset of hot, painful swelling of the affected gland. Milk is watery and contains clots. Systemic involvement is usually not obvious. Streptococcus spp. are commonly isolated.

TREATMENT: Therapy should be based on the guidelines in the section on acute and subacute bovine mastitis, p. 125.

Chronic Mastitis

CAE/OPP. Bilateral induration of the udder ("hard udder"), with a concomitant decrease in milk yield is associated with caprine arthritis and encephalitis (CAE) in goats and ovine progressive pneumonia (OPP, maedi-visna) in sheep. Milk from infected udders is a source of infection for lambs and kids. Considered to be a cause of growth retardation in lambs and kids.

Control

1. Pasteurize milk prior to feeding.
2. Cull infected animals.

CORYNEBACTERIUM INFECTION. (*Corynebacterium pseudotuberculosis*) Mastitis may develop due to extension of supramammary lymph node abscessation. Affected animals should be culled.

PIGS

Acute Mastitis

Signs include sudden onset of fever, depression, and anorexia, in association with hot, painful swelling of the mammae. The milk is purulent, and the sow resists attempts by the piglets to suck; therefore, they rapidly lose condition. Sows may die from toxemia and cardiovascular collapse.

Coliform organisms are the common cause, particularly *Klebsiella* spp. and *Escherichia coli*. Sawdust bedding may be a predisposing factor.

T R E A T M E N T: Administer systemic antibiotics: broad-spectrum agents, such as potentiated sulphonamides. Administer antiinflammatory drugs, such as flunixin meglumine. Provide cardiovascular support, including fluid administration, if practical.

MASTITIS, METRITIS, AGALACTIA SYNDROME. Signs develop within 2–3 days of parturition and include fever, inappetance, and depression, initially. Endotoxemia is believed to cause the clinical signs, although gram-negative metritis or mastitis may not always be present.

T R E A T M E N T: Administer broad-spectrum parenteral antibiotics and corticosteroids to decrease inflammation. Oxytocin should be administered frequently to promote milk let-down.

Chronic Mastitis

The affected glands are swollen and painful; pus can be expressed. *Staphylococcus aureus, Actinomyces (Corynebacterium) pyogenes* and streptococci are among the common causes.

T R E A T M E N T: Systemic antibiotic therapy is indicated; however, animals with refractory infections should be culled.

6

Musculoskeletal System

"We see only what we know."
Goethe

HORSES

Myopathies

CLOSTRIDIAL MYOSITIS. (*Clostridium perfringens, C. septicum, C. chauvoei, C. fallax*) Associated with injections and wounds. Signs include fever, depression, colic, lameness or generalized stiffness, swelling of affected area, and laminitis occasionally. Usually sudden in onset. Often fatal.

T R E A T M E N T: Administer parenteral penicillin and analgesics. Provide supportive care. May require surgical drainage.

ENZOOTIC MUSCULAR DYSTROPHY. (vitamin E/selenium deficiency) Affects foals in the first few months of life. Signs include muscle weakness, incoordination, and stiffness, leading to recumbency. Animal may die. Affected foals do not suckle or if ambulatory have reduced milk intake.

T R E A T M E N T: Administer vitamin E and selenium to affected foals. Control by treating mares during gestation.

EXERTIONAL RHABDOMYOLYSIS: TYING-UP, MONDAY MORNING DISEASE. Occurs in adult horses after heavy exercise. Signs include stiffness, reluctance to move, colic signs, sweating, swelling over affected areas (often involves gluteals and longissimus muscles). Myoglobinuria may be observed and usually indicates severe muscle damage.

T R E A T M E N T: Administer analgesics and antiinflammatories. Ensure adequate hydration. Administer mannitol (0.25 g/kg, i.v.) in severe cases; repeat 2–3 times during the first 24 hours.

POSTANESTHETIC MYOSITIS. Ischemic damage to muscle due to prolonged recumbency on hard surfaces. Signs include localized swelling and loss of limb function.

T R E A T M E N T: Administer analgesics and antiinflammatories. Administer mannitol (0.25 g/kg, i.v.) in severe cases and repeat 2–3 times during the first 24 hours. Maintain hydration.

TRAUMA. May result in muscle damage.

T R E A T M E N T: Depends on the type of injury sustained.

HYPERKALEMIC PERIODIC PARALYSIS. Rare. Mainly seen in young, male Quarter horses. The entire body trembles, often after exercise. Yawning and flicking of third eyelid may be followed by recumbency and tetany and later flaccidity. Increased serum potassium concentration during these episodes.

T R E A T M E N T: None successful.

BOTULISM. See Chapter 8.

MYOTONIA. (cause unknown) Rare. Reported in several breeds. Signs include prominent hindlimb muscles, stiff gait, dimpling following percussion of muscle.
T R E A T M E N T: None specific.

MONENSIN POISONING. Monensin is an ionophore feed additive for ruminants. Accidental feeding to horses produces muscle damage, primarily to the cardiac muscle. Signs include sweating, arrhythmias, and respiratory distress. Animal may be found dead. Occasionally myoglobinuria is evident.
T R E A T M E N T: Provide supportive care.

FIBROTIC OR OSSIFYING MYOPATHY. Sequel to trauma, usually involves restrictive lesion of muscles of hindlimb and, rarely, forelimb. A congenital form has been described. Semitendinosus, semimembranosus, and biceps femoris most commonly involved.
T R E A T M E N T: Myectomy of the semitendinosus has been performed in some cases.

Joint Diseases

Consult texts on lameness for recommendations on diagnoses and treatment of specific conditions outlined here.

SEPTIC ARTHRITIS. Common in neonates, sequel to bacterial septicemia. May occur concurrently with fever or other signs of systemic illness or may occur without premonitory signs in 6–8-week-old foals. Signs include lameness and distension of joint capsule and periarticular area. Also occurs in adults, secondary to an open wound, intra-articular injections, and less commonly to septicemia.
T R E A T M E N T: Administer parenteral antibiotics and antiinflammatories. Lavage joint.

IDIOPATHIC SYNOVITIS: WINDPUFFS, BOG SPAVIN. Chronic synovial effusion in joint, without associated lameness. Signs restricted to joint distension.
T R E A T M E N T: No specific therapy required.

VILLONODULAR SYNOVITIS. Affects the fetlock. Generally occurs in racing animals. Lameness, if present, is accentuated by flexion. Joint effusion is evident. Soft tissue mass is palpable at dorsal attachment of joint capsule.
T R E A T M E N T: Surgical excision of mass.

TRAUMATIC ARTHRITIS. Follows single or continuous episodes of trauma.

Synovitis/Capsulitis

Acute. Signs include obvious lameness, swollen joint, and pain on palpation.

Chronic. Signs include subtle lameness (exacerbated by exercise) and decreased range of motion due to fibrosis and thickening of joint capsule.

Ligamentous Damage. Examples are sprain and tearing or stretching of ligaments. Signs vary depending on severity of lesion. Rupture of ligaments may lead to joint instability or luxation.

Intraarticular Fractures. Most commonly affects carpus and fetlock. Chip fractures occur more frequently in these joints; in other joints fracture extends from articulating long bones to involve articular surface.

Meniscal Damage. Affects stifle joint. Infrequent injury. Usually affects medial meniscus and may be accompanied by tearing of medial collateral ligament. Signs are those of nonspecific lameness.

DEGENERATIVE JOINT DISEASE: DJD

Acute. Affects young horses in training. Occurs frequently in carpus and fetlocks and joints with a large range of motion. Synovitis/capsulitis occurs prior to degeneration of articular cartilage.

Chronic. Frequently seen in intertarsal and pastern joints (joints with small range of motion, high load), e.g., ringbone and bone spavin.

Incidental. Found at necropsy. Clinical significance doubtful.

DJD Secondary to Articular Damage. Includes septic arthritis, fractures, and osteochondrosis.

Chondromalacia. Cartilaginous damage, specifically a lesion on articular surface of patella.

OSTEOCHONDROSIS, OSTEOCHONDRITIS.
Defective endochondral ossification with necrosis in deep cartilage layers. Young horses are affected. Stifle, hock, and shoulder most commonly affected. Signs include joint distension, moderate or no lameness, and often an asymmetrical gait.

DEFECTIVE OSSIFICATION. Uneven pressure on immature cartilage may lead to abnormal ossification. Carpal or tarsal joints are affected. There is angular deformity of carpus or flexural deformity of tarsus. Prematurity is a predisposing factor.

Carpal Form. There is generally no pain or swelling. Deformity is present from birth and may progress. Valgus or varus forms occur.

Tarsal Form. Signs include sickle-shaped hocks.

SYNOVIAL OSTEOCHONDROMATOSIS. Islets of cartilage or bone may develop in synovium. Can detach and become free in joint and may resemble osteochondrosis fragments or chip fractures.

SYNOVIAL HERNIA. Defect in joint capsule, with herniation of synovial membrane. Manifests as subcutaneous swelling. Fluctuates on pressure.

IMMUNE-MEDIATED JOINT DISEASE. Very rare in horses.

Diseases of Bones

TRAUMA. May involve any area. Fractures may result and signs of external trauma may be evident. There is usually severe lameness when long bones or foot is involved.

OSTEITIS. Inflammation of bone originating in periosteum. Frequently involves extremities where there is little soft tissue coverage. If skin penetration occurs, infection may result. Sequestrum formation may occur in presence of infection and fistulation.

OSTEOMYELITIS. Inflammation commences in medullary cavity.

Hematogenous. Usually occurs in neonates subsequent to septicemia. Often accompanied by systemic disease, including pneumonia and umbilical infection.

Trauma-Associated. Follows open fracture, internal fixation, or a penetrating wound. Phlegmon or cellulitis may also be evident. Often results in severe lameness.

T R E A T M E N T: Administer antibiotics and analgesics. Response is generally poor. Curettage of lesion may be helpful. Overall the prognosis is poor and if the condition is hematogenous in origin, multiple joints may be affected.

OSTEOPOROSIS
Localized. Reduction of bone matrix usually without loss of mineral content. Frequently seen during external immobilization of limbs. More common in young animals due to rapid bone turnover. Condition predisposes to fracture.

Generalized. Rare. May be associated with poor nutrition.

OSTEODYSTROPHY. Abnormal bone development or metabolism. Associated with some angular limb deformities in foals.

FLUOROSIS. Rare. Can cause osteoporosis. Signs include exostosis formation, intermittent lameness, and discoloration of teeth.

HEREDITARY MULTIPLE EXOSTOSES. Signs are usually noticeable at birth and include bilaterally symmetrical, firm, bony enlargements that affect long bones, ribs, and pelvis. Lameness is caused by interference with tendon and muscle movement.

CALCINOSIS CIRCUMSCRIPTA. A granulomatous mass, secondary to deposition of calcium in the subcutis. Usually occurs over lateral aspect of stifle.

OSTEODYSTROPHIA FIBROSA: BRAN DISEASE. Rare. "Big head" is the classic form, with enlargement of mandible and facial bones, associated with a diet high in bran.

T R E A T M E N T: Correct dietary imbalances.

HYPERTROPHIC OSTEOPATHY: MARIE'S DISEASE. Associated with space-occupying thoracic lesions. Signs include periosteal hyperostoses with thickening of long bones and "pallisade" formation and pain and swelling of soft tissues.

EPIPHYSITIS. Common. This dysplasia of the growth plate is usually self-limiting and disappears as growth plate closes. Signs include enlargement of ends of long bones, particularly distal end of the radius, tibia, and third metacarpal. Lameness, heat, and pain over affected area occur in severe cases.

ANGULAR LIMB DEFORMITIES. Causes include

1. Disparity of growth rate between medial and lateral aspects of growth plate
2. Joint laxity
3. Defective endochondral ossification of carpal and splint bones
4. Traumatic luxation or fracture of carpal bones.

Carpal valgus is the most common flexural deformity.

CATTLE

Myopathies

Infectious Causes

CLOSTRIDIAL MYOSITIS. (*Clostridium chauvoei, C. septicum, C. novyi type B, C. sordelli, C. perfringens*) Two clinical presentations have been described.

Blackleg. Signs include fever, anorexia, depression, emphysematous swelling over the affected muscles, rapid course, and high mortality. Frequent cause of sudden death.

Malignant Edema. Signs include fever, anorexia, depression, and edematous, painful swelling accompanying a local wound. May be emphysematous. May affect vulvar area after calving.

T R E A T M E N T: Administer parenteral penicillin and analgesics. Provide fluid therapy. May require tissue debridement.

SARCOCYSTOSIS. (*Sarcocystis cruzi, S. hirsuta*)

Acute. Protozoan myositis. Signs include transient fever, decreased production, nasal discharge, salivation, hemorrhagic vaginitis, and abortion.

Chronic. Signs include muscle twitching, emaciation, submandibular edema, and agalactia.

T R E A T M E N T: No specific therapy, although ionophores have been used with some success. Eliminate contamination of cattle feed by dog feces.

BOVINE EPHEMERAL FEVER. (rhabdovirus) Occurs in Asia, Africa, and Australia. Signs include fever, anorexia, stiffness and lameness, nasal and ocular discharge, excessive salivation, head shaking, and swelling around joints. Animals may become recumbent. Subcutaneous emphysema is sometimes present. Usually not a fatal disease.

T R E A T M E N T: No specific therapy. Analgesics may be indicated.

THROMBOEMBOLIC MENINGOENCEPHALITIS. *(Haemophilus somnus)* Muscle hemorrhages and joint involvement lead to stiffness in gait. Accompanied by fever, depression, retinal hemorrhages, and neurologic signs.

T R E A T M E N T: Administer parenteral tetracyclines, penicillins, or other broad-spectrum antibiotics. Administer short course of corticosteroids (dexamethasone).

Metabolic Diseases and Nutritional Imbalances

VITAMIN E/SELENIUM DEFICIENCY

White Muscle Disease. Subacute enzootic muscular dystrophy is the most common form. Early signs include stiffness, trembling, and weakness. May progress to lateral recumbency. Respiratory muscle involvement may cause labored breathing. Fever and muscle soreness are also seen. In later stages ill-thrift, knuckling of fetlocks, and dysphagia are evident.

T R E A T M E N T: Administer parenteral vitamin E and selenium. Rest is important.

Acute Enzootic Muscular Dystrophy. Mainly seen in hand-reared calves on vitamin E/selenium–deficient diet. Sudden death is a feature. May be seen with peracute respiratory distress, frothy nasal discharge, and irregular heart rate with rapid onset of death.

Miscellaneous Conditions

PARALYTIC MYOGLOBINURIA. Recorded in older cattle. Evident after sudden exercise following prolonged confinement. Associated with marginal blood selenium concentration. Signs include myoglobinuria, muscle stiffness, and recumbency. Some may die.

T R E A T M E N T: Confine animals and administer parenteral vitamin E/selenium. Fluid therapy is required in severe cases.

TRAUMA. May cause muscle damage. Other signs of injury, such as hair loss or skin damage, may be seen.

T R E A T M E N T: Provide supportive care and administer analgesics.

EXERTIONAL MYOPATHY. Independent of vitamin E/selenium deficiency. Follows severe exercise in many species, including cattle. Signs similar to those for paralytic myoglobinuria.

T R E A T M E N T: Confine animal and provide supportive care.

ISCHEMIC MYONECROSIS. Associated with prolonged recumbency, including downer cows.

T R E A T M E N T: None specific. Administer analgesics and antiinflammatories.

Toxicities

ENZOOTIC CALCINOSIS: MANCHESTER WASTING DISEASE, ENTEQUE SECO. Chronic condition involving calcification of blood vessels, lungs, ligaments, and tendons, and paleness of muscle. Signs include stiffness, weight loss, and shifting of weight on limbs. Related to chronic intake of *Cestrum*, *Trisetum flavescens*, *Solanum malacoxylon*, which have vitamin D_3-like activity.

T R E A T M E N T: None specific. Remove animals from source.

IONOPHORE POISONING. (monensin, lasalocid) Overdosage leads to cardiac muscle damage and signs of heart failure, including weakness, muscle tremors, tachycardia, and decreased ruminal activity. Later signs include distended jugular veins, ascites, brisket edema, and death.

T R E A T M E N T: None specific.

Joint Diseases

Inflammatory Condition

SEPTIC ARTHRITIS. Common.

Calves. (coliforms, *Staphylococcus* spp., *Fusobacterium* spp., occasionally *Mycoplasma* spp.) Often sequel to septicemia, accompanied by other signs, such as fever, respiratory signs, and omphalitis.

T R E A T M E N T: Administer parenteral antibiotics and antiinflammatories. Perform joint lavage.

Weanlings–Adults. (*Mycoplasma agalactia* var. *bovis*) Outbreaks in feedlot cattle. Signs include fever, depression, lameness or stiffness, and distension of joints and tendon sheaths, frequently accompanied by pneumonia. Pleuritis and pericarditis may also be evident.

T R E A T M E N T: Administer parenteral tetracyclines, tylosin, or lincomycin.

SUPPURATIVE ARTHRITIS. Occasionally results from infection with *Actinomyces pyogenes*.

T R E A T M E N T: Administer penicillin and lavage joint.

LOCALIZED JOINT INFECTION. Extension of local infection into joint, for example, septic pedal arthritis secondary to foot abscess or a penetrating wound.
T R E A T M E N T: Administer parenteral antibiotics and nonsteroidal antiinflammatory drugs. Joint lavage is advisable.

THROMBOEMBOLIC MENINGOENCEPHALITIS. (*Haemophilus somnus*) Outbreaks common in feedlots. Signs include fever, respiratory and neurologic signs, and retinal hemorrhages. Joint effusion and muscle hemorrhages also occur, leading to stiffness of gait.
T R E A T M E N T: Parenteral penicillins, tetracyclines, or sulfonamides are effective.

BRUCELLOSIS. (*Brucella abortus*) Infection in cows or vaccination of calves with strain 19 may produce arthritis, especially of carpi. Reportable disease.
T R E A T M E N T: Slaughter clinical cases.

BOVINE EPHEMERAL FEVER. (rhabdovirus) Occurs in Australia and Africa. May produce joint effusion. Signs include fever, anorexia, stiffness, and head shaking.
T R E A T M E N T: None specific. Oral aspirin may provide some relief from discomfort.

TRAUMATIC ARTHRITIS. Inflammation of joint is secondary to synovial trauma, to ligamentous or meniscal damage, or to intraarticular fractures.
T R E A T M E N T: Administer nonsteroidal antiinflammatories, preferably aspirin or phenylbutazone. Provide rest and immobilize the limb. Repair fracture.

Degenerative Joint Disease

DEGENERATIVE COXOFEMORAL ARTHROPATHY. Affects beef bulls. Acetabulum is shallow. Occurs especially in rapidly growing cattle. Stiffness or lameness may be seen.
STIFLE DEGENERATION. Trauma or aging leads to degeneration of cartilage and osteoarthritis. Meniscal or ligamentous damage may instigate degenerative changes. Joint instability may lead to rupture of the cranial cruciate, thus presenting as an acute severe lameness.
OSTEOCHONDROSIS. Affects young, rapidly growing animals. Manifests as a disturbance of maturation of joint cartilage and growth plates. Fissures or ulcerations occur in articular cartilage, precipitating

synovial inflammation. Multiple lesions are common and are often bilaterally symmetrical. Stifle is frequently affected. Lameness may be present.

SPONDYLITIS AND ANKYLOSIS. Fusion of lumbosacral vertebrae. In mature bulls and older cows, fracture at point of fusion produces signs of stiff gait and difficulty in rising.

T R E A T M E N T: Administer analgesics, e.g., aspirin or phenylbutazone. Confine the animal. Surgical repair is possible for cruciate rupture.

COLLATERAL LIGAMENT DAMAGE (STIFLE)

Lateral Collateral Ligament. Damage to this ligament is relatively uncommon. Affected animals tend to walk with limb abducted, thus placing more weight on medial toe. May palpate lateral "gaping" of joint on adduction.

Medial Collateral Ligament. Traumatic damage to this ligament is quite common in dairy heifers. May involve medial meniscus. Signs include excessive medial meniscal mobility and lengthening of ligament. "Gaping" of joint occurs medially on abduction of limb. Lameness is usually evident.

T R E A T M E N T: Administer analgesics and provide rest.

Diseases of Bones

Osteomyelitis

ACTINOMYCOSIS. (*Actinomyces bovis*) Rarifying granulomatous osteomyelitis with no systemic involvement. Usually found in the mandible (lumpy jaw), less commonly in maxilla. Firm, painful swelling may discharge to surface. Interferes with mastication.

T R E A T M E N T: Iodides, sulfonamides, and some other antibiotics may be effective. Surgical resection may be considered in severe cases.

MISCELLANEOUS CAUSES. (*Staphylococcus* spp., *Streptococcus* spp., *Fusobacterium* spp., *Actinomyces pyogenes*) Common in calves, owing to hematogenous spread, or subsequent to local severe bacterial infection. May be accompanied by septicemia, or signs may be restricted to fever and lameness. Common sites include long bones and vertebrae.

T R E A T M E N T: Administer parenteral antibiotics, analgesics. When possible, curettage affected bone. Prognosis is poor.

Nutritional Imbalances

RICKETS. (vitamin D deficiency) Affects young growing animals. Inadequate mineralization of bone, secondary to low dietary vitamin

D and calcium. Bowing of long bones, enlargement of epiphyses and costochondral junctions, and separation of tendinous insertions from bones may occur, leading to lameness and generalized stiffness.

T R E A T M E N T: Correct deficiency and allow animals access to sunlight.

OSTEOMALACIA. Demineralization of bone. Dairy cows are affected. Results from low phosphorus intake or calcium-deficient diets. May lead to stiffness, lameness, and a high incidence of fractures.

T R E A T M E N T: Ensure proper dietary calcium-phosphorus ratio.

COPPER DEFICIENCY. Causes ill-thrift in cattle, often accompanied by coat changes, diarrhea, and anemia. Calves develop skeletal changes, firm swelling of epiphyses, bowing of legs, arched back, and flexor tendon contracture. "Falling disease" with acute heart failure occurs in southern hemisphere.

T R E A T M E N T: Copper may be supplied orally as mineral mix or may be spread on pasture. Parenteral administration is also used.

MANGANESE DEFICIENCY. Calves are born with limb deformities: enlargement of joints and knuckling of fetlocks.

T R E A T M E N T: Ensure adequate dietary concentrations of manganese.

FLUOROSIS. Chronic fluorine intoxication. Pigmentation or spotting of teeth occurs. In osteofluorosis, outbreaks of lameness and stiff gait may occur.

VITAMIN A DEFICIENCY. Causes abnormal bone development, particularly of skull.

T R E A T M E N T: Supplementation of diet.

Congenital Disorders

INHERITED OSTEOARTHRITIS. Two types are described:

1. Gradual onset in older cattle of both sexes. Stifle joints are the most severely affected. Occasionally only one joint is involved. Signs include stiff gait.

2. A degenerative arthropathy of the hip joint.

INHERITED MULTIPLE ANKYLOSIS. Congenital defect affecting Holstein calves. Signs include short neck and ankylosed vertebrae. Few affected calves are born alive. Dystocia is common.

INHERITED ARTHROGRYPOSIS. Multiple tendon contracture. Joint surface is not affected. Rigid extension or flexion of limbs results in dystocia. Several forms of the disease occur.

INHERITED SPLAYED DIGITS. Progressive spreading of claw begins at

2–3 months of age. Lameness develops at this stage. Later, animals spend long periods in recumbency.

INHERITED HYPERMOBILITY IN JOINTS. Extreme joint flexibility. Many joints are involved.

OSTEOGENESIS IMPERFECTA. Affects Holstein-Friesian cattle. Pink teeth, due to lack of dentine and enamel, and joint laxity of limbs are characteristic in neonates. Various other defects may occur.

INHERITED DWARFISM

Snorter Dwarfs. Mainly affects Angus breed. Signs include short legs, wide head, protruding lower jaw, protrusion of forehead, and abnormal maxilla. This leads to respiratory difficulty.

Bulldog Calves. Affects Channel Island breeds and Dexter cattle. Signs include prominent forehead, protruding tongue, short thick neck, and short legs. Miscellaneous other forms occur.

ARTHROGRYPOSIS. Akabane virus and bovine viral diarrhea virus are recognized causes. There are also many cases of unknown etiology. Intrauterine infection leads to deformities of limbs and vertebral column, resulting in failure of muscle development and in joint flexure. Presentation may include hydranencephaly.

CROOKED CALF SYNDROME. Associated with lupin ingestion by pregnant cows. Calf is born with excessive flexion, malalignment, and rotation of limbs.

MANGANESE DEFICIENCY. Calves are born with limb deformities, enlargement of joints, and knuckling of fetlocks.

***ASTRAGALUS* TOXICITY.** (*Astragalus* spp.) Skeletal abnormalities include flexor tendon contracture, hypermobility of hock, and carpal flexure.

SHEEP AND GOATS

Myopathies

CLOSTRIDIAL MYOSITIS. (*Clostridium chauvoei, C. septicum, C. novyi* type B, *C. sordelli, C. perfringens*)

True Blackleg. Not common in sheep. Signs are similar to those in cattle. Subcutaneous emphysema is not generally seen before death.

Malignant Edema. Commonly a result of wound infection with clostridia (e.g., shearing, castration, or trauma to vulva at parturition). Signs include high fever, depression, lameness or stiffness, and swelling around affected area. High mortality.

T R E A T M E N T: Administer parenteral penicillin and provide supportive care. Local debridement or drainage if necessary.

BIG HEAD. (*Clostridium novyi* type B) Signs include edema of the head and periorbital area, spreading to the neck. Commonly seen in rams. Associated with trauma.

T R E A T M E N T: Parenteral penicillin or tetracyclines are effective.

EXERTIONAL MYOPATHY. Unrelated to vitamin E/selenium status. Follows severe exercise, as occasioned by being chased by dogs. Signs include stiff gait, recumbency, and myoglobinuria. May be fatal.
T R E A T M E N T: Administer analgesics and provide supportive care.

WHITE MUSCLE DISEASE. (vitamin E/selenium deficiency) Signs include mild fever, stiff gait, muscle tremors, and occasionally, diarrhea. Usually a herd problem.
T R E A T M E N T: Correct dietary deficiency. Administer parenteral vitamin E/selenium.

TRAUMA. May cause muscle damage. Skin lesions or wool loss may reflect site of injury.
T R E A T M E N T: Administer analgesics and provide supportive care.

ISCHEMIA. Animals trapped in dorsal recumbency, or recumbent due to disease, e.g., pregnancy toxemia, may develop ischemic myonecrosis.
T R E A T M E N T: Provide supportive care and administer analgesics.

IONOPHORE POISONING. (monensin, lasalocid) These ionophores are feed additives for ruminants. Overdosage may lead to skeletal muscle damage, with inappetence, incoordination, and tremors leading to recumbency. Cardiac muscle may also be affected. Myoglobinuria may occur.
T R E A T M E N T: Provide supportive care. Remove animals from source.

CASSIA POISONING. (coffee senna, wild coffee) Occurs in southern USA in tropical areas. Signs include weakness, anorexia, and occasionally diarrhea.
T R E A T M E N T: None specific.

IXIOLAENA BREVICOMPTA POISONING. Cardiomyopathy, nephrosis, hepatosis, and CNS degeneration are evident postmortem.
T R E A T M E N T: None specific.

Diseases of Joints and Bones

TICK PYEMIA. Reported only in UK in sheep. Causes *Staphyloccus aureus* septicemia in lambs 2–12 weeks old. Fever, arthritis, meningitis, and depression commonly occur.

T R E A T M E N T: Parenteral penicillin is effective.

ERYSIPELAS. *(Erysipelothrix rhusiopathiae)*
Acute Form. Occurs during first month of life. Causes a nonsuppurative arthritis after minor surgeries or umbilical infection. High herd incidence. Joints may remain swollen. Lameness and weight loss are common.

Chronic Form. Occurs in animals 2–6 months old. There is multiple joint involvement and severe lameness. Has been associated with use of pig slurry on pasture.

Laminitis. Affects adults. Associated with dipping or wet, contaminated surfaces. Signs include heat and swelling below carpus or tarsus. Several legs may be affected. Other signs are severe lameness and edema and hemorrhage within the hoof.

T R E A T M E N T: Administer parenteral antibiotics, especially penicillin. Administer analgesics and provide supportive care.

MYCOPLASMA SEROSITIS/ARTHRITIS

Goats. In California and Australia goats are affected. Signs include fever, joint swelling, pain on palpation, polyserositis, and occasionally meningitis.

Sheep and Goats. *(M. capricolum)* May cause septicemia with pneumonia and arthritis. *M. mycoides* var. *mycoides* causes acute arthritis in young kids with fever, diarrhea, lameness, and recumbency.

T R E A T M E N T: Macrolides (e.g., tylosin) or tetracyclines, and analgesics are indicated.

SEPTIC ARTHRITIS. In neonates, failure of passive antibody transfer is associated with septicemia and joint involvement, with fever, depression, and other signs of septicemia. Septic arthritis in adults is secondary to trauma, hoof abscess, or local phlegmon, but rarely to septicemia. See under calves, p. 135.

T R E A T M E N T: Administer parenteral antibiotics, and provide supportive care.

HAEMOPHILUS AGNI INFECTION. Disease of weanling lambs. Septicemia is usually fatal. Survivors may develop polyarthritis.

T R E A T M E N T: Parenteral, broad-spectrum antibiotics are indicated.

CHLAMYDIAL ARTHRITIS. Probably caused by *Chlamydia psittaci.* Common. Polyarthritis in feedlot lambs. Low mortality. Signs include depression, fever, lameness, stiffness, conjunctivitis, pneumonia, and occasionally CNS signs.

T R E A T M E N T: Parenteral tetracyclines may be effective.

CAPRINE ARTHRITIS-ENCEPHALITIS: CAE. (lentivirus) Goats are affected. Causes arthritis in mature animals. Onset is insidious and carpal joints are most frequently affected. Animals are afebrile and gradually lose condition. Other signs of CAE include posterior ataxia (encephalitis) in kids, chronic indurated mastitis, and chronic interstitial pneumonitis in adults.
T R E A T M E N T: Measures are only palliative. Analgesics are indicated for arthritis.

COPPER DEFICIENCY. Osteoporosis of the long bones may develop with copper deficiency. Bones have a tendency to fracture.
T R E A T M E N T: Provide dietary supplement or administer copper salts orally. Parenteral copper may also be administered.

CALCIUM DEFICIENCY. Affects lactating ewes and suckling lambs. Lameness is frequently seen, associated with bone demineralization. Fractures are uncommon.
T R E A T M E N T: Supplement diet.

Inherited and Congenital Disorders

AKABANE VIRUS INFECTION. Causes congenital arthrogryposis, hydranencephaly, and microencephaly. Severity of disease varies with stage of pregnancy at which viremia occurs in the dam.
ARTHROGRYPOSIS
Goats. Congenital disease, possibly inherited. May be due to lysosomal storage defect.
Sheep and Goats. Toxic plants including lupins, tobacco, and Jimson weed have been associated with congenital arthrogryposis.
ARTHROGRYPOSIS: MULTIPLE TENDON CONTRACTURE. Inherited disease. Affects Corriedale and Merino breeds. Brachygnathia inferior and spinal column abnormalities may also be evident in Corriedales.
INHERITED CONGENITAL MYOTONIA. Abnormality of muscle fibers. Signs include sudden onset of stiffness and recumbency on exertion, followed by recovery. Familial in goats.
SPIDER LAMBS: HEREDITARY CHONDRODYSPLASIA. Suffolk and Hampshire lambs are affected. May be present at birth or become obvious later. Diagnosis is based on physical findings and radiographic features, which include irregular and widened growth plates. The olecranon has multiple areas of ossification in the cartilage. The changes begin before 3 weeks of age.
INHERITED AGNATHIA. Absence of lower jaw. Occurs in sheep.
INHERITED BRACHYGNATHIA. Merino and Rambouillet breeds affected. Shortening of mandible occurs.
CRANIOFACIAL DEFORMITY. Border Leicester lambs are affected. Signs include cerebral defects with nasomaxillary deformity.

OSTEOGENESIS IMPERFECTA. Affects sheep. Normal size at birth. Abnormal production of bone matrix. Bones are fragile, and fractures result.

PIGS

Myopathies

TRAUMA. Crushing of piglets by sow, or injection myositis (e.g., iron-dextrans) may be causes of muscle damage.
T R E A T M E N T: Provide supportive therapy.

SPLAYLEG. Observed within a few hours of birth. Signs include splaying of hindlimbs. Piglets are unable to stand. Higher incidence in males. Inherited disease. Affects mainly Pietrain and Landrace breeds. Lesion is a myofibrillar hypoplasia. Up to 50% mortality. Survivors recover in 7–10 days.
T R E A T M E N T: None specific.

PIETRAIN CREEPER SYNDROME. Rare. Progressive familial myopathy, with myofibrillar degeneration. Occurs in Pietrain and Landrace breeds. Onset within 3 weeks of birth. Both sexes affected. High incidence, up to 30%, within litter. Signs include tremor of fore and hindlimbs.
T R E A T M E N T: None.

WHITE MUSCLE DISEASE. (vitamin E deficiency) Aggravated by high fat diet, low cysteine and methionine intake. Signs include sudden death with cardiac form (mulberry heart); muscle tremor, staggering, and weakness (white muscle disease); poor growth or sudden death from hepatosis dietetica; anemia; and infertility.
T R E A T M E N T: Correct dietary deficiencies, and administer parenteral vitamin E.

PORCINE STRESS SYNDROME: MALIGNANT HYPERTHERMIA. Common. Inherited trait. Many breeds are affected, especially Pietrain, Poland-China, and some strains of Landrace. Stress-associated. Abnormal muscle metabolism leads to sustained muscle contracture, lactic acidosis, hyperkalemia, hyperthermia, and death.
T R E A T M E N T: Not cost effective. Prevent by reducing stress.

BACK MUSCLE NECROSIS. Affects growing pigs. Similar pathogenesis to porcine stress syndrome. Signs include difficulty in walking and pain and swelling over affected longissimus dorsi muscles. Can be fatal.

T R E A T M E N T: Control by avoiding stress.

ASYMMETRICAL HINDQUARTER SYNDROME. (genetic etiology suspected) Uncommon disease. Onset at 2–3 months of age. Asymmetry of one hindlimb, with abnormal muscle and fat distribution.
 T R E A T M E N T: None.

IONOPHORE POISONING. (monensin, lasalocid, salinomycin) Used as feed additive. Overdosage leads to skeletal and cardiac myopathy. Signs include anorexia, paresis, myoglobinuria, diarrhea, and death.
 T R E A T M E N T: Provide supportive care.

CLOSTRIDIAL MYOSITIS. *(Clostridium septicum, C. chauvoei)* Rare in pigs. Gas gangrene has been reported.
 T R E A T M E N T: Administer parenteral penicillin and provide supportive care.

Infectious Arthritis

STREPTOCOCCAL INFECTION
Streptococcus suis **type I.** Affects piglets prior to weaning. Signs include fever, depression, polyarthritis, and meningitis. High mortality rate.
 T R E A T M E N T: Administer parenteral antibiotics (e.g., penicillin) or potentiated sulfonamides.

Streptococcus suis **type II.** Mainly affects 3–12-week age group. Signs include fever initially, then septicemia and neurologic signs. Arthritis may occur when meningitis does not develop. High mortality.
 T R E A T M E N T: Administer parenteral penicillin or potentiated sulfonamides.

GLASSER'S DISEASE. *(Haemophilus parasuis)* Usually affects pigs 4–16 weeks old. High herd incidence of meningitis, polyserositis, and polyarthritis. Signs include fever, anorexia, depression, respiratory distress, and lameness with stiff gait, swollen joints, tenosynovitis, and tenovaginitis, in addition to nervous signs. In susceptible pigs, meningitis, cyanosis, reluctance to move, and edematous ears are pathognomonic. Occasionally chronic arthritis develops in recovered animals.
 T R E A T M E N T: Administer parenteral antibiotics, e.g., penicillins or sulfonamides. Control: Vaccination may be effective.

ACTINOBACILLOSIS. *(Actinobacillus suis, A. equuli)* Causes septicemia in piglets prior to weaning. Signs include fever, depression, skin hemorrhage, and swollen joints. Sudden death may occur.

T R E A T M E N T: Administer parenteral antibiotics (e.g., tetracyclines).

MYCOPLASMAL ARTHRITIS. *(Mycoplasma hyosynoviae, M. hyorhinis)* Affects pigs 3–12 weeks old. Signs include fever (mild), lameness, and joint swelling (which may become chronic). Nonsuppurative. Peritonitis, pericarditis, and pleuritis also occur with *M. hyorhinis* but *not* with *M. hyosynoviae.*
   T R E A T M E N T: Administer tetracyclines (orally or parenterally), tylosin, or tiamulin.

ERYSIPELAS. *(Erysipelothrix rhusiopathiae)* Polyarthritis may develop acutely during septicemia. Any joint can be affected, but the most commonly affected joints are knee, stifle, hock, elbow, and spinal column. Lameness and stiffness are evident. Chronic suppurative arthritis without prior signs may also occur, usually in older pigs.
   T R E A T M E N T: Administer parenteral penicillin.

MISCELLANEOUS CONDITIONS. *(Escherichia coli, Staphylococcus* spp., *Pasteurella* spp., and others) May cause arthritis or osteomyelitis, leading to lameness.
   T R E A T M E N T: Administer parenteral antibiotics.

Metabolic Diseases and Nutritional Imbalances

RICKETS. (vitamin D deficiency) Affects young pigs. Uncommon. Characterized by low serum calcium and phosphorus concentrations. Signs include decreased growth rate, lameness, and mild fever. Swollen joints and bone deformities develop. Champing of jaws is common. An inherited form of rickets occurs due to a specific defect in intestinal calcium uptake.
   T R E A T M E N T: Ensure proper balance of dietary calcium, phosphorous, and vitamin D.

CONGENITAL HYPEROSTOSES: THICK FORELEGS. Signs include thickening of forelegs below elbows, and stretching and discoloration of skin. High mortality. Lesion probably results from separation of periosteum from bone.
   T R E A T M E N T: None specific.

OSTEOMALACIA. Chronic bone-calcium depletion secondary to low dietary calcium, vitamin D, and phosphorus. Pathologic fractures lead to lameness.
   T R E A T M E N T: Administer calcium borogluconate parenterally, and correct dietary imbalance.

VITAMIN A DEFICIENCY
Congenital Form. Piglets are stillborn or weak. Hindlimb deformities may occur.

Acquired Form. Occurs in adults with spinal cord demyelination.

T R E A T M E N T: Ensure adequate dietary concentration of vitamin A. Parenteral supplementation may be indicated in some cases.

Foot Lesions

TRAUMA. Sole erosions, bruising, and hoof-wall cracks may result from poor flooring or bedding. All ages may be affected.

T R E A T M E N T: Correct underlying causes.

BIOTIN DEFICIENCY. Sows are particularly affected. Signs include hoof-wall cracks, sole and heel erosions, and poor reproductive performance.

T R E A T M E N T: Correction of dietary deficiency.

FOOT-AND-MOUTH DISEASE. (picornavirus) Extremely contagious. Signs include fever, depression, coronary band vesicles with severe lameness (acute), and lingual ulcers. Hoof may be shed. Sudden death may occur in piglets. Other species are affected, especially cattle, but also other cloven-hoofed animals.

T R E A T M E N T: Isolation and slaughter to control outbreaks. Notifiable.

SWINE VESICULAR DISEASE. (enterovirus) Vesicles on coronary bands and supernumerary digits. Occasionally the horn is shed. Less commonly, lesions occur on the snout and oral mucosa, and rarely, on the abdomen and legs. Neurologic signs have been reported in some outbreaks. Other species are not affected.

T R E A T M E N T: None specific.

CLAW DEFORMITIES. Associated with lack of exercise. Adult pigs usually affected. Congenital forms also occur.

LAMINITIS. May be sequel to toxemia. Signs include lameness, bounding digital pulses, and pain on digital pressure.

T R E A T M E N T: Treat underlying disease (e.g., metritis or mastitis) in addition to providing supportive care.

Miscellaneous Conditions

INTERVERTEBRAL DISC DISEASE. Lameness may be seen in sows and boars with disc disease. Kyphosis may develop following discospondylitis and spondylosis.

T R E A T M E N T: None specific. Culling may be indicated.

OSTEOCHONDROSIS. (etiology unknown) Defective ossification of cartilage resulting in abnormal bone development. Signs include stiffness of hindlimbs, especially after rising, abnormal stance, and shortened stride. Separation of femoral head (epiphysiolysis) may occur.
T R E A T M E N T: No specific therapy. Exercise and attention to balancing of dietary nutrients is recommended.

FRACTURES. Trauma leading to fractures can cause lameness. Luxation of the tuber ischii is seen in adult sows. Recumbency results.
T R E A T M E N T: None specific. Culling is indicated.

NEW WORLD CAMELIDS

Myopathies

WHITE MUSCLE DISEASE. New World camelids require more vitamin E/selenium than other species. All ages are susceptible. Signs include stiffness, lameness, weakness, and recumbency.
T R E A T M E N T: Administer parenteral injections of vitamin E/selenium, and correct dietary deficits. Confine affected animals.

CLOSTRIDIAL MYOSITIS. (*Clostridium chauvoei, C. septicum, C. perfringens*) Should be considered in febrile, lame animals, especially if crepitant swelling at puncture wound or injection sites is noted.
T R E A T M E N T: Administer parenteral penicillin. Debride affected areas.

Diseases of Joints and Bones

SEPTIC ARTHRITIS. Primarily affects neonates. Sequel to hypogammaglobulinemia and septicemia. Other signs include fever and pneumonia. May occur in single joints as an extension of local infection.
T R E A T M E N T: Administer antibiotics, joint lavage, supportive care.

COCCIDIOIDOMYCOSIS. (*Coccidioides immitis*) Occurs on the west coast of the USA. Signs include dermatitis, osteomyelitis, periarthritis, and CNS involvement.
T R E A T M E N T: None successful.

FRACTURES. Long-bone fractures are common. Occasionally sacral fractures are encountered.
T R E A T M E N T: Stabilization is indicated.

Congenital Disorders

ANGULAR LIMB DEFORMITIES. Many congenital deformities are reported, including carpal valgus and varus. Other deformities include shortening of femur, medial patellar luxation, polydactyly, and scoliosis.

T R E A T M E N T: Valgus or varus deformities may be corrected by application of casts in young animals. Surgical correction may be attempted before closure of growth plates.

DWARFISM. Uncommon.
AGENESIS OF FACIAL BONE. Uncommon.
BRACHYGNATHIA. May affect mandible or maxilla.

Ophthalmology

"He had but one eye and the popular prejudice runs in favour of two."

Charles Dickens, *Nicholas Nickleby*

CONGENITAL OCULAR DEFECTS

Congenital ocular defects include anophthalmia, microphthalmia, cyclopia (in sheep, associated with ingestion of skunk cabbage [Veratrum californicum]), dermoid cysts, entropion, ectropion, agenesis of eyelids, corneal opacities, hypoplasia of iris, hypopigmentation of iris (heterochromia iridis), persistent pupillary membrane, cataracts, aphakia (absence of lens), microphakia, ectopic lens, glaucoma, and retinal agenesis.

CONJUNCTIVITIS

Conjunctivitis is inflammation of the conjunctiva.

Clinical Signs

1. Chemosis—edema of the conjunctiva.
2. Injection of blood vessels in conjunctiva.
3. Ocular discharge
   a. Serous, e.g., mechanical irritation or viral infection
   b. Mucous, e.g., dry eye
   c. Purulent, e.g., bacterial infection
4. Hyperplasia of conjunctiva.
5. Lymphoid follicular hyperplasia—especially in chronic conjunctivitis.
6. Blepharospasm.

Causes

General Causes

1. Bacterial, viral, or mycotic infections. The normal conjunctiva has a microflora; however, culturing large numbers of organisms from an affected eye should be considered significant.

2. Parasitic infections, e.g., Thelazia spp.

3. Direct trauma to the conjunctiva from foreign bodies, dust, or ectopic cilia.

4. Focus of infection, e.g., infected tooth root or lacrimal or meibomian gland adenitis.

5. Allergies.

6. Conjunctival desiccation, poor lid apposition (occasionally seen in neonates), or keratoconjunctivis sicca (uncommon in large animals).

7. Neoplasia—squamous cell carcinoma in cattle ("cancer eye") and horses. This is relatively rare.

8. Secondary to ocular diseases, e.g., ulcerative keratitis or intra-ocular disease.

9. Secondary to dermatitis, e.g., seborrhea or demodicosis.

10. As a manifestation of systemic disease, e.g., infectious bovine rhinotracheitis or malignant catarrhal fever.

Specific Causes (See pp. 152–153.)

Diagnosis

Most cases of conjunctivitis are mild, and those caused by bacterial infections respond well to short duration treatment with antibiotics. After a general physical examination and a thorough examination of the eye, the following tests may be performed, especially in the more severe and chronic inflammations.

CULTURE AND SENSITIVITY. Most frequently, bacterial tests are performed; less frequently, fungal or viral tests are performed. Culture and sensitivity are indicated, e.g., if the inflammation is not responding to the antibiotic therapy or if an agent other than a bacterium is suspected of causing the conjunctivitis. It is important to obtain this material before the instillation of any eye medications.

CYTOLOGIC EXAMINATION OF THE CONJUNCTIVA. Cytologic examination detects the presence of neutrophils, bacteria, etc. Chronic bacterial infections may cause significant increases in the mononuclear cell count. Biopsy of the conjunctival tissue may be performed.

NASOLACRIMAL SYSTEM. Evaluate for patency. Fluorescein dye instilled into the conjunctival sac should appear at the nasolacrimal opening within 5 min.

T R E A T M E N T:

1. Remove physical irritants, e.g., parasites, particulate matter, ectopic cilia. Surgery is necessary to remove ectopic cilia.

2. Treat infectious causes, e.g., with broad-spectrum antibiotics (before obtaining sensitivity results if deemed necessary). Instill drugs into conjunctival sac every 4–6 h. If chlamydial organisms are suspected, tetracyclines are usually efficacious. To achieve maximal drug effect, discharges should be flushed from the eye before drug is administered.

3. Treat associated systemic diseases, e.g., dermatologic conditions.

KERATITIS AND CONJUNCTIVITIS

Keratitis is inflammation of the cornea. Keratoconjunctivitis is inflammation of the cornea and conjunctiva.

Clinical Signs

Clinical signs include corneal edema, loss of corneal transparency, ocular discharge, neovascularization of cornea (later stages), evidence of pain (blepharospasm or epiphora), secondary iridocyclitis.

Causes

General Causes

INFECTION. Most organisms can adhere to the cornea only if there is damage to the corneal epithelium. Exceptions are *Moraxella bovis* and herpesviruses.

DRY EYE. This is not a common cause. Unlike the dog, large animals rarely have a primary reduction in tear production. Lid dysfunction or facial nerve damage (e.g., trauma or listeriosis) may result in a dry eye and keratitis.

BASEMENT MEMBRANE DEFECT. This is occasionally seen in aged horses and results in separation of the stroma from the epithelial layer.

ULCERATIVE KERATITIS. Causes include trauma, e.g., foreign body or entropion. Corneal ulcer may be (a) uncomplicated or (b) complicated by bacterial (often gram-negative) and/or fungal infection. Enzymatic keratomalacia commonly occurs in complicated keratitis, as a result of collagenase and proteases released from damaged corneal and inflammatory cells. The ulcer can be detected and delineated by staining the eye with fluorescein dye.

CORNEAL STROMAL ABSCESSES. A sequel to corneal epithelial penetration or to trapping of bacteria after healing of punctate corneal lesions. A distinct opacity is visible in corneal stroma.

Specific Causes of Keratitis and Conjunctivitis

HORSES

Moraxella equi. Conjunctivitis, ocular discharge, and epithelial erosions at the canthi are present.

Habronema spp. Raised, yellow granular particles are present in the conjunctiva.

Thelazia lacrimalis. Spirurid worm, 10–20 mm long, may cause irritation; located in conjunctival sac.

Onchocerca spp. Microfilaria may cause conjunctivitis.

Equine Herpesvirus. Signs include corneal ulceration (pinpoint) and edema, photophobia, and lacrimation.

Equine Viral Arteritis. (togavirus) Signs include fever, vasculitis, lacrimation, and limb and preputial edema; occasionally, corneal opacity and photophobia.

Trauma. Trauma is a common cause of keratoconjunctivitis because of the prominent position of the eye.

CATTLE

Moraxella bovis. Keratitis or conjunctivitis caused by this organism is also called pink eye and New Forest disease. Usually occurs in summer months; outbreaks are common. Characterized by development of central corneal edema, a white spot, or a vesicle that may ulcerate. Recovery in most cases. Only disease causing outbreaks of corneal ulceration. Disease responds well to topical antibiotics (e.g., penicillin) if treated early.

Infectious Bovine Rhinotracheitis. (herpesvirus) Herd involvement common. Signs are mild and include corneal edema. Generally there is no ulceration.

Malignant Catarrhal Fever. (herpesvirus) Sporadic. Signs include severe uveitis, corneal edema, and neovascularization; no ulceration is present. Fever is accompanied by severe systemic disease.

Mucosal Disease. (pestivirus) In the acute form, excessive tearing and corneal edema may occur.

Theileria parva. Occurs in Africa and Asia. Signs include fever, depression, ocular and nasal discharge, and lymphadenopathy.

Thelazia spp. Spirurid worm. Worldwide distribution.

Miscellaneous. *Mycoplasma, Ureaplasma,* and *Chlamydial* spp. and trauma are other causes of conjunctivitis in cattle.

SHEEP AND GOATS

Chlamydia psittaci (ovis)—one of the most important infectious causes.

Mycoplasma conjunctivae—one of the most important infectious causes.

Acholeplasma oculi.

Branhamella ovis.

Rickettsia conjunctivae.

Infectious bovine rhinotracheitis—has been implicated in keratoconjunctivis outbreaks in goats.

Diagnosis

A thorough eye examination should be performed and the presence of entropion, ectopic cilia, distichiasis, or foreign bodies determined.

The blink reflex is evaluated, and the completeness of eyelid closure is noted. The anterior chamber should be examined, as deep ulcers often give rise to anterior uveitis. The degree of aqueous flare and the presence of synechiae and miosis should be determined.

CULTURE AND SENSITIVITY. These tests should be performed in cases of ulceration if economically justifiable. The edge of the ulcer should be cultured. Ideally, the procedure is performed without topical anesthesia; however, if this is not possible, proparacaine, which has the least bacteriostatic effects of available topical anesthetics, may be used.

CYTOLOGIC EXAMINATION OF CORNEA. Corneal scrapings should be collected, transferred to glass slides, and stained with Gram's and Wright's stains. A surgical blade may be used for this purpose, and the center and periphery of the ulcer should be scraped. Care should be exercised during this procedure to avoid corneal perforation. Adequate restraint of the animal is critical.

FLUORESCEIN DYE. Because the fluorescein dye is hydrophilic, it does not stain the intact corneal epithelium, which is lipid in nature. If the cornea is ulcerated, the stroma will retain the dye.

SCHIRMER'S TEAR TEST. This test is not used routinely but is indicated if keratoconjunctivitis sicca (dry eye) is suspected. In the horse, values of less than 5 mm/min indicate inadequate tear production. This test should be performed before the application of any medications to the eye.

ROSE BENGAL TEST. Devitalized tissue and mucus are stained. This test is not commonly used.

T R E A T M E N T:

1. **Cause.** Eliminate underlying cause when possible, e.g., foreign body.

2. **Antibacterial drugs.** With uncomplicated ulcers, a broad-spectrum antibiotic (e.g., combination of neomycin and polymixin) should be instilled into the conjunctival sac every 6–8 h until the ulcer has resolved. If the ulceration is more severe, progressive, or chronic or fails to respond to antimicrobial therapy, the choice of antibiotics should be based on the results of corneal culture and sensitivity. Cytologic examination of corneal scrapings may aid in the diagnosis. Scrapings should be examined for the presence of bacteria and fungi.

3. **Atropine sulphate.** To relieve the ciliary spasm and associated pain and to dilate the pupil and thereby reduce the possibility of synechiae, atropine sulphate may be administered topically (1–4% solution) every hour until the pupil dilates. Once the pupil is dilated, the frequency of atropine administration can be reduced to once daily or once every other day as a 1% solution. Long-term use in the horse can cause colic.

4. **Antifungal agents.** If fungal keratitis is suspected or confirmed, antifungal agents may be administered. Available antifungal agents include pimaricin, miconazole, amphotericin B, and nystatin. Fungal infection should be suspected if an ulcerative keratitis deteriorates during antibiotic therapy. Predisposing causes include long-term antibiotic and/or corticosteroid therapy. Prolonged use of antibiotics changes the normal flora from being predominantly gram-positive to one that is mainly gram-negative and fungal. The cornea may be bubbly in appearance.

5. **Anticollagenase therapy.** Acetylcysteine is commonly included in ulcer solutions for its anticollagenase activity. It has the disadvantage of being an irritant. It is not indicated for superficial ulcers.

Note: For convenience of administration, the aforementioned drugs are usually combined and diluted with methylcellulose (artificial tears). In cases in which therapy is of long duration and the nature of the animal makes treatment difficult or impossible, a nasolacrimal or subpalpebral lavage system should be inserted.

6. **Systemic nonsteroidal antiinflammatories**. These may be administered to reduce discomfort associated with corneal ulceration and anterior uveitis. Available nonsteroidal antiinflammatories include phenylbutazone, flunixin meglumine, and aspirin.

7. **Protection of ulcerated area**. Conjunctival or third eyelid flaps can be created. Conjunctival flaps are more difficult to create, but have the advantage of providing antimicrobial and anticollagenolytic elements. They provide good support because they are fixed to the limbus and do not impede movement of the globe. Although tarsorrhaphies and third eyelid flaps protect the cornea, they do little to promote healing.

Subconjunctival Injections

The conjunctival route can be used to deliver drugs to the eye. Antimicrobials and atropine can be injected in volumes up to 1.0 mL, preferably into the bulbar conjunctiva.

UVEITIS

Uveitis is an inflammation of the uveal tract, which consists of the iris, ciliary body, and choroid. On clinical grounds, uveitis can be divided into anterior uveitis (iridocyclitis) and posterior uveitis (choroiditis). Choroiditis is diagnosed less commonly, perhaps owing to the difficulty of examining the posterior segment in the presence of iridocyclitis.

Types

EQUINE RECURRENT UVEITIS: PERIODIC OPHTHALMIA, MOON BLINDNESS. (*Onchocerca* and *Leptospira* spp. are implicated) Disease is usually unilateral, occasionally bilateral. Generally presents as an acute inflammatory episode. Signs include blepharospasm, photophobia, conjunctival hyperemia, congestion of episcleral vessels, miosis, corneal edema, and reduced intraocular pressure. Sequelae include vision deficit, anterior or posterior synechiae, cataracts, retinitis, and bulbar shrinkage.

T R E A T M E N T: Administer topical corticosteroids (if no corneal ulceration is present) and systemic antiinflammatory drugs (e.g., phenylbutazone and aspirin). Topical atropine may be used to dilate pupil.

BACTERIAL UVEITIS. Frequently occurs in neonates secondary to septicemia. Reported to occur in ewes fed silage, possibly caused by *Listeria monocytogenes.* Also occurs as a sequel to keratitis.

T R E A T M E N T: Administer topical and systemic (if septicemia is suspected) antibiotics, topical atropine, and systemic antiinflammatories (e.g., phenylbutazone).

CLOUDY EYE

Animals may be presented for evaluation of a "cloudy" or opaque eye.

Cloudy eye may be caused by the following:

1. Epithelial corneal edema caused by ulcerative keratitis
2. Endothelial corneal edema caused by recurrent uveitis, stromal abscess (may have an epithelial component), or glaucoma
3. Corneal fibrosis caused by scarring of old corneal wounds
4. Lipid deposition in cornea (rare)
5. Anterior chamber abnormalities such as aqueous flare, a sequel to protein and cellular effusion in uveitis
6. Lens abnormalities such as cataracts
7. Vitreous abnormalities such as cellular/proteinaceous material in posterior chamber, a sequel to inflammation

T R E A T M E N T: Depends on underlying cause.

RED EYE

Inflammation that results in hyperemia of blood vessels imparts a red appearance to the eye. It can be extra- or intraocular in origin.

EXTRAOCULAR DISEASE. Extraocular disease is generally accompanied by injection of superficial blood vessels. These vessels move when the conjunctiva is lifted and run parallel to the limbus. Blood flow is from fornix to limbus.

INTRAOCULAR DISEASE. Intraocular disease is accompanied by injection of deep episcleral/ciliary vessels. These vessels run perpendicular to the limbus and do not move when the conjunctiva is lifted.

Blood flow is from limbus to fornix. Causes include uveitis and glaucoma (rare). Bracken fern poisoning is potentially a cause of intraocular hemorrhage in cattle.

T R E A T M E N T: Depends on underlying cause.

BLINDNESS/VISION IMPAIRMENT

Horses

Congenital Ocular Diseases

RETINAL AGENESIS. Rare.
RETINAL DYSPLASIA.
T R E A T M E N T: None.

GLAUCOMA. Congenital. Usually occurs in association with buphthalmos.
T R E A T M E N T: None successful.

ANOPHTHALMIA/MICROPHTHALMIA. Anophthalmia is extremely rare. Microphthalmia can be unilateral or bilateral.
T R E A T M E N T: None needed.

CONGENITAL CATARACT. Unilateral or bilateral. Accounts for 30% of congenital ocular defects.
T R E A T M E N T: Surgical removal.

NIGHT BLINDNESS. Occurs in Appaloosa breed. The severity of the condition varies greatly. No histologic or anatomical lesion.
T R E A T M E N T: None.

OTHER CONGENITAL CONDITIONS. Dermoids, optic nerve hypoplasia, strabismus.

Plant Toxicities

LEUKOENCEPHALOMALACIA: MOLDY CORN POISONING. (*Fusarium moniliforme*) Moniliformin, a toxin found in moldy corn, causes pharyngeal paralysis, blindness, and other neurologic signs.
T R E A T M E N T: None successful.

AFLATOXICOSIS. (*Aspergillus flavus*) Caused by mycotoxins in feed.
T R E A T M E N T: None successful.

BLIND STAGGERS. (*Astragalus* spp.) Chronic selenium toxicity. Signs include blindness, ataxia, head pressing, and aimless wandering.
T R E A T M E N T: None successful.

Infectious Causes

VIRAL ENCEPHALITIS. Rabies (rhabdovirus), Western/Venezuelan/Eastern equine encephalitis (togavirus). May cause blindness.
T R E A T M E N T: None specific. Provide supportive care and antiinflammatories. Rabies cases should not be treated.

BACTERIAL MENINGOENCEPHALITIS. Causes include strangles and other systemic infections, especially neonatal septicemia.
T R E A T M E N T: Administer broad-spectrum antibiotics and corticosteroids. Provide supportive care.

Miscellaneous Causes

TRAUMA. Can be unilateral or bilateral; causes peripheral or central damage to optic nerve.
T R E A T M E N T: Administer antiinflammatories.

PITUITARY NEOPLASIA. Pressure on optic chiasm by pituitary adenoma may cause blindness.
T R E A T M E N T: An attempt to reduce the tumor size with drug therapy may help. However, once nerve damage occurs the prognosis is poor. Cyproheptadine and pergolide have been used to treat these tumors, with limited success.

KERATITIS. May result from infection or trauma.
T R E A T M E N T: See Treatment, pp. 154–155.

RECURRENT UVEITIS: MOON BLINDNESS. Can be unilateral or bilateral. Causes temporary or permanent blindness.
T R E A T M E N T: See Equine Recurrent Uveitis, pp. 155–156.

Cattle

Congenital Ocular Diseases

STRABISMUS. Has been observed in cattle with neurologic disease. An inherited form has also been reported.
T R E A T M E N T: Surgical correction can be done in selected cases.

ECTOPIC LENS AND CATARACT. Congenital inherited defect in Jerseys. Severe vision deficits.
T R E A T M E N T: None.

INHERITED CONGENITAL BLINDNESS. Lenticular shrinking and opacity. Occurs in Brown Swiss cattle.

TREATMENT: None.

CONGENITAL CORNEAL OPACITY. Corneal edema, leading to cloudiness. Occurs in Holstein breed.
TREATMENT: Usually not undertaken.

CONGENITAL BLINDNESS IN SHORTHORNS. Blindness appears to be linked to coat color. Retinal detachment, cataracts, and other changes are present.
TREATMENT: None.

Systemic Diseases in Calves (0–3 Months)

HYDROCEPHALUS. Genetic etiology suspected in Holsteins, Herefords, Charolais, and Ayrshire. Viral etiologies suspected in other cases. Signs include blindness, bawling, and recumbency.
TREATMENT: None.

LEAD POISONING. The acute form is more common in calves. Signs include blindness, wandering, staggering, muscle tremors, rolling of the eyes, and bellowing. Pupils may be dilated. Palpebral reflex is diminished or absent.
TREATMENT:

1. Supportive care and seizure control.
2. Chelation therapy
   a. CaNa$_2$ EDTA (50 mg/kg/day in divided doses, *slow* i.v.); may need to continue for 3–5 days.
   b. Dimercaprol (4 mg/kg every 4–6 h initially) may be given in association with CaNa$_2$ EDTA. (Irritant to muscle.)
   c. D-penicillamine is too expensive for routine use.
3. Administration of thiamine (10 mg/kg every 4–6 h for 2 days) improves outcome in cases of lead toxicity.

HYPOVITAMINOSIS A. Congenital form. Lesion due to compression of optic nerve or sequel to abnormal cranial bone development. Blindness, seizures, facial nerve paralysis, weakness, and ataxia may develop.
TREATMENT: None.

SPACE-OCCUPYING LESIONS. Includes brain abscessation and neoplasia.
TREATMENT: Poor response to antibiotic therapy in abscessation.

OPTIC NEURITIS. Secondary to meningitis. Blindness is a prominent finding, with depression, lateral recumbency, and opisthotonus as accompanying signs.

T R E A T M E N T: Administer broad-spectrum antibiotics and corticosteroids, control seizures and provide supportive care.

DEHORNING INJURIES. Thermal injury due to excessive cautery of horn bud and damage to underlying cortex. May cause blindness and other cortical signs.

T R E A T M E N T: Control seizures, administer corticosteroids, and provide supportive care.

TRAUMA. Cranial trauma is rare in cattle.

T R E A T M E N T: Depends on severity of condition. Administer antiinflammatories (e.g., dexamethasone), control seizures, and provide supportive care.

SALT POISONING. Uncommon. Regurgitation, diarrhea, blindness, and ataxia are common signs.

T R E A T M E N T: See p. 161.

Systemic Diseases in Weanlings and Adults

POLIOENCEPHALOMALACIA. (thiamine deficiency) Signs include absence of fever, blindness, active palpebral and corneal relexes, wandering, and ataxia, leading to recumbency, opisthotonus, and extensor spasms.

T R E A T M E N T: Disease is usually responsive to thiamine administration (10 mg/kg, i.v. or i.m.). Repeat 3–4 times at 6 to 8-h intervals.

VITAMIN A DEFICIENCY. Occurs in cattle age 1–3 years. Associated with lack of green feed. Signs include night blindness, syncope, convulsions, paralysis, and corneal cloudiness.

T R E A T M E N T: Early cases may respond to vitamin A supplementation.

THROMBOEMBOLIC MENINGOENCEPHALITIS. (*Haemophilus somnus*) Mainly an autumn and winter disease. Signs include fever, depression (marked), extension of head, ataxia, and lingual paralysis. Blindness and circling are sometimes seen. Retinal hemorrhage and strabismus may be present.

T R E A T M E N T: Disease shows good response to antibiotics (e.g., penicillin or tetracyclines) if treated early.

INFECTIOUS BOVINE RHINOTRACHEITIS. (herpesvirus) Encephalitic form may affect calves under 6 months. Blindness, fever, depression, and seizures may result.

T R E A T M E N T: None specific. Provide supportive care.

MALIGNANT CATARRHAL FEVER. (herpesvirus) Signs include fever, lymphadenopathy, nasal and ocular discharge, corneal opacity, hypopyon, and meningoencephalitis, leading to blindness in some cases. High mortality rate.

T R E A T M E N T: None specific.

TRAUMA. Damage to optic nerve tracts (skull fracture, etc.) is rare in cattle.

T R E A T M E N T: Depends on severity of condition. Administer antiinflammatories (e.g., dexamethasone), control seizures, and provide supportive care.

SPACE-OCCUPYING LESIONS. Examples include brain abscesses and neoplasms. Circling, head pressing, seizures, and blindness may be features of this condition.

T R E A T M E N T: Poor response to antibiotic treatment in cases of abscessation.

RETROBULBAR MASSES. Examples are bovine leukosis, abscessation, and sinusitis (frontal/maxillary). May cause unilateral or bilateral blindness.

T R E A T M E N T: Surgical drainage of sinuses or abscesses.

HEAVY METAL POISONING. Examples include lead and mercury. Blindness, ataxia, and head pressing occur in mercury poisoning. Acute lead poisoning may cause blindness, with muscle twitching, champing of the jaws, and nystagamus. More common in calves than adults.

T R E A T M E N T: See Treatment of Lead Poisoning, p. 159.

NERVOUS FORM OF KETOSIS. Most common in adult, lactating dairy cows in early lactation or in beef cows on a poor plane of nutrition. Signs include hyperesthesia, abnormal behavior, champing of the jaws, salivation, circling, head pressing, and blindness. Diagnosis is based on milk and urinary ketone body content and clinical presentation.

T R E A T M E N T: Administer dextrose (500 mL of a 50% solution) i.v. Correct underlying cause.

GRAIN OVERLOAD. Signs include vision deficits, with decreased menace response and palpebral and pupillary light reflex in severe cases.

T R E A T M E N T: Empty rumen using a stomach tube or perform rumenotomy. Administer fluids i.v. and thiamine in severe cases.

SALT POISONING. Uncommon in older cattle. Regurgitation, diarrhea, blindness, and ataxia are common signs.

T R E A T M E N T: Remove source. Mildly affected animals should receive small volumes of water at frequent intervals initially.

For treatment of severe cases, intravenous fluid administration is necessary. (See Chapter 12.)

FOCAL SYMMETRICAL ENCEPHALOMALACIA. Sequel to chronic *Clostridium perfringens* type D enterotoxemia. Mainly seen in young adults and weanlings. Signs include blindness, ataxia, and paralysis.
T R E A T M E N T: None specific.

Plant Toxicities

ERGOT OF RYE. *(Claviceps purpurea)* Acute intoxication causes depression, deafness, intermittent convulsions, and staggering and can lead to comatose state. Intermittent blindness is a feature. In chronic form, gangrene of the extremities occurs.
T R E A T M E N T: None specific.

SELENIUM TOXICITY
Acute. Ingestion of selenium-accumulating plants. Apparent blindness in acute toxicity in association with head pressing. Signs include diarrhea, ataxia, tachycardia, and severe respiratory distress.
T R E A T M E N T: None specific. Provide supportive care.

Chronic. Usually sequel to consumption of locoweed *(Astragalus* spp.). Signs include "blind staggers," dullness, emaciation, pica, and blindness. Signs are a consequence of hepatic encephalopathy.
T R E A T M E N T: None specific.

MALE FERN. *(Dryopteris felix mas)* Signs include blindness secondary to degeneration of the optic nerve, depression, and ataxia.
T R E A T M E N T: None specific.

PYRROLIZIDINE ALKALOIDS. Encephalopathy due to chronic liver damage. Depression or excitement, ataxia, head pressing, blindness, convulsion, diarrhea, and tenesmus may be seen. Secondary to chronic ingestion of *Senecio* (ragwort), *Crotalaria,* and *Amsinckia* spp.
T R E A T M E N T: None specific.

RAPE OR KALE TOXICITY. *(Brassica* spp.) Signs include blindness, head pressing, mania. Pupillary light reflex may be intact. Most cases recover. May also occur with feeding of beets and beet pulp.
T R E A T M E N T: Poor response. Control seizures, provide supportive care.

YELLOW WOOD/IRONWOOD TOXICITY. Australia. Associated with ingestion of leaves. Signs include anorexia, dullness, and blindness.
T R E A T M E N T: Affected animals die in spite of treatment.

AFLATOXICOSIS. *(Aspergillus flavus)* Toxin produced by agent in moldy grain. Hepatotoxicosis leads to jaundice and central nervous system signs including circling, blindness, incoordination, and convulsions.

T R E A T M E N T: None specific.

Miscellaneous Causes

NEOPLASIA. For example, squamous cell carcinoma ("cancer eye"). Most common in Hereford cattle. May develop on eyelid or conjunctiva and spread to cornea.

T R E A T M E N T: Excision in early cases, or cryosurgery.

KERATITIS. (e.g., *Moraxella bovis*) Severe cases may result in vision impairment.

T R E A T M E N T: Penicillin topically or subconjunctivally in cases of *Moraxella bovis* infection.

Sheep and Goats

Toxicities

LEAD POISONING. Relatively uncommon. Signs include anorexia; constipation followed by passage of dark, foul-smelling feces; hyperesthesia; and convulsions. Blindness may be a feature. Palpebral reflex is absent or diminished.

T R E A T M E N T:

1. Supportive care and seizure control.
2. Chelation therapy
   a. CaNa$_2$ EDTA (50 mg/kg/day in divided doses, *slow* i.v.); may need to continue for 3–5 days.
   b. Dimercaprol (4 mg/kg every 4–6 h initially) may be given in association with CaNa$_2$ EDTA. (Irritant to muscle.)
   c. D-penicillamine is too expensive for routine use.
3. Administration of thiamine (10 mg/kg, i.v. or i.m., every 4–6 h for 2 days) improves outcome in cases of lead toxicity.

PREGNANCY TOXEMIA. Late (often twin) pregnancy. Associated with malnutrition or inanition. Signs include separation from flock, blindness, bruxism, tremors, and apparent confusion. Abortion is common; ewes often die.

T R E A T M E N T: For mild cases, reduce stress (e.g., provide shelter), offer supplementary carbohydrates, and administer propylene glycol (50 mL orally twice daily for 3–4 days). For severe cases, administer i.v. glucose, corticosteroids, and propylene glycol (50 mL orally twice daily). Induce parturition or perform cesarean. Provide supportive care.

RAPE OR KALE TOXICITY. (*Brassica* spp.) Sudden onset of blindness associated with recent ingestion of *Brassica* spp., e.g., rape or kale. Other signs include diarrhea, fever, and hemoglobinuria, usually more than one animal is affected.
T R E A T M E N T: None specific.

BEET TOXICITY. Feeding of fodder beet, sugar beet, or mangolds. May lead to blindness, in association with other neurologic signs.
T R E A T M E N T: None specific. Provide supportive care.

BRIGHT BLINDNESS. Bracken ingestion. Occurs in sheep over 1½ years of age.
T R E A T M E N T: None specific.

SELENIUM POISONING: BLIND STAGGERS. Blindness may be a manifestation of chronic ingestion of *Astragalus* spp. (selenium-converter plants).
T R E A T M E N T: None specific.

YELLOW WOOD/IRONWOOD TOXICITY. Occurs in Australia. Ingestion of leaves from these trees may cause blindness.
T R E A T M E N T: None successful.

PYRROLIZIDINE ALKALOIDS. Chronic toxicity leads to cirrhosis and hepatoencephalopathy. Sheep are more resistant to toxicity than cattle. Blindness may be a sign.
T R E A T M E N T: None specific.

Miscellaneous Causes

HYPOVITAMINOSIS A. Uncommon. Potential cause of blindness.

POLIOENCEPHALOMALACIA. Caused by thiamine deficiency. Common; worldwide distribution. Signs include blindness, incoordination, opisthotonus, nystagmus, and convulsions. Associated with dietary changes. Pupillary light reflex is intact.
T R E A T M E N T: Administer thiamine (10 mg/kg i.v. or i.m.); repeat 3–4 times at 8-h intervals.

GRAIN OVERLOAD. History of excessive grain intake. Signs include severe depression, abdominal pain, apparent blindness, incoordination, diarrhea, and recumbency.

T R E A T M E N T: Empty rumen using a stomach tube or perform rumenotomy. Administer thiamine and provide supportive care.

FOCAL SYMMETRICAL ENCEPHALOMALACIA. Sequel to chronic *Clostridium perfringens* type D enterotoxemia. Mainly seen in weaned lambs, occasionally adults. Signs include blindness, ataxia, and onset of paralysis.
T R E A T M E N T: None specific.

MENINGOENCEPHALITIS. *Escherichia coli* septicemia in neonatal lambs and listeriosis in adults are examples. Signs include severe depression with extension of neck initially; if untreated, ataxia, apparent blindness, nystagmus, recumbency, and convulsions may occur. High mortality rate. Listeriosis commonly affects cranial nerves 5, 7, and 8.
T R E A T M E N T: Administer broad spectrum antibiotics in neonatal septicemia. Administer penicillin or tetracyclines if listeriosis is suspected. Administer corticosteroids (short course) and provide supportive care.

SPACE-OCCUPYING LESIONS. Brain abscess, gid cyst (*Coenurus cerebralis*), and tumors. Gradual (sometimes acute) onset of circling, blindness, ataxia is common.
T R E A T M E N T: Apart from successful surgical excision of gid cysts, cases respond poorly to treatment.

Pigs

Toxicities

ARSANILIC ACID TOXICITY. Caused by overadministration of arsenicals used in the control of swine dysentery. Signs include muscle tremors, blindness, and incoordination. Paralysis and death can occur.
T R E A T M E N T: Administer sodium thiosulfate and provide supportive care.

SALT POISONING/WATER DEPRIVATION. Acute form follows ingestion of large amounts of water after a period of depletion. Signs include blindness, circling, walking backwards, convulsions, and death.
T R E A T M E N T: Remove source of salt. Supply water in small volumes frequently, in the initial stages following toxicity.

Infectious Causes

MENINGOENCEPHALITIS. Potential causes are *Streptococcus suis* type I in preweaning pigs, *S. suis* type II in weaned pigs, and neonatal septicemia. Signs include depression, fever, nystagmus, blindness, incoordination, and convulsions.

T R E A T M E N T: Administer penicillin, other broad-spectrum antibiotics, a short course of dexamethasone, and anticonvulsants if necessary.

BLUE EYE. (paramyxovirus) Occurs in Mexico. Seen in piglets 2–21 days of age. Corneal edema and encephalitis are signs.

T R E A T M E N T: None specific.

EDEMA DISEASE. (*Escherichia coli*) Mainly affects recently weaned pigs. Signs include edema of the gastrointestinal tract, palpebral edema, blindness, ataxia, head pressing, recumbency, convulsions, and death. High mortality rate.

T R E A T M E N T: Provide supportive care.

Miscellaneous Causes

THIAMINE DEFICIENCY. Reported to occur in sows kept outdoors. Associated with chronic ingestion of bracken. Signs include blindness, poor growth, and sudden death due to heart failure.

T R E A T M E N T: Administer thiamine (10 mg/kg, i.v. or i.m.) Repeat 3–4 times at 6-h intervals.

New World Camelids

Congenital Ocular Diseases

CATARACTS. Pupillary light response may be present, even in severe forms.

T R E A T M E N T: Surgical correction in selected cases.

RETINAL DEGENERATION. Unresponsive pupil.

T R E A T M E N T: None.

Systemic Diseases

EQUINE HERPESVIRUS TYPE 1. Has occurred in animals kept in association with horses. Blindness, retinal degeneration, and atrophy of optic disc are signs.

T R E A T M E N T: None specific.

MENINGITIS. (e.g., *Escherichia coli*) Sequel to neonatal sepsis. Blindness, fever, depression, and anorexia are signs.

T R E A T M E N T: Administer broad-spectrum antibiotics, short course of dexamethasone, and provide supportive care.

Nervous System

EVALUATION OF THE NERVOUS SYSTEM

"All the physicians and authors in the world could not give a clear account of his madness. He is mad in patches, full of lucid intervals."

Miguel Cervantes

For descriptive purposes, neurologic disorders are divided into diseases that involve (a) the brain, (b) the spinal cord, and (c) the peripheral nerves.

DISORDERS OF THE BRAIN

The Regions of the Brain

Clinically, the brain may be described as consisting of five regions:

1. Cerebrum or telencephalon—includes the cerebral cortex and subcortical nuclei (basal nuclei).
2. Diencephalon—consists of the thalamus and hypothalamus.
3. Brainstem—includes the midbrain, pons and medulla.
4. Cerebellum—includes the cerebellar cortex and cerebellar nuclei.
5. Vestibular system—includes the peripheral and central (vestibular nuclei) components.

Diseases of each of these regions shall be described in general before the specific neurologic diseases in horses, cattle, sheep and goats, pigs, and New World Camelids are discussed.

Cerebral Disease

Changes in neurologic status are variable, partly on the basis of the anatomical size of the cortex, but may include the following:

BLINDNESS. Results from lesions affecting the occipital (visual) cortex. If the optic nerve tract is normal, the pupillary light reflex should be intact.

BEHAVIOR CHANGES. Implies a lesion in the frontal lobe or limbic system. May include aimless wandering, head pressing, circling in wide circles (aversive syndrome). Circling implies that the lesion is unilateral or asymmetrical. Continuous yawning is often a feature of cerebral disease. Depression and stupor, or else seizures, may be present to varying degrees.

POSTURE/MOVEMENT. Posture is normal, but deficits in postural reactions (e.g., hopping) may be present. Deficits are contralateral to the lesion. The gait is usually normal, but a mild hemiparesis may be present contralateral to the lesion.

Thalamic/Hypothalamic Disease

Disorders of the diencephalon produce signs similar to those of cerebral disease and, in addition, may include signs of endocrine and autonomic dysfunction and deficits in optic nerve function.

Brainstem Disease

Signs may include the following:

1. Depression or coma.
2. Dysfunction of cranial nerves 3–12. One or more nerves may be affected.
3. Posture/movement—ataxia and hemi- or tetraparesis. The deficits may be ipsi- or contralateral to the lesion.
4. Respiratory and vasomotor centers—these are resistant to disease states. Occasionally neurogenic hyperventilation occurs in midbrain disease.

Cerebellar Disease

Signs may include the following:

1. Head or whole body tremors.
2. Dysmetria, especially hypermetria.
3. Deficient or absent menace response.
4. Vestibular signs (nystagmus).
5. Ataxia, wide base stance.
6. Absence of depression or muscle weakness.

Vestibular Disease

Lesions of the vestibular system are generally accompanied by head tilt. If vestibular disease is suspected but the lesions are subtle, blindfolding the animal may aid diagnosis. This should be done cautiously, because the affected animal may fall suddenly, causing injury to itself or attendants. Vestibular disease may be peripheral or central.

PERIPHERAL LESIONS. Signs include the following:

1. Head tilt (ipsilateral to the lesion).
2. Fast phase of nystagmus opposite to the side of the lesion and in any direction except vertical (nystagmus is generally *not* a feature of vestibular syndrome in the horse).
3. Loss of balance or awkward gait.

Over a period of 5–7 days the nystagmus resolves and the problem with balance becomes less severe. The head tilt remains.

CENTRAL LESIONS. Signs include the following:

1. Head tilt.
2. Nystagmus (horizontal, vertical, or rotatory).
3. Ataxia and a tendency to roll in one direction; deviation of the trunk (concavity toward the side of the lesion) and contralateral extensor tonus.
4. Depression.
5. Other cranial nerve (e.g., 5 and 7) deficits.
6. Circling to side of lesion (circles of short radii).

Cranial Nerves

Knowledge of the cranial nerve pathways is helpful in localizing brain lesions. With the exception of the olfactory and optic nerves, which terminate in the cortex, the cranial nerves terminate in the midbrain (nerves 3 and 4), pons, and medulla (nerves 5–12).

OLFACTORY NERVE. Originates in the nasal mucosa and terminates in the pyriform cortex.

Assessment. Its function is difficult to assess in animals.

OPTIC NERVE. Originates in retina and terminates in the lateral geniculate and pretectal nuclei, which are involved in vision and the pupillary light reflex, respectively.

Assessment

1. Menace response
2. Pupillary light reflex (PLR), direct and consensual.

Blindness in association with a *normal PLR* indicates a lesion in the lateral geniculate nuclei, optic radiation, or visual cortex. Blindness in association with an *abnormal PLR* indicates that the lesion is rostral to the lateral geniculate nuclei.

OCULOMOTOR NERVE. Originates in midbrain, at the level of the caudal colliculus. Provides motor innervation to dorsal, ventral, and medial recti, to ventral oblique, and to pupillary constrictor muscles.

Assessment

1. PLR
2. Normal nystagmus in association with cranial nerves 4 and 6.

TROCHLEAR NERVE. Originates in midbrain at level of caudal colliculus. Provides motor innervation to dorsal oblique muscle.

Assessment. Lesions of trochlear cause abnormal nystagmus. Dorsomedial strabismus is occasionally seen in ruminants with polioencephalomalacia.

TRIGEMINAL NERVE. Motor fibers originate in pons. Provides motor innervation to muscles of mastication. Provides sensory innervation through ophthalmic, maxillary, and mandibular branches to rostral medulla.

Assessment

1. Motor innervation—jaw tone and ability to close mouth.
2. Sensory innervation—(a) ophthalmic branch—palpebral reflex (upper lid); (b) maxillary branch—nasal mucosal and facial sensation and palpebral reflex (lower lid); (c) mandibular branch—response to skin pinch on mandible.

ABDUCENT NERVE. Originates in rostral medulla. Provides motor innervation to lateral rectus and retractor bulbi muscles.

Assessment. Lesions of abducent cause medial strabismus and inability to retract the globe.

FACIAL NERVE. Motor fibers originate in rostral and ventrolateral medulla. Provides motor innervation to muscles of facial expression. Provides sensory innervation to rostral two-thirds of tongue.

Assessment

1. Motor innervation—facial asymmetry, ear droop, ptosis, and muzzle deviation. Absence of palpebral and/or menace response.
2. Sensory innervation—more difficult to assess. Lack of sensation in rostral part of tongue.

VESTIBULOCOCHLEAR NERVE. Provides sensory function to inner ear. Cell body in rostral medulla.

Assessment. Peripheral vestibular disease (e.g., otitis interna), head tilt, nystagmus, and loss of balance. Middle ear lesions usually produce only a head tilt. Hearing—response to noise (handclap).

GLOSSOPHARYNGEAL NERVE. Motor fibers originate in caudal medulla. Provides motor innervation to pharynx and palate. Provides sensory innervation to pharynx, palate, and caudal one-third of tongue.

Assessment. Dysphagia, diminished gag reflex.

VAGUS NERVE. Motor fibers originate in nucleus ambiguus in the caudal medulla. Provides innervation to pharynx and larynx. Provides sensory innervation to larynx, pharynx, abdominal and thoracic viscera, esophagus, and trachea (visceral sensory).

Assessment. No gag reflex; laryngeal and pharyngeal paralysis (if bilateral).

ACCESSORY SPINAL NERVE. Originates in nucleus ambiguus in the caudal medulla and first 5 or 6 cervical cord segments; exits the skull in the jugular foramen. Provides motor innervation to trapezius, sternocephalicus, and brachiocephalicus muscles.

Assessment. Atrophy of aforementioned muscles.

HYPOGLOSSAL NERVE. Originates in hypoglossal nucleus in the caudal medulla and exits the skull via the hypoglossal canal. Innervates the muscles of the tongue.

Assessment. Tongue tone, presence of atrophy.

Examples of Neurologic Deficits

1. A depressed steer with a head tilt to the right (cranial nerve 8) has a lesion in the rostral medulla (right side).

2. A depressed horse with right dorsomedial strabismus (cranial nerve 4) and right facial paralysis (cranial nerve 7) probably has multifocal disease, since the midbrain and medulla are affected.

Nystagmus

An involuntary rhythmical movement of the eyeballs. Physiologic nystagmus can be elicited by turning the head from side to side and is characterized by the presence of a rapid phase in the direction of the gaze. A postrotatory nystagmus normally occurs after rapid rotation of the animal.

Normal or Physiologic Nystagmus

Often referred to as a "doll's eye response" or the "oculocephalic reflex." Cranial nerves 3, 4, 6 (Fig. 8–1), and 8, the vestibular nuclei, and the medial longitudinal fasciculus are responsible for the normal nystagmus. Nystagmus allows the animal to maintain visual contact on stationary objects as the body moves. It may be vertical, horizontal, rotatory, or mixed. Pendular nystagmus has no fast and slow components and may be of ocular origin due to poor vision or may be congenital. A pendular nystagmus is occasionally seen in cattle, and calves may be born with the condition; it is not associated with vestibular disease.

Abnormal Nystagmus

Usually results from a lesion in the vestibular system. Control of the ocular muscles is primarily a function of the semicircular canals. Toxic nystagmus may follow treatment with certain drugs, such as

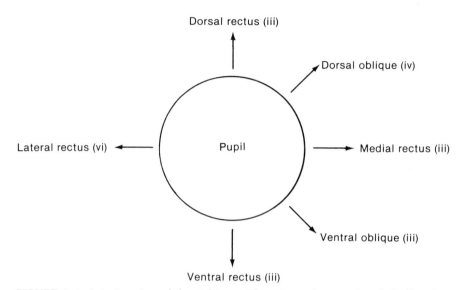

FIGURE 8–1. Anterior view of the right eye. The extraocular muscles, their direction of pull (arrow), and innervation are indicated. The retractor bulbi (vi), which retracts the eyeball, is not represented.

barbiturates. The direction of the slow phase generally indicates the side of the lesion; i.e., a slow phase to the right indicates a lesion on the right side.

Peripheral Vestibular Disease

The nystagmus is either horizontal or rotatory but not vertical, and the rapid phase is opposite to the side of the lesion; it does not change in direction with variation of head position. The nystagmus is accompanied by head tilt and loss of balance.

Central Vestibular Disease

The nystagmus may be in any direction and may vary with changes in head position. Accompanying signs include head tilt, depression (reticular formation), hemi- or tetraparesis, and a tendency to roll in *one* direction.

Circling

Circling may be the result of lesions in many different areas of the brain and therefore is not itself localizing.

If the lesion is in the cerebral cortex, other signs such as depression or wandering are evident. Cerebral lesions cause animals to make wide circles. Tight circling with head tilt is associated with vestibular disease.

Circling has been associated with the following disease states.

BRAIN ABSCESS. Secondary to septicemia, results in pressure atrophy of neural tissue.

PARASITES. Gid in sheep, cerebral nematodiasis.

NEOPLASIA. Rare in all species.

SALT POISONING/WATER DEPRIVATION. Pigs particularly.

HAEMOPHILUS SOMNUS. Associated fever, depression and/or retinal hemorrhages, respiratory involvement.

LISTERIOSIS. *(Listeria monocytogenes)* Ruminants. Fever, depression, cranial nerve deficits, especially in the 7th and 8th cranial nerves.

MOLDY CORN POISONING. *(Fusarium moniliforme)* Horses. Associated depression, head pressing, and blindness.

POLIOENCEPHALOMALACIA. Thiamine deficiency. Ruminants. Signs are blindness, ataxia, wandering, and opisthotonus.

DISORDERS OF THE SPINAL CORD

Localization of Spinal Cord Lesions

Lower Motor Neuron System

The lower motor neuron (LMN) comprises (a) a cell body located in the ventral horns of the gray matter of the spinal cord and in the nuclei of cranial nerves (3–7 and 9–12) and (b) an axon (by way of the peripheral nerves) to the motor end plate.

FUNCTION. The LMN is the final common pathway by which nerve impulses reach the muscle.

SIGNS. Signs of LMN disease include flaccid paralysis, diminished or absent reflexes, and muscle atrophy (not in acute phase).

Upper Motor Neuron System

The cell bodies of the upper motor neuron (UMN) system arise in the cerebral cortex, particularly the motor area, and descend through the internal capsule, brainstem, and spinal cord.

The UMN network is divided into the pyramidal (e.g., corticospinal tract) and extrapyramidal (e.g., rubrospinal tract) systems. The latter is more important in domestic animals.

FUNCTIONS. The UMN influences the motor nuclei of the LMNs in the brainstem (cranial nerves) and spinal cord. The UMN exerts control over muscle tone by influencing the α and γ motor neurons in the brainstem and spinal cord.

SIGNS

1. Paresis/paralysis, the severity of which increases as the location of the lesion descends the tract.

2. Normal or increased muscle tone (spasticity), due to loss of inhibitory influence of UMN. Decerebrate rigidity is the result of total loss of the inhibitory influence of the UMN. Severe head trauma, resulting in separation of the brainstem and higher centers, and seizures are examples of how this may occur.

3. Reflexes may be normal or hyperreflexic.

Spinal Cord

Spinal cord segments are referred to as cervical, thoracic, lumbar and sacral.

SIGNS

Cervical Region (C_1–C_6). UMN signs to thoracic and pelvic limbs.

Cervicothoracic (C_7–T_2). Affects LMN to thoracic limbs (brachial plexus), resulting in weakness and hyporeflexia of thoracic limbs. Muscle atrophy. Affects UMN to pelvic limbs, resulting in paresis/paralysis. Reflexes may be normal or hyperreflexia.

Thoracolumbar (T_3–L_3). Thoracic limbs are normal; UMN to pelvic limbs is affected.

Lumbosacral (L_4–S_2). Thoracic limbs are normal; LMN to pelvic limbs is affected, i.e., weakness and hyporeflexia.

Sacral (Caudal to S_2). Atony of urinary bladder, reduced tail tone, and hypoesthesia of perineum are present.

Evaluation of the Spinal Cord in Large Animals

After a general physical examination and assessment of brain and cranial nerve function, evaluation of the neck, thoracic limbs, trunk, pelvic limbs, and sacrococcygeal region is undertaken. Particular attention is given to skeletal and muscle symmetry, tail and anal tone, localized sweating (e.g., Horner's syndrome), and areas of hypoesthesia and hypoalgesia.

Postural reactions such as hemiwalking and wheelbarrowing can be tested only in small or neonatal animals; for this reason, in large animals much emphasis is placed on evaluation of gait.

Evaluation of Gait

A normal gait implies an intact ascending sensory tract and descending motor tract. The gait can be examined more thoroughly if the animal is used to being led and being put through maneuvers such as backing and turning. Of primary importance in evaluation of gait is

to determine whether a particular gait abnormality is due to a neurologic deficit or a musculoskeletal lesion.

The gait is evaluated for the presence of ataxia, weakness, dysmetria, and spasticity.

ATAXIA. Results from a loss of proprioceptive sense in the extremities and manifests as poor coordination of limbs and body. The animal
may have poor foot placement and on circling will circumduct the
outside limb. The ataxia may be exacerbated by raising the animal's
head while walking on a slope. Ataxia is more pronounced at speeds
greater than a walk and may be especially obvious if the animal has
to stop suddenly.

WEAKNESS. Can result from UMN or LMN lesions. If the UMN is
involved, weakness is present in the limbs caudal to the lesion.
Weakness in one limb is indicative of LMN disease. The animal may
be unable to bear weight on the affected limb, or the limb may tremble.
The animal's strength can be tested by applying pressure over the
lumbar area or shoulder and pulling on the tail during the walk.

DYSMETRIA. An inability to control the range of voluntary movement may result in hypo- or hypermetria. In cerebellar disease, hypermetria without weakness is a common finding.

SPASTICITY. An increase in normal muscle tone. The maintenance
of normal muscle tone is dependent on normal functioning of the
motor cortex, subcortical nuclei, midbrain, vestibulum, spine, and
neuromuscular system. The affected animal moves with a stiff gait,
and the affected limbs have minimal flexion.

Cutaneous (Panniculus) Reflex

Cutaneous sensations from each dermatome enter the spinal cord
and synapse with the lateral thoracic nerve (C_8–T_1). The latter innervates the cutaneous trunci. This reflex is not as obvious in large
animals as in dogs and cats. Lesions that involve only single nerve
roots are not likely to be detected, since each dermatome is supplied
with three spinal nerves. To check this reflex, the skin is pinched with
a hemostat in a caudal to cranial direction.

DISEASES OF PERIPHERAL NERVES

With few exceptions, peripheral nerve diseases are uncommon in
large animals and generally are a result of trauma and inflammation.
The following are examples of peripheral nerve injury.

OBTURATOR PARALYSIS. Associated with injury during calving.

RADIAL NERVE PARALYSIS. Results from direct trauma to the area
or is secondary to pressure damage during general anesthesia.

FACIAL NERVE PARALYSIS. E.g., damage sustained during general
anesthesia, from the head collar, or from a hard surface (horse).

SUPRASCAPULAR NERVE PARALYSIS. The suprascapular nerve may be damaged due to harness or when the animal collides with a door jamb.

HORNER'S SYNDROME. Subsequent to guttural pouch mycosis.

VESTIBULAR NERVE (UNILATERAL). Often subsequent to head trauma involving the petrous temporal area of the cranium.

GLOSSOPHARYNGEAL PARALYSIS. Often subsequent to guttural pouch mycosis.

Horner's Syndrome

Lesions involving the sympathetic nerve supply to the eye may result in Horner's syndrome.

TYPES

First-Order Horner's Syndrome. Involves lesions in the spinal cord prior to synapse of sympathetic fibers with cell bodies in the ventral gray matter at T_1–L_3. Causes include brainstem, cervical, and thoracic cord lesions. Accompanied by other clinical signs. If the ventral roots or the proximal part of the spinal nerves are affected, ipsilateral LMN signs are evident.

Second-Order Horner's Syndrome. Caused by lesions of the preganglionic sympathetic fibers between the ventral gray matter at T_1–L_3 and the cranial cervical ganglion. Examples include mediastinal neoplasia, brachial plexus injury, perineural inflammation (e.g., extravascular injection of irritants or guttural pouch mycosis), and trauma to neck (e.g., surgery or puncture wound).

Third-Order Horner's Syndrome. Damage to sympathetic nerve between cranial cervical ganglion and the motor end plate. Examples are middle ear disease and retrobulbar masses.

SIGNS

Ptcsis of Upper Eyelid and Flaccidity of Lower Eyelid. Due to denervation of smooth muscle.

Miosis. Paralysis of iridal radial muscle fibers.

Enophthalmos. Paralysis of periorbital smooth muscle allows sinking of globe into orbit.

Prominence of the Third Eyelid. Due to lack of smooth muscle tone.

Profuse Ipsilateral Sweating (Horse). Follows pre- or postganglionic sympathetic damage, due to sweat gland stimulation by increased blood flow.

NEUROLOGIC DISEASES IN HORSES

FOALS (0–4 WEEKS)

Congenital Abnormalities

NEONATAL MALADJUSTMENT. Associated with fetal distress and hypoxia during delivery. Cerebral hemorrhage and edema occur, leading to neurological signs. Foals may remain normal for 6–12 h after birth. Loss of suck reflex is an early sign, followed by disorientation, wandering, apparent blindness; may emit a barking sound; may progress to recumbency, nystagmus, seizures. Must be distinguished from septicemia—usually afebrile before onset of seizures.

T R E A T M E N T: Provide supportive care, control seizures, administer i.v. mannitol.

NARCOLEPSY/CATAPLEXY. Sleep attacks (narcolepsy) and lack of muscle tone (cataplexy) have been reported in many breeds and all ages, including neonates.

T R E A T M E N T: May respond to antidepressants.

HYDROCEPHALUS. Occasionally seen. Features are ventral deviation of eyes, varied neurologic signs, domed skull.

T R E A T M E N T: None advised.

CEREBELLAR ABIOTROPHY. Affects Arabian, Swedish Gotland, Oldenberg foals. Signs develop from birth to a few months of age and include symmetrical spasticity of all limbs, hypermetria, ataxia, intention tremor, absence of menace response. Condition is progressive and believed to be hereditary.

T R E A T M E N T: None.

ATLANTO-OCCIPITAL MALFORMATION. Inherited malformation in Arabian foals. May be evident at birth, or onset of signs may be delayed for weeks or months. Subluxation of atlanto-occipital joint leads to pressure on spinal cord; ataxia, paresis, and recumbency follow. May see extension of neck, abnormal vertebrae palpable; clicking of neck may be heard during flexion/extension.

T R E A T M E N T: Surgery could be attempted to stabilize the joint.

Infectious Diseases

BACTERIAL MENINGITIS. (*Escherichia coli* and *Klebsiella* spp., *Pseudomonas* spp., etc.) Common. Sequel to placentitis, failure of passive transfer of antibodies, other stresses leading to septicemia. Portals of infection include umbilical, respiratory, alimentary routes. Signs include fever, anorexia, loss of suck reflex, profound depression, weakness, recumbency, seizures, nystagmus, opisthotonus. May be accompanied by enteritis, swollen joints, pneumonia, anterior uveitis, umbilical swelling.

T R E A T M E N T: Provide supportive care; administer broad-spectrum antibiotics, short course of corticosteroids (dexamethasone).

BOTULISM: SHAKER FOAL. *(Clostridium botulinum)* Signs include severe muscle weakness, recumbency, dysphagia, pupillary dilation, severe tremors if animal is assisted to stand. Characterized by elaboration of toxin in necrotic tissue (e.g., umbilical infection, liver necrosis) or formation of toxin in and absorption from the gut. Prognosis is guarded.

T R E A T M E N T: Provide supportive care. Administer antiserum if available. Prognosis is guarded.

Miscellaneous Conditions

HYPOGLYCEMIA. May result from inadequate intake of milk, low environmental temperature, concurrent disease (e.g., septicemia). Signs include weakness, incoordination, recumbency, seizures, death if untreated.

T R E A T M E N T: Provide supportive care and oral feeding. Control seizures, administer i.v. dextrose (5 or 10%) in severe cases.

TRAUMA. Uncommon in neonates. Animal may have history of injury, sudden onset of signs, which vary with severity of lesion.

T R E A T M E N T: Depends on severity of signs. Reduce brain edema, (corticosteroids, mannitol), control seizures, provide supportive care.

WEANLING AND ADULT HORSES

Parasitic Diseases

VERMINOUS ENCEPHALITIS. Many different parasites may undergo aberrant migration through central nervous system. Nervous signs depend on site of migration.

T R E A T M E N T: Administer ivermectin (0.2 mg/kg, p.o.) and dexamethasone parenterally.

EQUINE PROTOZOAL MYELOENCEPHALITIS. *(Sarcocystis* spp.) Most common in young Standardbreds. Causes focal myeloencephalitis.

Signs may include ataxia (often one limb affected); paresis; cranial nerve signs including head tilt, dysphagia, unilateral facial paralysis; signs of brain involvement including circling, depression. Poor prognosis.

T R E A T M E N T: Administer potentiated sulfonamides, pyrimethamine, and antiinflammatories (nonsteroidal).

Toxicities

MOLDY CORN POISONING. Toxicity due to *Fusarium moniliforme*. Signs include acute onset of ataxia, hyperexcitability, head pressing, blindness, circling, sweating. High mortality rate. Toxin may also cause liver damage, with icterus, hepatoencephalopathy, swelling of lips, petechiation of mucous membranes. Prognosis is poor.

T R E A T M E N T: Provide supportive care.

AFLATOXICOSIS. Caused by ingestion of grain contaminated with *Aspergillus flavus*. May cause central nervous system edema, liver, kidney necrosis. Neurologic signs develop. Prognosis is poor.

T R E A T M E N T: Provide supportive care.

YELLOW-STAR THISTLE POISONING. (*Centaurea* spp.) Occurs in summer. Toxin causes nigropallidal encephalomalacia. Signs include smacking movement of lips and failure to prehend food or move it to pharyngeal area. Animal can swallow but may die from starvation. Prognosis is poor.

T R E A T M E N T: Provide supportive care.

BLIND STAGGERS. (*Astragalus* spp.) Caused by selenium converter plants ingested under drought conditions. Occurs in southern USA. Signs include ataxia, blindness, maniacal behavior.

T R E A T M E N T: None specific. Provide supportive care.

PYRROLIZIDINE ALKALOIDS. (*Senecio, Crotalaria,* and *Amsinckia* spp.) Occurs in midwestern and southern USA. Cirrhosis of the liver develops following prolonged exposure. Signs of hepatoencephalopathy ensue, including yawning, blindness, circling, ataxia, behavioral changes. Death occurs days to weeks after onset of signs.

T R E A T M E N T: None successful.

LEAD POISONING. Chronic lead poisoning may occur near smelters. Signs include dysphagia, laryngeal paralysis, weakness, recumbency.

T R E A T M E N T:

1. Supportive care and seizure control.
2. Chelation therapy

   a. CaNa$_2$ EDTA (50 mg/kg/day in divided doses, *slow* i.v.); may need to continue for 3–5 days.

   b. Dimercaprol (4 mg/kg every 4–6 h initially) may be given in association with CaNa$_2$ EDTA. (Irritant to muscle.)

   c. D-penicillamine is too expensive for routine use.

3. Administration of thiamine (10 mg/kg every 4–6 h for 2 days) improves outcome in cases of lead toxicity.

Infectious Diseases

EASTERN/WESTERN/VENEZUELAN ENCEPHALITIS. (togavirus) Usually occurs in young unvaccinated animals. Seasonal incidence (insect transmission), usually late summer or fall. Signs initially include fever and moderate hyperesthesia, followed by severe depression, blindness, circling, dysphagia, head pressing, ataxia, and recumbency followed by seizures. Rapid progression to complete paralysis in most cases, death in 1–5 days. Eastern equine encephalitis (EEE) may produce a significant viremia in the horse. The highest mortality rate is associated with EEE.

   T R E A T M E N T: Provide supportive care.

RABIES. (rhabdovirus) Various presentations. Behavioral changes including aggression, excessive whinnying, dysphagia, ataxia, progressing to recumbency and death. Short course.

   T R E A T M E N T: None.

SNOWSHOE HARE VIRUS. (California serogroup) Insect transmission (mosquito). Reported in Canada. Signs include hyperesthesia, somnolence, twitching of muscles, hypermetria, ataxia; usually recovery occurs over several days.

   T R E A T M E N T: Provide supportive care.

BORNA VIRUS. (unclassified virus) Occurs in Germany. Low morbidity, high mortality. Mild fever, followed by pharyngeal paralysis, muscle tremors, later flaccid paralysis, and recumbency. Death usually occurs within 3 weeks of onset of signs.

   T R E A T M E N T: None specific. Provide supportive care.

LOUPING ILL. (flavivirus) Occurs in Europe. Fever, muscle tremors, bounding (louping) gait, ataxia, progressing to recumbency, convulsions, death. Diffuse meningoencephalitis.

   T R E A T M E N T: None specific. Provide supportive care.

JAPANESE ENCEPHALITIS. (flavivirus) Occurs in Malaysia. Disease of humans; may be transmitted to horses. May be mild, with fever, jaundice, recovery. Severe form includes fever, hyperesthesia, muscle tremors, ataxia, recovery in 5–7 days.

T R E A T M E N T: None specific.

EQUINE INFECTIOUS ANEMIA. (lentivirus) Rare cause of ataxia and weakness in horses.

T R E A T M E N T: None specific.

OTHER VIRAL ENCEPHALITIDES. Cache Valley virus, St. Louis encephalitis virus, Jamestown Canyon virus, Powassan virus.

T R E A T M E N T: Provide supportive care.

BACTERIAL MENINGOENCEPHALITIS. May be due to brain abscessation or may be a complication of strangles (Streptococcus equi). Signs of diffuse meningoencephalitis. Usually fatal. Foals older than 6–8 weeks may develop septic meningitis due to E. coli, Salmonella, Klebsiella, and Actinobacillus spp.

T R E A T M E N T: Provide supportive care; administer broad spectrum antibiotics, corticosteroids (dexamethasone).

Bacterial Toxins

TETANUS. (Clostridium tetani) Sequel to deep wound. Signs include stiffness, hyperesthesia, trismus (lockjaw), prominence of third eyelid, development of saw-horse stance, recumbency, tetanic limbs, death from respiratory paralysis.

T R E A T M E N T: Administer penicillin, tetanus antitoxin; control muscle spasm (valium, acepromazine); perform wound debridement if indicated; provide general supportive care.

BOTULISM. (Clostridium botulinum) Onset of flaccid paralysis, followed by dysphagia, recumbency, death due to respiratory failure. Has been associated with big-bale silage feeding. Prognosis is guarded.

T R E A T M E N T: Provide supportive care. Administer antiserum, if available.

Miscellaneous Conditions

TRAUMA. Sudden onset of neurologic signs after trauma to the cranium. Usually a history of falling over backwards. Severe trauma may result in recumbency, convulsions, nystagmus. Prognosis poor in these cases.

T R E A T M E N T: Provide supportive care, control seizures, reduce brain edema (corticosteroids, mannitol).

THIAMINE DEFICIENCY. Caused by ingestion of thiaminase-containing plants (bracken fern, horsetails). Signs include ataxia, muscle tremors, depression, bradycardia, recumbency.

T R E A T M E N T: Administer thiamine (10.0 mg/kg, slow i.v. or i.m.) every 6–8 h for 2 days.

NARCOLEPSY/CATAPLEXY. Sleep attacks (narcolepsy) and lack of muscle tone (cataplexy) have been reported in many breeds and all ages, including neonates.

T R E A T M E N T: May respond to antidepressants.

LACTATION TETANY. Associated with hypocalcemia and occasionally with hypomagnesemia. Most common in postpartum period, often associated with stress (transport, weaning). Animals with mild form recover. Animals with severe form have tachypnea, mild fever, muscle fasciculation, diaphragmatic "thumps," stiffness, trismus, and decreased fecal and urinary output and may die if untreated.

T R E A T M E N T: Administer calcium borogluconate (5–10 g, slow i.v.). $MgSO_4$ (100 ml of 20% solution) may be added to the calcium solution.

NEURITIS OF THE CAUDA EQUINA. Adults affected. Signs are urinary incontinence with bladder and anal sphincter atony, and perineal analgesia, often accompanied by cranial nerve signs including facial nerve paralysis, vestibular signs, and trigeminal involvement. Prognosis is poor.

T R E A T M E N T: Administer corticosteroids, provide supportive care.

NEOPLASIA. Central neurologic signs may be seen with intracranial tumors, such as melanoma, cholesteatoma, pituitary adenoma.

T R E A T M E N T: None usually attempted.

ATAXIA IN HORSES

EQUINE PROTOZOAL MYELOENCEPHALITIS. (*Sarcocystis* spp.) Signs may include ataxia (often one limb affected); paresis; and cranial nerve signs including head tilt, dysphagia, unilateral facial paralysis. Signs are asymmetric. Poor prognosis.

T R E A T M E N T: Administer potentiated sulfonamides, pyrimethamine, and antiinflammatories (nonsteroidal).

NEURITIS OF THE CAUDA EQUINA. Adults affected. Signs are urinary incontinence with bladder and anal sphincter atony, and perineal analgesia, often accompanied by cranial nerve signs including facial nerve paralysis, vestibular signs, and trigeminal involvement. Prognosis is poor.

T R E A T M E N T: Administer corticosteroids; provide supportive care.

EQUINE DEGENERATIVE MYELOPATHY. Common. Seen in horses from birth to several years old. Associated with vitamin E/selenium deficiency. Often gradual onset. Signs include spastic, jerking movements, mainly in the hindlimbs. Signs are generally symmetric. Ataxia on circling; no cranial nerve deficits. Severe cases may have forelimb involvement, and animals may "dog-sit."

T R E A T M E N T: Some success reported with administration of vitamin E to clinical cases and pregnant mares.

CERVICAL VERTEBRAL MALFORMATION. Mainly seen in young adult horses. Slow, progressive onset. Occurs frequently in rapidly growing males. Stenosis (functional/mechanical) of vertebral canal, most commonly at C_3–C_4 or C_4–C_5, leading to pressure on cord. Bilateral ataxia and paresis are the main signs. No cranial nerve involvement.

T R E A T M E N T: Conservative: reduce nutritional level; implement stall rest. Surgical: stabilize affected vertebrae.

EQUINE HERPESVIRUS MYELOENCEPHALOPATHY. (equine herpesvirus type 1) Herd outbreaks. Hindlimb ataxia, with lack of bladder, anal, tail tone; may be preceded by fever. Paresis of the limbs may also occur, usually symmetrical. Signs usually progress rapidly and then stabilize.

T R E A T M E N T: Corticosteroids are indicated in early stages. Provide supportive care. Physical support (slinging) in selected cases.

ABERRANT PARASITE MIGRATION. Signs depend on site of lesion. Diagnosis is difficult; cerebrospinal fluid analysis is helpful (eosinophils).

T R E A T M E N T: Administer anthelmintics and corticosteroids; provide supportive care.

VASCULAR LESIONS OF CORD. E.g., hemorrhage, thromboembolic lesions.

T R E A T M E N T: Administer antiinflammatories, allow rest, and provide supportive care.

NEOPLASIA. Rare.
T R E A T M E N T: None usually attempted.

TRAUMA. Signs depend on site of injury.
T R E A T M E N T: Depends on cause and severity of lesion. Administer antiinflammatories, allow rest, and provide supportive care.

ATLANTO-OCCIPITAL MALFORMATION. Inherited malformation in

Arabian foals. May be evident at birth, or onset of signs may be delayed for weeks or months. Subluxation of atlanto-occipital joint leads to pressure on spinal cord; ataxia, paresis and recumbency follow. May see extension of neck, abnormal vertebrae palpable; clicking of neck may be heard during flexion/extension. The foal may resent palpation of the poll.

T R E A T M E N T: Surgery could be attempted to stabilize the joint.

RABIES. (rhabdovirus) The paralytic or spinal cord form of rabies is characterized by an ascending paralysis, with loss of tail and anal sphincter tone. The disease may progress to involve the brain stem (dumb form), resulting in depression. Hyperesthesia may be a feature of the disease and is intermittent in some cases. The paralytic form may be preceded by a variety of clinical signs, including colic and behavioral changes (aggression, compulsive circling, and abnormal vocalization). Fever is a feature in approximately half of these animals. Once signs appear, the survival time is less than 7 days.

T R E A T M E N T: None.

NEUROLOGIC DISEASES IN CATTLE

CONGENITAL/HEREDITARY DISEASES

BOVINE VIRAL DIARRHEA. (pestivirus) Some calves may be stillborn. Others may be born weak, be uncoordinated, have fine head tremors, or be unable to stand due to cerebellar hypoplasia. Arthrogryposis may be part of this presentation.
T R E A T M E N T: None.

HYDROCEPHALUS. Seen in neonates. Genetic hydrocephalus, associated with Holstein, Hereford, Ayrshire, Charolais breeds. Born dead or weak, bawling constantly, unable to stand. Dyschondroplasia also present. In utero bovine viral diarrhea virus infection also may cause internal hydrocephalus.
T R E A T M E N T: None.

AKABANE VIRUS. Seen in neonates. Occurs primarily in Southern Hemisphere. Viral infection in utero may cause hydranencephaly and arthrogryposis. Cortical signs predominate; cortex and cerebellum may be involved. Destruction of neuronal tissue by virus in developmental stages.
T R E A T M E N T: None.

BLUETONGUE. (orbivirus) Mainly a disease of sheep (neonates). Fetal calf may develop hydranencephaly with cerebral and cerebellar degeneration. Cerebral signs predominate.
T R E A T M E N T: None.

CEREBELLAR HYPOPLASIA. Genetic basis confirmed in Holsteins, Herefords, Shorthorns. Signs include inability to stand, incoordination. Bovine viral diarrhea virus is also a cause of in utero infection.
T R E A T M E N T: None.

CEREBELLAR ABIOTROPHY. Has a genetic basis in Holsteins. Signs include ataxia, intention tremors, dysmetria.
T R E A T M E N T: None.

CEREBELLAR HYPOMYELINOGENESIS. Affects Herefords, Angus, Shorthorns, Jerseys. Progressive ataxia develops.
T R E A T M E N T: None.

PROGRESSIVE ATAXIA. Affects Charolais breed.
T R E A T M E N T: None.

WEAVER SYNDROME. Affects Brown Swiss. Signs develop at 5–8 months most commonly. Symmetric hindlimb ataxia, normal motor and sensory reflexes, weaving gait. Disease progresses over 12–18 months.
T R E A T M E N T: None.

SPASTIC PARESIS: ELSO HEEL. Occurs in younger cattle. Signs include unilateral or, less commonly, bilateral hindlimb spasticity. Extended hock and pastern may be present due to extensor spasm during motion.
T R E A T M E N T: Palliative surgery may be performed.

SPASTIC SYNDROME. Occurs in mature cattle. Chronic progressive disorder of Holsteins, Channel Island breeds primarily. Sudden spasm of both hindlimbs, back, neck.
T R E A T M E N T: None.

HEREDITARY NEURAXIAL EDEMA: MAPLE SYRUP URINE DISEASE. Rapid onset of recumbency within a few days of birth in polled Herefords.
T R E A T M E N T: None.

GANGLIOSIDOSIS. Mainly affects Friesian calves. Signs develop within a few weeks to months of birth. Progressive ataxia, recumbency, and death follow.
T R E A T M E N T: None.

MANNOSIDOSIS. Affects Angus, Galloway, Simmental, Murray Grey breeds. Caused by mannosidase deficiency. Signs include ataxia, aggression, head tremor. Signs usually develop with a few months of birth. The condition is fatal.
T R E A T M E N T: None.

METABOLIC DISEASES

HYPOGLYCEMIA. Affects neonates most commonly. Signs include depression, weakness, ataxia, seizures, coma, and death.
T R E A T M E N T: Administer i.v. glucose. Control seizures.

POLIOENCEPHALOMALACIA. Thiamine deficiency. Usually affects younger ruminants. Frequently sequel to dietary change. Signs include ataxia, wandering, blindness, opisthotonus, seizures, dorsomedial strabismus. Normal pupillary light reflex. Diarrhea is sometimes seen.
T R E A T M E N T: Early cases respond rapidly to thiamine (10 mg/kg i.v. or i.m. every 6/8 h for 4–5 treatments). Administer a short course of corticosteroids (e.g., dexamethasone).

VITAMIN A DEFICIENCY. Affects calves 3–10 months old. Common in feedlot calves. Early signs include night blindness progressing to total blindness, xerophthalmia, seizures, and paralysis. In neonates, a congenital form is seen, with blindness, seizures, facial nerve paralysis, and corneal cloudiness.

TREATMENT: Early cases may respond to vitamin A injections (500 I.U./kg) and dietary supplementation.

HYPOMAGNESEMIC TETANY. Affects adult cows, suckling calves, lactating cows, and calves grazing lush pastures. Common. Signs include an anxious expression, bellowing, hyperesthesia, excitement, and muscle tremors, followed by convulsions and sudden death.

TREATMENT: Animals show good response to infusion of $MgSO_4$ slow i.v. or s.c. See Chapter 12.

HYPOCALCEMIA: PARTURIENT PARESIS, MILK FEVER. Affects dairy cows (usually), mostly within 24 hours of calving. Signs include hyperexcitability, ataxia, and weakness, with inappetance and decreased urination and defecation. Sternal recumbency follows, with the head held against the flank. Tachycardia and a decrease in body temperature occur, followed by muscle flaccidity, recumbency, bloat, and dilated pupils. If untreated, death may occur during convulsive episode.

TREATMENT: Responds to i.v. calcium in most instances. See Chapter 12.

TRANSIT TETANY. Affects all ages. Usually, but not exclusively, associated with late pregnancy. Also appears after or during transport. In early stages, restlessness, hyperesthesia, trismus, bruxism, ataxia, gastrointestinal stasis may be seen. Paddling may occur after recumbency. Posterior paralysis may be seen.

TREATMENT: May respond to treatment with an i.v. combination of Ca/Mg and glucose.

KETOSIS. Occurs in heavy lactation or starvation states. Signs include weight loss, salivation, licking at coat, circling, ataxia, occasionally blindness, and head pressing. Behavioral abnormalities are seen; animal may be aggressive. Accompanied by fatty liver.

TREATMENT: Administer propylene glycol (200 g, p.o. b.i.d.) for 2–4 days. Administer glucose infusions, e.g., 500 ml of a 50% solution, i.v.; may need to be repeated. Corticosteroids, e.g., dexamethasone (15 mg for average cow).

SALT POISONING/WATER DEPRIVATION. Affects all ages, but usually calves. Regurgitation, diarrhea, opisthotonus, blindness, weakness, ataxia, and knuckling at fetlocks are signs.

T R E A T M E N T: Administer fluids. For choice of fluids, see Chapter 12.

PARASITIC DISEASES

NERVOUS COCCIDIOSIS. (*Eimeria* spp.) Affects young cattle. Fever, diarrhea, or dysentery may be accompanied by muscle tremors, hyperesthesia, nystagmus, opisthotonus, and convulsions. Mortality is high, even with supportive care. Pathogenesis uncertain, but neurotoxins have been implicated.
T R E A T M E N T: Provide supportive care. Control convulsions.

ABERRANT PARASITE MIGRATION. (*Hypoderma* spp., *Parelaphostrongylus tenuis*, *Coenurus cerebralis*, *Taenia multiceps*, and *Setaria* spp.) May cause neurologic signs.
T R E A T M E N T: Corticosteroids and ivermectin (0.2 mg/kg) may be helpful.

PLANT TOXICITIES

PYRROLIZIDINE ALKALOIDS. (*Senecio* and *Crotalaria* spp.) Pyrrolizidine alkaloids cause chronic hepatic fibrosis. Hepatoencephalopathy, typified by depression, head pressing, apparent blindness, convulsions. Severe diarrhea and tenesmus may be present. Jaundice and photosensitization may be seen. Prognosis is poor.
T R E A T M E N T: No specific antidote. Provide supportive care.

ASTRAGALUS, CANARY GRASS, AND MALE FERN. (*Astragalus, Phalaris*, and *Dryopteris* spp.) Signs include drowsiness, blindness, ataxia. Recovery is common.
T R E A T M E N T: No specific antidote.

POISON HEMLOCK. (*Conium maculatum*) Signs include dysentery, excessive salivation, frequent regurgitation; may be followed by ataxia, convulsions, death. Hay and fresh standing plant are sources of toxin.
T R E A T M E N T: No specific antidote. Provide supportive care.

LABURNUM. (*Cytisus laburnum*) Cytisine is the toxic principle. Signs include excitement, ataxia, convulsions, death.
T R E A T M E N T: No specific antidote. Provide supportive care.

LUPINS. *(Lolium perenne)* Alkaloids in seeds are toxic principle. Ataxia, convulsions, excessive salivation, recumbency are seen. Prognosis is poor.

T R E A T M E N T: No specific antidote. Provide supportive care.

RHODODENDRON/MOUNTAIN LAUREL. *(Andromeda* spp./*Kalmia* spp.) Andromedotoxin is the active principle. Signs include hyperexcitability, ataxia, and paralysis; regurgitation may be seen. Recovery in 48–72 h in mild cases. Severely affected animals may die.

T R E A T M E N T: No specific antidote. Provide supportive care.

OLEANDER. *(Nerium oleander)* Signs include excitement, convulsions, frequent urination, and defecation. Prognosis is poor.

T R E A T M E N T: No specific antidote. Provide supportive care.

MYCOTOXINS

AFLATOXINS. *(Aspergillus flavus)* Occurs in adult cattle. Pigs also affected. Signs include decreased milk yield, jaundice, blindness, and convulsions due to hepatoencephalopathy.

T R E A T M E N T: None specific.

ERGOT. *(Claviceps paspali)* Cerebellar ataxia may be seen. Hypersensitivity to noise, muscle tremors.

T R E A T M E N T: None specific. Remove from pasture.

ERGOT OF RYE. *(Claviceps purpurea)* Sporadic occurrence. Acute toxicity causes neurologic signs including drowsiness and ataxia. Intermittent blindness also occurs. Seizures may be followed by paralysis and coma.

T R E A T M E N T: None specific.

BLUE-GREEN ALGAE. (e.g., *Microcystis* spp.) May cause ataxia, opisthotonus, and death.

T R E A T M E N T: None specific.

PERENNIAL RYEGRASS. *(Lolium perenne)* Occurs mainly in New Zealand, also UK and Australia. Similar to disease in sheep. Endophytic fungus *Acremonium lolii* produces tremorgenic toxins. Signs are tetanic spasms, stiffness, especially noticeable during movement. Prognosis is poor.

T R E A T M E N T: No specific antidote. Provide supportive care.

CHEMICAL TOXINS

LEAD

Acute Form. Affects calves most commonly. Short course (less than

24 h). Signs include hyperesthesia, blindness, champing of jaws, and snapping of eyelids.

Subacute Form. Affects older cattle. Animals live several days. Signs include blindness, ataxia, profound depression, fetid diarrhea, bruxism, and recumbency.

Chronic Form. Rare. Signs include weakness, ataxia, and seizures.

T R E A T M E N T:

1. Supportive care and seizure control.
2. Chelation therapy
   a. CaNa$_2$ EDTA (50 mg/kg/day in divided doses, slow i.v.); may need to continue for 3–5 days.
   b. Dimercaprol (4 mg/kg every 4–6 h initially) may be given in association with CaNa$_2$ EDTA. (Irritant to muscle.)
   c. D-penicillamine is too expensive for routine use.
3. Administration of thiamine (10 mg/kg i.v. or i.m. every 4–6 h for 2 days) improves outcome in cases of lead toxicity.

ARSENIC. Occurs at any age. Signs include colic, diarrhea, muscle tremors, ataxia, and blindness. High mortality rate.

T R E A T M E N T: Generally unsatisfactory, especially in acute cases. Dimercaprol (see Lead) and sodium thiosulfate (20–30 g in 10% solution, p.o.) may be beneficial.

MERCURY. Occurs at any age. Signs include diarrhea, stomatitis, incoordination, blindness, hyperesthesia, recumbency, and convulsions.

T R E A T M E N T: Remove mercury from gut by use of purgatives. Dimercaprol may be helpful if administered early in the course of disease.

SELENIUM. Affects grazing animals. Acute toxicity results in respiratory distress, blindness, head pressing, and difficulty in eating and drinking.

T R E A T M E N T: Sodium thiosulfate (20–30 g in a 10% solution, p.o.) has been used, though response is poor.

ORGANOPHOSPHATES. Signs include salivation, tremors, pupillary constriction, and ataxia; may lead to coma and death. History of a recent deworming with an organophosphate may support diagnosis.

T R E A T M E N T: Provide supportive care; administer atropine (0.05–0.50 mg/kg, i.v. or i.m.). Repeat as necessary.

NOTE: Many other chemicals including certain insecticides, molluscides, herbicides may cause neurologic signs.

BACTERIAL TOXINS

TETANUS. *(Clostridium tetani)* Affects all ages. Sporadic occurrence. Signs include onset of limb stiffness, trismus (lockjaw), prolapse of third eyelid, marked hyperesthesia, bloat, "pump-handle" tail, and wide stance. Death due to respiratory paralysis. Some animals recover over weeks to months.

T R E A T M E N T: Perform wound debridement if applicable. Administer parenteral antitoxin in early cases, tetanus toxoid, penicillin, antispasmodics (e.g., valium), or tranquilizers (e.g., phenothiazines). Provide supportive care.

BOTULISM. *(Clostridium botulinum)* Sporadic occurrence. Affects all ages. Herd outbreaks may occur. Signs include muscle weakness followed by dysphagia, recumbency, respiratory failure, and death.

T R E A T M E N T: Provide supportive care. Administer antitoxin if available. Muscarinic drugs (e.g., neostigmine) may be helpful, but these have a very short duration of action and undesirable side effects.

FOCAL SYMMETRICAL ENCEPHALOMALACIA. *(Clostridium perfringens* type D) Affects young cattle and yearlings. Signs include salivation, excitement, depression later, bruxism, apparent blindness, opisthotonus, seizures, and coma. Characterized by sudden onset and quick course.

T R E A T M E N T: None specific.

INFECTIOUS DISEASES

NEONATAL SEPTICEMIA. *(Escherichia coli* and *Salmonella, Streptococcus,* and *Staphylococcus* spp.) Signs include fever, depression, neck rigidity, opisthotonus, nystagmus, and coma. May be associated with diarrhea, navel ill.

T R E A T M E N T: Administer antibiotics and short course of corticosteroids; provide supportive care.

BRAIN ABSCESS. *(Actinomyces pyogenes* and *Staphylococcus* and *Streptococcus* spp.) Gradual onset of unilateral or bilateral blindness, depression, circling. Usually reflects unilateral involvement. Frequently afebrile. Prognosis is guarded.

T R E A T M E N T: Poor response to antibiotics.

LISTERIOSIS. *(Listeria monocytogenes)* Usually adult bovines. Facial, trigeminal, vestibulocochlear nerves frequently affected; brainstem involvement. Fever may be present. Hemiparesis and circling are common.

T R E A T M E N T: Administer oxytetracycline (10 mg/kg, i.v.) twice daily or procaine penicillin (20,000 I.U./kg, i.m.) twice daily; treat for 7–10 days. Other antibiotics may be effective. Corticosteroids (dexamethasone) may be beneficial in early cases.

THROMBOEMBOLIC MENINGOENCEPHALITIS. *(Haemophilus somnus)* Affects mainly feedlot cattle. Rapid course. Signs include fever, depression, coma, retinal hemorrhages, or cranial nerve deficits. Blindness, circling and opisthotonus are also seen.

T R E A T M E N T: Responds to antibiotics if treated early; penicillin or tetracyclines are efficacious. Corticosteroids may be beneficial in early stages.

INFECTIOUS BOVINE RHINOTRACHEITIS. Neurologic form (bovine herpesvirus) Usually affects calves and young cattle. Signs include conjunctivitis, upper and lower respiratory disease, excitement followed by circling, ataxia, depression, onset of paralysis, and recumbency. Pruritus may be a feature. May resemble pseudorabies. High mortality rate.

T R E A T M E N T: None specific; provide supportive care.

PSEUDORABIES. (herpesvirus) Affects all age groups. Direct or fomite contact with swine is a prerequisite. Signs include intense pruritus, self-mutilation, fever, excessive salivation, maniacal or aggressive behavior. Bellowing may be a feature. A spinal form is also recognized, with paraplegia and a dog-sitting posture. Death is usual.

T R E A T M E N T: None successful.

MALIGNANT CATARRHAL FEVER. (herpesvirus) Usually affects adults. Associated with sheep or wildebeest. Signs include depression, incoordination, ataxia, tremors, and shivering; occasionally bellowing, bruxism, and aggression. These neurologic signs are accompanied by fever, diarrhea or constipation, respiratory signs, and hypopyon. High mortality rate.

T R E A T M E N T: Administer antibiotics; provide supportive care.

RABIES. (rhabdovirus) Affects all ages. Signs include variable behavior, depression or excitement, bellowing (hoarseness), sexual excitement, and aggression. May see cranial nerve deficits, loss of tongue tone, inability to swallow. Diagnosis is difficult. Ascending paralysis is frequently seen.

T R E A T M E N T: Not recommended. Verify by postmortem examination.

LOUPING ILL. (flavivirus) Affects all ages. Occurs in the UK; possibly a similar disease in eastern Europe (Russian spring-summer encephalitis). Tick-borne disease. Signs include high fever, up to 42° C; stiff "louping" or jerky movements; muscle tremors; ataxia. Recovery is followed by immunity.
T R E A T M E N T: None specific.

BOVINE SPONGIFORM ENCEPHALOPATHY. Affects adult cows 3–6 years, usually dairy breeds. Reported primarily in the UK. Slow onset of behavioral changes; apprehensiveness; later tremors, hypermetria, ataxia, progressing to recumbency and death. Suspected to be a slow virus disease, similar to scrapie in sheep.
T R E A T M E N T: None. Affected herds are slaughtered.

SPORADIC BOVINE ENCEPHALOMYELITIS. (*Chlamydia* spp.) Seen especially in calves younger than 6 months. Signs include fever, nasal discharge, respiratory difficulty, salivation, and stiffness in early stages; followed in some cases by ataxia, circling, and occasionally opisthotonus. Many animals recover, but mortality is up to 30%.
T R E A T M E N T: May respond to tetracycline therapy.

HEART WATER DISEASE. (*Cowdria ruminantium*) Present in tropical and subtropical areas. Peracute and acute forms occur. Peracute cases usually die quickly. Acute form: ataxia, blindness, circling, recumbency, convulsions, and death.
T R E A T M E N T: Administer tetracyclines.

MISCELLANEOUS CONDITIONS

TRAUMA. Occurs at any age. A variety of clinical signs including coma and seizures may accompany central nervous system trauma.
T R E A T M E N T: Provide supportive care. Administer drugs as indicated, e.g., i.v. mannitol, corticosteroids, dimethylsulfoxide.

NEUROLOGIC DISEASES IN SHEEP AND GOATS

LAMBS (0–3 MONTHS)

Congenital Diseases

BORDER DISEASE. (pestivirus) Hairy Shakers; small, weak lambs. Usually a flock problem, with abortions and infertility. Signs include tremors, stunted skeletal growth, narrow face, prominent hairs.
TREATMENT: None effective.

CONGENITAL SWAYBACK. Affects lambs 0–7 days. Copper deficiency. Signs include blindness and spasticity.
TREATMENT: None effective.

DELAYED-ONSET SWAYBACK. Usually occurs at 1–2 months. Hindlimb weakness and ataxia are characteristic, exacerbated by exercise.
TREATMENT: Poor response to copper supplementation; ewes should be supplemented in midpregnancy.

DAFT LAMB DISEASE. Recessive trait in Corriedale and Border Leicester. Characterized by cerebellar cortical atrophy and muscular dystrophy. Wide stance, staggering are seen.
TREATMENT: None. Euthanasia is recommended.

CONGENITAL HYDRANENCEPHALY. Akabane, bluetongue, and border disease virus infections in utero may cause hydranencephaly.
TREATMENT: None effective.

Infectious Diseases

BACTERIAL MENINGOENCEPHALITIS. (e.g., *Escherichia coli* and *Staphylococcus* and *Streptococcus* spp.) Entry via umbilicus, intestinal, pharyngeal, or respiratory route. Signs include fever, depression, anorexia, recumbency, rigid neck, extensor spasms, and coma.
TREATMENT: Administer broad-spectrum antibiotics (e.g., potentiated sulfonamides) and corticosteroids, e.g., dexamethasone (0.1–1.0 mg/kg, short course).

BRAIN ABSCESS. Can be single or multiple. Multiple abscesses are often a sequel to tick-borne septicemia. Single abscess is more commonly associated with castration and tail docking. Blindness, circling, ataxia are common signs. Spinal abscess may cause posterior paralysis.

T R E A T M E N T: Poor response to antibiotic therapy.

LISTERIOSIS. *(Listeria monocytogenes)* Commonly, but not invariably, associated with silage feeding. Brainstem signs include facial paralysis (unilateral most common), circling, depression, and coma.
T R E A T M E N T: Administer oxytetracycline (10–15 mg/kg, i.v., i.m.) twice daily or procaine penicillin (20,000 I.U., i.m.) twice daily. Other antibiotics may also be effective. Corticosteroids, e.g., dexamethasone (0.1–1.0 mg/kg, short course), may be administered.

LOUPING ILL. (flavivirus) Occurs in the UK. Lambs may die without exhibiting neurologic signs. Signs include tremor of neck muscles, generalized muscle rigidity, hyperesthetic reaction to noise, and incoordination of pelvic limbs. May proceed to paralysis, recumbency, and death.
T R E A T M E N T: None specific.

PSEUDORABIES. (herpesvirus) Linked with close contact with pigs or with fomites. Signs include intense focal pruritus, pharyngeal paralysis, and death (sometimes sudden). High mortality rate. May occur in outbreaks.
T R E A T M E N T: None successful.

RABIES. (rhabdovirus) Affects all ages. Dumb form most common. Signs include tenesmus, ataxia, paralysis, and death.
T R E A T M E N T: Not recommended. Confirm diagnosis by postmortem examination.

Bacterial Toxins

TETANUS. *(Clostridium tetani)* Organism enters through umbilicus or surface wounds. Slow onset of extensor rigidity, extension of neck, hyperesthesia, recumbency, and trismus (lockjaw). Death usually results from respiratory paralysis.
T R E A T M E N T: Perform wound debridement if applicable. Administer parenteral antitoxin, tetanus toxoid, penicillin, antispasmodics (e.g., diazepam). Provide supportive care.

CLOSTRIDIAL ENTEROTOXEMIA. *(Clostridium perfringens* type D) Signs include convulsions, bruxism, depression, and sudden death. Prognosis is poor.
T R E A T M E N T: Administer antitoxin and oral penicillin. Provide supportive care.

FOCAL SYMMETRICAL ENCEPHALOMALACIA. *(Clostridium perfrin-*

gens type D) All ages affected. A manifestation of chronic infection. Head pressing may occur.

T R E A T M E N T: None effective.

Miscellaneous Conditions

TRAUMA. Signs depend on site of lesion.

T R E A T M E N T: Administer antiinflammatories and provide supportive care.

HYPOGLYCEMIA. May result from inadequate intake of milk or from concurrent disease (e.g., septicemia). Signs include weakness, incoordination, recumbency, seizures, and death, if untreated.

T R E A T M E N T: Provide supportive care and oral feeding in mild cases. In severe cases, control seizures; administer glucose, i.v. or intraperitoneally.

ADULT SHEEP

Metabolic Diseases

POLIOENCEPHALOMALACIA/CEREBROCORTICAL NECROSIS. Caused by thiamine deficiency. Associated with changes in diet, anthelmintic use. Animal is afebrile, occasionally has diarrhea. Blindness, star gazing, normal pupillary light reflex, and dorsomedial strabismus are commonly present; leads to recumbency, with paddling and opisthotonus.

T R E A T M E N T: Good response to thiamine (10 mg/kg, i.v. or i.m., every 4 h, for four to five treatments) administration in early stages. Provide supportive care. Steroids (e.g., dexamethasone) may be administered to reduce brain edema.

PREGNANCY TOXEMIA. Affects ewes in late pregnancy. Related to poor nutritional status and twin or triplet pregnancy. Animal separates from flock, may appear blind, with head pressing and star gazing; later becomes depressed, recumbent; may remain so for 2–4 days. Ketone odor may be detectable on the breath. Fetal death may lead to abortion or toxemia, or to improvement in some cases.

T R E A T M E N T: For mild cases, reduce stress (e.g., provide shelter), offer supplementary carbohydrates, and administer propylene glycol (50 ml twice daily for 3–4 days). For severe cases, administer i.v. glucose, corticosteroids, propylene glycol (50 ml twice daily). Induce parturition or perform cesarean. Provide supportive care.

HYPOMAGNESEMIA. Signs include muscle tremors and ataxia in early stages, followed by stamping of feet, limb spasticity, and convulsions.

T R E A T M E N T: $MgSO_4$ (25 ml of a 20% solution, s.c.; or 15–25 ml of a 20% solution added to 0.5–1.0 g of calcium borogluconate, slow i.v. or s.c.).

HYPOCALCEMIA. Affects ewes in late pregnancy and early lactation.

Signs include muscle tremors in early stages, followed by sternal recumbency, constipation, decreased to absent ruminations, and depression. Death may follow if untreated.

T R E A T M E N T: Calcium borogluconate (0.5–1.0 g as a 20% solution, s.c. or slow i.v.).

LIVER DISEASE. (pyrrolizidine alkaloids [Senecio and Crotalaria spp.], chronic copper poisoning, aflatoxins [Aspergillus spp.] and lupins) Hepatic failure may lead to hepatoencephalopathy.

T R E A T M E N T: None successful.

Parasitic Diseases

PARASITIC MIGRATION: WHITE-TAILED DEER WORM. (Parelaphostrongylus tenuis) Seasonal occurrence, fall to winter. Aberrant migration through central nervous system may cause ataxia and other signs.

T R E A T M E N T: Administer corticosteroids, e.g., dexamethasone (0.1–1.0 mg/kg, i.m. or i.v.) and ivermectin (0.2 mg/kg, s.c.).

GID. (Coenurus cerebralis) Intermediate stage of dog tapeworm (Taenia multiceps). Following ingestion of contaminated feed, cyst develops in cranial cavity. Signs include blindness, circling (to affected side), and softening of calvarium.

T R E A T M E N T: Surgical removal of the cyst is possible in many cases.

Toxicities

HEAVY METAL POISONING. Occurs in all ages. Lead, arsenic, mercury may cause neurologic signs: ataxia, incoordination.

T R E A T M E N T:

Lead
1. Supportive care and seizure control.
2. Chelation therapy
   a. CaNa$_2$ EDTA (50 mg/kg/day in divided doses, slow i.v.); may need to continue for 3–5 days.
   b. Dimercaprol (4 mg/kg every 4–6 h initially) may be given in association with CaNa$_2$ EDTA. (Irritant to muscle.)
   c. D-penicillamine is too expensive for routine use.
3. Administration of thiamine (10 mg/kg every 4–6 h for 2 days) improves outcome in cases of lead toxicity.

Arsenic

Arsenic may be treated with dimercaprol. Sodium thiosulfate (3–5 g in 100 ml of water, p.o.), based on cattle dosage, may be beneficial.

ORGANOPHOSPHATE (OP) POISONING. Usually follows topical administration of OP anthelmintic. Signs include salivation, increased muscarinic activity (e.g., bradycardia and constriction of pupils), ataxia, and drowsiness. Delayed toxicity, up to 1 month, has been associated with haloxon administration. Signs of delayed toxicity involve the pelvic limbs and include paresis and ataxia.

T R E A T M E N T: If topical OP is the source, washing the excess from the fleece may be helpful. Administer atropine (0.05–0.50 mg/kg parenterally) as needed to control the adverse muscarinic side effects. Anticonvulsants (e.g., diazepam) may be indicated.

TOXIC PLANTS. Locoweed (*Astragalus* and *Oxytropis* spp.) and lupins (*Lupinus* spp.). Signs of lupin poisoning include ataxia, convulsions, and frothing at the mouth.

T R E A T M E N T: None specific.

Infectious Diseases

LISTERIOSIS. (*Listeria monocytogenes*) Commonly associated with silage feeding. Signs include ptosis, circling, and unilateral facial paralysis; animal may have dropped jaw, ataxia, and head tilt. Occasionally "dry eye" and keratitis are present. Recumbency and death occur if untreated.

T R E A T M E N T: Administer oxytetracycline (10–15 mg/kg, i.v. or i.m.) twice daily, or procaine penicillin (20,000 I.U., i.m.) twice daily, for 7–10 days. Corticosteroids (dexamethasone) may be administered in early stages.

BRAIN ABSCESS. (*Actinomyces pyogenes* and *Staphylococcus, Pasteurella, Streptococcus* spp.) Hematogenous or direct spread (head wounds). Usually slow onset of signs, which may include blindness, circling to the affected side.

T R E A T M E N T: Poor response to antibiotics.

SCRAPIE. Affects adults more than 2 years of age. Signs include pruritus, loss of fleece, weight loss, nibbling movements in response to cutaneous stimulation, and ataxia. Affected animals invariably die.

T R E A T M E N T: None.

LOUPING ILL. (flavivirus) Associated with ticks. Confined to the UK. Similar condition occurs in Russia and central Europe. Signs include fever; ataxia; muscle tremors; jerky, bounding gait; and hypersensitivity to noise.

T R E A T M E N T: None specific. Vaccine available for use in enzootic areas.

MAEDI-VISNA: OVINE PROGRESSIVE PNEUMONIA. Retroviral disease of adult sheep. A separate syndrome from progressive pneumonia. Signs include locomotor weakness, stumbling, and weight loss.

T R E A T M E N T: None specific.

PSEUDORABIES. (herpesvirus) Close contact with pigs or with fomites necessary. Signs include intense focal pruritus, pharyngeal paralysis, and death (sometimes sudden). High mortality rate. May occur in outbreaks.

T R E A T M E N T: None successful.

RABIES. (rhabdovirus) Affects all ages. Dumb form most common. Signs include tenesmus, ataxia, paralysis, and death. Spread by bites from infected animals.

T R E A T M E N T: Not recommended. Confirm diagnosis by postmortem examination.

Bacterial Toxins

CLOSTRIDIAL ENTEROTOXEMIA. (*Clostridium perfringens* type D) Adults may develop staggering, salivation, and champing of the jaws and become obtunded. Death occurs in 12–24 h. Prognosis is poor.

T R E A T M E N T: Administer antitoxin; provide supportive care.

FOCAL SYMMETRICAL ENCEPHALOMALACIA. (*Clostridium perfringens* type D) All ages affected. A manifestation of chronic infection. Head pressing may occur.

T R E A T M E N T: None effective.

TETANUS. (*Clostridium tetani*) Organism enters through umbilicus or surface wounds. Slow onset of extensor rigidity, extension of neck, hyperesthesia, recumbency, trismus (lockjaw). Death usually results from respiratory paralysis.

T R E A T M E N T: Perform wound debridement if applicable. Administer parenteral antitoxin, tetanus toxoid, penicillin, antispasmodics (e.g., diazepam). Institute supportive care.

BOTULISM. (*Clostridium botulinum*) Initial signs include ataxia, incoordination; followed by limb paralysis, respiratory muscle paralysis, and death. Prognosis is poor.

T R E A T M E N T: Provide supportive care.

Miscellaneous Conditions

SPINAL ABSCESS. Sporadic. May be a sequel to navel ill and bacteremia. Ataxia, posterior/tetraparesis, and recumbency are signs.

T R E A T M E N T: Poor response to antibiotic therapy.

NEOPLASIA. Signs depend on location.
T R E A T M E N T: None effective.

CEROID LIPOFUSCINOSIS. Occurs in young adults of South Hampshire breed. Genetic condition. Signs include behavior changes, blindness, twitching of eyelids, and locomotor abnormalities including ataxia.
T R E A T M E N T: None effective.

TRAUMA. E.g., head butting in rams. Acute onset. Signs may include ataxia and depression.
T R E A T M E N T: Depends on extent of damage. Administer corticosteroids (e.g., dexamethasone). Provide supportive care.

KANGAROO GAIT. Cause unknown. Occurs in nursing ewes. Affected animals have a characteristic gait, weak and uncoordinated forelimbs with weight bearing on hindlimbs.
T R E A T M E N T: None specific. May resolve after weaning.

KIDS (0–3 MONTHS)

Congenital Abnormalities

CONGENITAL MALFORMATIONS. E.g., vertebral anomalies. Presentation depends on location of lesion.
T R E A T M E N T: None.

β-MANNOSIDASE DEFICIENCY. Affects Nubian goats. Signs include recumbency, nystagmus, head tremor, deafness, flexural deformities of limbs, and doming of skull.
T R E A T M E N T: None.

MYOTONIA. Observed soon after birth. Involves most of striated skeletal muscles. On exertion, the animal falls on its side with extensor rigidity of the limbs. Function returns rapidly.
T R E A T M E N T: None.

Infectious Diseases

BACTERIAL MENINGOENCEPHALITIS. Usually occurs in neonates, predisposed by inadequate colostrum intake. Organisms enter via gut, pharyngeal, respiratory, or umbilical route. Fever, depression, anorexia, recumbency, extensor spasms, coma occur.

T R E A T M E N T: Administer broad-spectrum antibiotics (e.g., potentiated sulfonamides) and corticosteroids, e.g., dexamethasone (0.1 mg/kg, short course).

BRAIN ABSCESS. Usually a sequel to septicemia, tail docking, or castration. Signs include blindness, circling, and ataxia. Spinal abscess may cause posterior paralysis.

T R E A T M E N T: Poor response to antibiotic therapy.

CAPRINE ARTHRITIS/ENCEPHALITIS. (lentivirus) Encephalitis form usually occurs in kids under 6 months of age. Predilection for joints, central nervous system, lung, udder. Signs may resemble those of swayback; pelvic limb paresis; occasionally blindness and brainstem signs. Usually progresses to recumbency. Recovery is rare.

T R E A T M E N T: None effective.

PSEUDORABIES. (herpesvirus) Rapid death, preceded by vocalizing, restlessness, sweating; pruritus may be a feature of the disease. Affected animals usually have had close contact with swine.

T R E A T M E N T: None effective.

RABIES. (rhabdovirus) Affects all ages. Signs include sudden behavioral changes, including sexual hyperactivity, aggression, self-mutilation, and lower motor neuron signs including flaccid paralysis.

T R E A T M E N T: Not recommended. Diagnosis confirmed by postmortem examination.

TOXOPLASMOSIS. (*Toxoplasma gondii*) Can cause diffuse encephalitis in kids. Usually fatal.

T R E A T M E N T: Administer potentiated sulfonamides and pyrimethamine, in addition to supportive care.

Bacterial Toxins

CLOSTRIDIAL ENTEROTOXEMIA. (*Clostridium perfringens* type D) Signs include convulsions, bruxism, depression, and sudden death. Death in 12–24 h.

T R E A T M E N T: Provide supportive care. Administer oral penicillin, hyperimmune serum.

TETANUS. (*Clostridium tetani*) All ages susceptible. Usually associated with wounds, e.g., castration. Signs include a slow onset of extensor rigidity, extension of neck, hyperesthesia, recumbency, and trismus (lockjaw). Death usually results from respiratory paralysis.

T R E A T M E N T: Perform wound debridement if applicable.

Administer parenteral antitoxin, tetanus toxoid, penicillin, antispasmodics (e.g., diazepam). Provide supportive care.

Miscellaneous Conditions

TRAUMA. Sudden onset. There may be physical evidence of injury. Thermal injury to the brain may result from the overzealous use of dehorning irons. Prognosis is guarded for most cases of thermal injury.

T R E A T M E N T: Mild cases may respond to supportive care, steroids, and anticonvulsants.

SWAYBACK. Results from copper deficiency. Occurs in kids up to 4 months of age. Characterized by pelvic limb paralysis that progresses to involve thoracic limbs.

T R E A T M E N T: Poor response to copper therapy.

HYPOGLYCEMIA. See under Lambs, p. 198.

ADULT GOATS

Infectious Diseases

LISTERIOSIS. *(Listeria monocytogenes)* Affects all ages. Fever initially, unilateral brainstem signs include head tilt, facial paralysis, dropped jaw.

T R E A T M E N T: Administer oxytetracycline (10–15 mg/kg, i.v. or i.m. twice daily) or procaine penicillin (20,000 I.U. twice daily). Treat for 7–10 days. Give corticosteroids (e.g., dexamethasone) in early stages.

BRAIN ABSCESS. Slow onset of signs, which may include blindness, circling to the affected side. May result from hematogenous or direct spread (head wound).

T R E A T M E N T: Poor response to antibiotics.

SCRAPIE. Affects adults over 2 years of age. Not as common as in sheep. Signs include pruritus, loss of hair, weight loss, nibbling movements in response to cutaneous stimulation, and ataxia. Affected animals invariably die.

T R E A T M E N T: None effective.

LOUPING ILL. (flavivirus) Signs similar to those of disease in sheep. Fever, tremors, muscle rigidity, high-stepping gait, incoordination, followed by paralysis and recumbency.

T R E A T M E N T: None specific.

CAPRINE ARTHRITIS/ENCEPHALITIS. (lentivirus) Encephalitic form can occur in goats up to 6 months of age. Predilection for joints, central nervous system, lung, and udder. Signs may resemble those of swayback; pelvic limb paresis; occasionally blindness and brainstem signs. Usually progresses to recumbency. Recovery is rare.

T R E A T M E N T: None effective.

PSEUDORABIES. (herpesvirus) Rapid death, preceded by vocalizing, restlessness, sweating; pruritus may be a feature of the disease. Affected animals usually have had close contact with swine.

T R E A T M E N T: None effective.

RABIES. (rhabdovirus) Affects all ages. Signs include sudden behavioral changes, including sexual hyperactivity, aggression, self-mutilation, and lower motor neuron signs including flaccid paralysis.

T R E A T M E N T: Not recommended. Diagnosis confirmed by postmortem examination.

Miscellaneous Conditions

For the following conditions the presenting signs in adult goats are similar to those in adult sheep, and the relevant section should be consulted.

CLOSTRIDIAL ENTEROTOXEMIA. (p. 201)

TETANUS. (p. 201)

BOTULISM. (p. 201)

POLIOENCEPHALOMALACIA/CEREBROCORTICAL NECROSIS. (p. 198)

PREGNANCY TOXEMIA. (p. 198)

HYPOMAGNESEMIA. (p. 198)

HYPOCALCEMIA. (p. 198)

LIVER DISEASE. (p. 199)

HEAVY METAL POISONING. (p. 199)

TOXIC PLANTS. (p. 200)

ORGANOPHOSPHATE POISONING. (p. 199)

PARASITE MIGRATION. (p. 199)

SPINAL ABSCESS. (p. 201)

NEOPLASIA. (p. 202)

TRAUMA. (p. 202)

NEUROLOGIC DISEASES IN PIGS

PREWEANING PIGS (<6 WEEKS)

Congenital Abnormalities

CONGENITAL SPLAYLEG. Signs are observed within a few hours of birth—splaying of hindlimbs, inability to stand. Mainly Pietrain and Landrace affected. Higher incidence in males. Lesion is a myofibrillar hypoplasia.

CONGENITAL TREMORS

A1: Myoclonia Congenita. (swine fever virus [SFV] infection in early gestation) All breeds and both sexes affected. High incidence and mortality in litter. Signs include tremor, ataxia, and inability to stand.

A2: Myoclonia Congenita. Etiology unknown. Worldwide distribution. Distinguished from A1 by lack of SFV involvement and low mortality.

A3: Congenital Cerebrospinal Hypomyelinogenesis. Occurs in male Landrace piglets. Signs include coarse tremors of forelimbs and head, swaying of hindlimbs; aggravated by cold and forced movement. Tremors absent during sleep. Few litters are afflicted; up to 25% of piglets in a litter are affected.

A4: Hereditary Tremor. Occurs in British Saddleback pigs. Low percentage of litters involved; affects up to 25% of piglets in a litter.

A5: History of exposure to organophosphates in midgestation. High proportion of litters and of piglets within litters are afflicted. High mortality rate.

B: Cause unknown. No lesions found consistently, but cerebellar hypoplasia is seen in some cases.

VITAMIN A DEFICIENCY (CONGENITAL FORM). Microphthalmia, cleft palate, herniation of spinal cord, internal hydrocephalus may be seen in newborn piglets. Piglets may be stillborn, weak, or clinically normal. Weak pigs exhibit recumbency and paddling due to increased cerebrospinal fluid pressure.

T R E A T M E N T: None effective.

Infectious Diseases

Viral Meningoencephalitis

PSEUDORABIES. (porcine herpesvirus) Usually occurs in piglets younger than 2 weeks. Ataxia, weakness, depression, disorientation followed by death. Spread by adult carriers. Almost always fatal.

T R E A T M E N T: None effective.

CYTOMEGALOVIRUS ENCEPHALITIS. Causes viral septicemia and encephalitis (same virus as inclusion body rhinitis). Pigs often found dead; may see incoordination, ataxia, recumbency.
T R E A T M E N T: None effective.

HEMAGGLUTINATING ENCEPHALOMYELITIS: VOMITING AND WASTING DISEASE. (coronavirus) Seen in piglets younger than 21 days old. Usually fever, vomiting, anorexia; some animals show neurologic signs, which include staring, apparent blindness, ataxia, hindlimb paralysis, recumbency, and death.
T R E A T M E N T: None effective.

BLUE EYE. (paramyxovirus) Recently identified in Mexico. Affects piglets 2–21 days old. Corneal edema (blue eye) and encephalomyelitis occur. Other signs are fever, depression, ataxia, incoordination, and death. High mortality rate.
T R E A T M E N T: None specific.

POLIOENCEPHALOMYELITIS: TESCHEN/TALFAN DISEASE. (enterovirus) Severe form in central Europe (Teschen). Signs include fever, progressive ataxia, recumbency, death in 3–5 days. Mild form occurs in North America and Australia (Talfan). Fever, ataxia, paresis, "dog-sitting." Death is uncommon.
T R E A T M E N T: None specific. Provide supportive care.

HOG CHOLERA: SWINE FEVER. (pestivirus) Signs include depression, anorexia, fever, huddling, vomiting, diarrhea or constipation, and conjunctivitis. Neurologic signs, including circling and tremors may occur early in disease course. High mortality rate. A variant strain of the virus produces a form of the disease in which nervous signs predominate.
T R E A T M E N T: None specific.

AFRICAN SWINE FEVER. (iridovirus) Signs include fever, dullness, inappetance, blotching of skin, vomiting, diarrhea, respiratory distress, and coughing. Incoordination may be seen. High mortality rate.
T R E A T M E N T: None specific.

Bacterial Meningoencephalitis

***STREPTOCOCCUS SUIS* TYPE I MENINGITIS.** Affects piglets 10–20 days old. Signs include fever, anorexia, depression, incoordination, seizures, opisthotonus, convulsions, and death.
***STREPTOCOCCUS SUIS* TYPE II MENINGITIS.** Mainly seen in piglets between 3 weeks and 3 months. Depression follows anorexia and fever, leading to neurologic signs.

T R E A T M E N T: Provide supportive care; administer parenteral penicillin and corticosteroids.

GLASSER'S DISEASE. *(Haemophilus parasuis)* Polyserositis of pigs 2–16 weeks old. Joint effusion, pleuritis, peritonitis, and meningoencephalitis. Recumbency follows fever, depression, stiff gait, central nervous system signs follow (outstretched neck, ataxia, nystagmus, incoordination), death ensues if untreated.
T R E A T M E N T: Broad-spectrum antibiotics and corticosteroids.

Miscellaneous Bacterial Conditions

MIDDLE EAR DISEASE. Infection may spread to involve cranial nerve 8; peripheral or central neurologic signs may ensue. Other signs are head tilt and nystagmus with peripheral disease. Loss of coordination and ataxia are seen if brainstem is involved.
T R E A T M E N T: Broad-spectrum antibiotics with a short course of corticosteroids may be beneficial.

TETANUS. *(Clostridium tetani)* Signs include onset of hyperesthesia, stiff gait, progressing to recumbency, erectness of ears and tail, extension of the neck. Death occurs from respiratory arrest.
T R E A T M E N T: Administer penicillin i.m. and tetanus antitoxin, control seizures, provide supportive care.

Miscellaneous Conditions

HYPOGLYCEMIA. Secondary to malnutrition. Signs include confusion, disorientation, ataxia, quadriplegia, seizures.
T R E A T M E N T: Oral or parenteral glucose.

HYPOTHERMIA. Neurologic signs may be evident.
T R E A T M E N T: Slow warming (e.g., using hot air heater, not directly applying heat).

SCIATIC NEURITIS. Sciatic nerve damage is often caused by injection injury. Pig is unable to extend the hock joint.
T R E A T M E N T: Administer corticosteroids or nonsteroidal antiinflammatories.

TRAUMA. E.g., damage to spinal column from overlying by sow.
T R E A T M E N T: Administer corticosteroids and antiinflammatories. Provide supportive care.

WEANED AND ADULT PIGS

Many of these diseases are common to all age groups. Refer to previous section where appropriate.

Deficiency States

COPPER. Uncommon. Seen in growing pigs 4–6 months old. Posterior ataxia leading to paralysis.
T R E A T M E N T: Poor response to copper supplementation.

PANTOTHENIC ACID. Rare. Hypermetria/goose stepping, progressing to posterior paralysis. Diarrhea and alopecia are also observed.
T R E A T M E N T: Calcium pantothenate, 0.5 mg/kg/day in the diet.

VITAMIN A. Seen in growing pigs. Signs include incoordination, head tilt, hindlimb paresis leading to paralysis. May be accompanied by skin changes and splitting of tips of bristles. Reproductive problems include stillborn or weak piglets; microphthalmia in piglets.
T R E A T M E N T: Supplementation of diet with vitamin A; parenteral injections of vitamin A in severe cases.

NIACIN/NICOTINIC ACID. Signs include anorexia, diarrhea, dermatitis, and posterior paralysis.
T R E A T M E N T: Supplementation of diet with nicotinic acid.

Toxicities

ORGANOPHOSPHATE POISONING. Signs include nystagmus, salivation, incoordination, and recumbency. Delayed onset of posterior paralysis has been reported 2–3 weeks after exposure. Associated with congenital tremors in newborns.
T R E A T M E N T: Administer atropine (0.05–0.50 mg/kg, i.m.); provide supportive care.

ARSENICALS. Used to prevent swine dysentery. Tremors, incoordination, paralysis, blindness, and death have been recorded. Toxicity appears to be associated with decreased water intake. Withdrawal of drug at onset of signs may resolve problem.
T R E A T M E N T: Generally unsatisfactory, especially in acute cases. Dimercaprol (4 mg/kg every 4–6 h initially) and sodium thiosulfate (20–30 g in 10% solution, p.o.) may be beneficial.

FURAZOLIDONE. Signs include ataxia, paresis, vomiting, and anorexia at high doses.

T R E A T M E N T: None specific; provide supportive care.

SELENIUM TOXICITY. Focal symmetric poliomyelomalacia. Has been associated with paralysis. Source is excessive dietary supplements or contaminated water.
T R E A T M E N T: None specific.

MERCURIALS. Fungicides in seed grain may contain mercury. Signs include blindness, ataxia, dysphagia, persistent walking, convulsions, and death.
T R E A T M E N T: None specific.

SALT POISONING/WATER DEPRIVATION
Acute Form. Ingestion of large amounts of salt causes gastroenteritis and neurologic signs, including prostration, blindness, head pressing, death.
Chronic Form. Sequel to decreased water intake on normal to high-salt diet. Sudden access to unlimited water supplies may precipitate signs, which include blindness, ataxia, head pressing, convulsions, and death.
T R E A T M E N T: Administer fluids. For choice of fluids, see Chapter 12.

Viral Diseases

POLIOENCEPHALOMYELITIS: TESCHEN/TALFAN DISEASE. (enterovirus) Severe form in central Europe (Teschen). Signs include fever, progressive ataxia, recumbency, death in 3–5 days. Mild form occurs in North America and Australia (Talfan). Fever, ataxia, paresis, "dog-sitting." Death is uncommon.
T R E A T M E N T: None specific. Provide supportive care.

PSEUDORABIES. (porcine herpesvirus)
Growing Pigs (3–5 months). Fever, anorexia, and depression may be followed by ataxia, muscle tremors, and convulsions. Deaths may occur, lower mortality than in neonatal infection. Respiratory disease may also be observed.
T R E A T M E N T: None specific.

Adult Pigs. Usually mild (inappetance) or subclinical. Central nervous system signs rare. Reproductive failure and agalactia often seen.
T R E A T M E N T: None specific.

HOG CHOLERA: SWINE FEVER. (pestivirus). Adult sows may abort in acute phase of disease. Fetal resorption may occur. Posterior ataxia has been seen in 4-month-old pigs born to sows infected with a low-virulence strain of the virus during gestation.

T R E A T M E N T: None specific.

AFRICAN SWINE FEVER. (iridovirus) Signs include fever, dullness, inappetance, blotching of skin, vomiting, diarrhea, respiratory distress, and coughing. Incoordination may be seen. High mortality rate.

T R E A T M E N T: None specific.

SWINE VESICULAR DISEASE. (picornavirus) Mild or unnoticed in adult sows. High herd incidence. Low mortality. Signs include fever; inappetance; lameness; and ulcers on coronary band, oral mucosa, snout, and occasionally skin. Resembles foot and mouth disease. Occasionally central nervous system signs are recorded, including ataxia, head pressing, paralysis.

T R E A T M E N T: None specific.

RABIES. Rare in pigs under modern management conditions. Signs include incoordination, salivation, twitching of snout, chewing movements, recumbency, and death. Signs vary widely.

T R E A T M E N T: Not advised. Brain tissue submitted for post-mortem diagnosis.

Bacterial Diseases

EDEMA DISEASE. (specific strains of *Escherichia coli*) Mainly seen postweaning. Vasculitis is the primary lesion; sudden death often is recognized initially. In other cases signs include dullness, blindness, incoordination; may result in recumbency and death. Edema of eyelids, snout, and larynx (with high-pitched vocalizations) can occur.

T R E A T M E N T: Provide supportive care; administer corticosteroids or nonsteroidal antiinflammatories.

CEREBROSPINAL ANGIOPATHY. (*Escherichia coli* [proposed]) Seen up to 5 weeks after weaning, occasionally in older pigs. Signs include depression, incoordination, aimless wandering, circling, and visual deficits; may lead to death.

T R E A T M E N T: None specific.

Bacterial Meningoencephalitis

***STREPTOCOCCUS SUIS* TYPE 2.** Meningitis in pigs from 3 weeks to 3 months. Occasionally in older pigs.

T R E A T M E N T: Provide supportive care; administer parenteral penicillin and corticosteroids.

GLASSER'S DISEASE. *(Haemophilus parasuis)* Polyarthritis, polyserositis, and meningitis in pigs 2–16 weeks old.
T R E A T M E N T: Adminster broad-spectrum antibiotics and corticosteroids.

MIDDLE EAR DISEASE. *(Actinomyces pyogenes* and *Pasteurella Streptococcal* spp.)
T R E A T M E N T: Broad-spectrum antibiotics with a short course of corticosteroids may be beneficial.

EPIDURAL ABSCESSES. Tail biting is commonly associated with abscess formation in the epidural tissues, resulting in signs of posterior paresis/paralysis.
T R E A T M E N T: Broad-spectrum antibiotics may be administered, although response is usually poor.

LEPTOSPIROSIS. The acute phase of infection *(Leptospira icterohaemorrhagiae* or *L. canicola)* occasionally produces neurologic signs.
T R E A T M E N T: Administer streptomycin, dihydrostreptomycin, or oxytetracycline parenterally.

Miscellaneous Conditions

HEAT STROKE. Stress or transport in warm conditions may lead to hyperthermia, convulsions, coma.
T R E A T M E N T: Implement cold hosing. Administer corticosteroids, nonsteroidal antiinflammatory drugs. Provide supportive care.

TRAUMA. Signs reflect the degree of trauma. External signs of bruising or lacerations may be evident.
T R E A T M E N T: Provide supportive care and appropriate wound management.

BRAIN ABSCESSATION. Abscesses in the brain may cause blindness, circling, depression, opisthotonus, convulsions, death.
T R E A T M E N T: Poor response to antibiotics.

TETANUS. *(Clostridium tetani)* Occasionally seen in postweaning pigs, usually following castration or umbilical infections. Signs include progressive stiffness of the muscles, with erect ears, and later recumbency and death.
T R E A T M E N T: Give antitoxin and penicillin. Perform wound debridement. Provide supportive care.

NEUROLOGIC DISEASES OF NEW WORLD CAMELIDS

Parasitic Diseases

PARASITE MIGRATION. (*Parelaphostrongylus tenuis*, the meningeal worm of white-tailed deer) Migration in camelids may cause neurologic disease involving spinal cord or brain. Paralysis is common.

T R E A T M E N T: Administer corticosteroids and ivermectin.

TICK PARALYSIS. Neurotoxin injected by engorging tick leads to paralysis and death. Ticks often located in axillary region. Recovery usually follows their removal.

T R E A T M E N T: None specific.

Infectious Diseases

BACTERIAL MENINGITIS. Septicemia in the neonatal period, predisposed to by hypothermia, hypoglycemia, and failure of passive antibody transfer. May lead to meningitis. Signs include fever, anorexia, depression; later neck stiffness, seizures, death.

T R E A T M E N T: Administer broad-spectrum antibiotics and corticosteroids; provide supportive care.

LISTERIOSIS. (*Listeria monocytogenes*) Infection leads to inflammation of brainstem. Signs include unilateral facial paralysis (ear droop, ptosis of eyelid, nostril paralysis), drooling, and circling.

T R E A T M E N T: Administer antibiotics (e.g., penicillin, tetracyclines) and corticosteroids (in early phase).

RABIES. (rhabdovirus) Diffuse encephalitis and a variety of clinical signs occur.

T R E A T M E N T: Not advised. Brain submitted for postmortem confirmation of diagnosis.

EQUINE HERPESVIRUS TYPE 1. North American outbreaks have been attributed to contact with zebras. Encephalitis may be a feature. Blindness, head tilt, ataxia are common findings.

T R E A T M E N T: Provide supportive care; give dimethylsulfoxide (1 g/kg i.v. in 5% solution) and dexamethasone.

COCCIDIOIDOMYCOSIS. (*Coccidioides immitis*) Endemic areas include arid areas of the west and southwest USA. Mainly disease of respiratory tract, but in disseminated form may cause meningitis, osteomyelitis, granuloma formation throughout the body including spinal cord. Skin form also occurs.

T R E A T M E N T: None successful.

Bacterial Toxins

TETANUS. *(Clostridium tetani)* Signs include initial hyperesthesia, followed by recumbency and continuous extensor spasm. Death may follow due to respiratory arrest. Associated with deep wounds.

T R E A T M E N T: Administer parenteral antitoxin, tetanus toxoid, and penicillin. Provide supportive care.

BOTULISM. *(Clostridium botulinum)* Main feature is onset of skeletal muscle paralysis, including dysphagia, ataxia, and respiratory paralysis, followed by death. Prognosis is guarded.

T R E A T M E N T: Provide supportive care. Give antitoxin if available.

ENTEROTOXEMIA. *(Clostridium perfringens* types A, C, and D) Associated with sudden death, or often preceded by depression, convulsions.

T R E A T M E N T: None specific.

Miscellaneous Conditions

BRAIN ABSCESS. Signs depend on location of abscess.

T R E A T M E N T: Poor response to antibiotic therapy.

FOXTAIL PENETRATION. Penetration of ear canal, nostril, or ocular region and tracking of plant awn to cranium may cause neurologic signs.

T R E A T M E N T: May be possible to remove awn in some instances.

TOXIC PLANTS. E.g., rhododendron, ragwort, black laurel, yew. Regional differences should be considered.

T R E A T M E N T: Provide supportive care.

TRAUMA. May cause neurologic signs, depending on area of brain or cord affected.

T R E A T M E N T: Administer antiinflammatories; provide supportive care.

TUMORS. Signs depend on the location of the lesion.

T R E A T M E N T: Usually not undertaken.

Hematopoietic System

ANEMIA

Anemia is a decrease in the total number of red blood cells and/or the hemoglobin concentration. Anemia usually occurs secondary to systemic disease.

Morphologic Classification

Macrocytic Anemia

In macrocytic anemia, mean corpuscular volume is increased.

A *transitory* macrocytic anemia occurs in response to acute loss of red cells through hemorrhage or hemolysis.

True *macrocytic anemia* occurs when the final stage of red blood cell maturation is bypassed, resulting in the release of large immature corpuscles. True macrocytic anemia is associated with vitamin B_{12} and folic acid deficiency.

Normocytic Anemia

Normocytic anemia is associated with chronic disease and depression of erythrocyte production. If chronic disease persists, cells may become microcytic.

Microcytic Hypochromic Anemia

Deficiency of iron or the body's inability to use it results in microcytic hypochromic anemia.

Etiologic Classification

Blood Loss Anemias

ACUTE BLOOD LOSS ANEMIA. Can be caused by the following:

1. Trauma, e.g., intra- or postoperative hemorrhage, collision with obstacles, or injuries sustained during fighting.
2. Gastric/abomasal ulcers or acute coccidiosis (especially in goats).
3. Umbilical hemorrhage in neonates, especially piglets.
4. Poisoning, e.g., coumarins (warfarin or sweet clover) or bracken fern toxicity.
5. Ruptured aneurysm, e.g., guttural pouch mycosis or cranial mesenteric artery aneurysm.
6. Neoplasms, e.g., ovarian tumors in horses.
7. Consumptive coagulopathies, e.g., disseminated intravascular coagulation or thrombocytopenic purpura.

CHRONIC BLOOD LOSS ANEMIA. Can be caused by the following:

1. Gastrointestinal ulcers.
2. Parasitism, e.g., ectoparasites—bloodsucking lice, ticks, and sheep keds *(Melophagus ovinus)*—or endoparasites—*Haemonchus contortus* and *Bunostomum* spp.

3. Coagulation disorders (rare).

Hemolytic Anemias

INTRAVASCULAR HEMOLYTIC ANEMIA. Can be caused by the following:

1. Babesiosis—cattle, horses.
2. *Clostridium perfringens* type A—sheep and cattle. *Cl. novyi* type D (bacillary hemoglobinuria)—cattle.
3. Acute leptospirosis—pigs, cattle, and sheep.
4. Chronic copper poisoning—especially sheep.
5. Postparturient hemoglobinuria—cows.
6. *Brassica* spp. and *Allium* sp. (onion).
7. *Mercurialis* spp. poisoning—sheep and cattle.
8. Water intoxication–calves.
9. Immune-mediated hemolytic anemia.
10. Snake venom poisoning.
11. Transfusion or drug reactions.

EXTRAVASCULAR HEMOLYTIC ANEMIA. Can be caused by the following:

1. Equine infectious anemia.
2. Eperythrozoonosis—cattle.
3. Anaplasmosis—cattle.
4. Isoerythrolysis of newborn—mainly foals and calves.
5. Autoimmune hemolytic anemia—rare.

Anemia Caused by Impaired Erythropoiesis

Impaired erythropoiesis can be caused by the following:

1. Chronic infectious disease.
2. Parasitism with nonbloodsucking parasites.
3. Nutritional imbalances, e.g., vitamin B_{12}, folate, cobalt, and copper deficiencies or molybdenum excess.
4. Toxins, e.g., chloramphenicol or chronic lead poisoning.
5. Miscellaneous causes, including neoplasia and chronic nephritis.
6. Bracken fern toxicity.

Regenerative Anemia

Reticulocytosis does not occur in the horse, but in ruminants it indicates red cell regeneration. In some cases in the horse, bone marrow regeneration may be indicated by an increase in the mean cell volume (MCV). Sequential measurement of the packed cell volume

(PCV) is a simple and practical way to measure the bone marrow response. Examination of bone marrow will aid in the evaluation of cases of nonregenerative anemia. The actual reticulocyte count is corrected for the magnitude of the anemia in one of two ways:

1. Absolute reticulocyte count = % Reticulocytes × Actual RBC number

2. Corrected % reticulocytes = % Reticulocytes × $\dfrac{\text{Actual PCV}}{\text{Normal PCV}}$

POLYCYTHEMIA (INCREASED HEMATOCRIT)

Primary polycythemia is very rare in large animals. Relative polycythemia may result from dehydration or splenic contraction in the horse in association with exercise. A compensatory polycythemia may occur in hypoxic conditions—e.g., in cardiac disease, at high altitudes, and in an animal with renal neoplasms that increase erythropoietin production.

NEUTROPHILIA

Neutrophilia is an increase in the number of neutrophils circulating in the blood due to a shift from the marginal neutrophil pool or increased production/release from bone marrow.

Etiologic Classification

1. Physiologic neutrophilia—transient and catecholamine induced. Physiologic neutrophilia is a consequence of mobilization of the marginal neutrophil pool. It is accompanied by lymphocytosis. There is no associated left shift.
2. Steroid-induced neutrophilia—exogenous administration or endogenous release of corticosteroids causes neutrophilia, lymphopenia, monocytosis, and eosinopenia. Neutrophilia is due to influx from the marginal pool to the circulating pool and decreased extravasation. Usually there is no left shift.
3. Responsive neutrophilia—due to influx of neutrophils from the marginal pool and bone marrow in response to stimuli, e.g., infection, neoplasia, or tissue necrosis. There may be an accompanying increase in circulating immature (band) neutrophils.

Specific Causes

1. Infectious disease—localized or generalized.
2. Neoplasia.

3. Increased corticosteroid concentrations (e.g., from Cushing's disease, stress, or exogenous administration).

4. Chemical toxicity.

5. Uremia.

6. Surgery.

7. Acute blood loss.

NEUTROPENIA

Neutropenia is a decrease in the number of circulating neutrophils to below the normal range. A left shift may sometimes be present.

Causes of neutropenia include

1. Increased consumption or destruction, e.g., overwhelming infection.

2. Decreased production as a result of some diseases (e.g., aplastic anemia) and certain drugs (e.g., sulfonamides, chloramphenicol, and phenylbutazone). No left shift occurs.

3. Sequestration, e.g., endotoxemia.

4. Immune mediated (rare).

LEFT SHIFT

A left shift may occur with neutrophilia or neutropenia. A left shift is an increase in the number of circulating immature (band) neutrophils. The left shift may be regenerative or degenerative. If it is *regenerative*, there is an increased total white cell count, with mature neutrophils outnumbering immature forms. If the left shift is *degenerative*, the total white cell count is normal or decreased, but there is a great increase in the number of immature cells, so that immature cells exceed mature neutrophils.

EOSINOPHILIA

Eosinophilia is an increase in the absolute number of eosinophils so that the number is above the normal range. Causes include

1. Parasitism—especially where migration through the tissues is occurring.

2. Allergic disorders, e.g., allergic dermatitis, certain tumors, and eosinophilic enteritis and dermatitis of horses.

EOSINOPENIA

Eosinopenia is a decrease in the absolute number of eosinophils so that the number is below the normal range. Eosinopenia may be

1. Physiologic—catecholamine induced.
2. Steroid induced—exogenous, due to corticosteroid administration, or endogenous, e.g., pituitary adenoma and secondary hyperadrenocorticism in the horse.

Periodic absence of eosinophils from the leukogram does not necessarily represent an abnormality.

MONOCYTOSIS

Monocytosis is an increase in the number of monocytes so that it is above the normal range. Causes include

1. Necrosis of tissue.
2. Chronic inflammation, e.g., abdominal abscessation.
3. Malignancy.
4. Stress.

Monocytosis is commonly associated with infection with intracellular organisms, e.g., brucellosis and chronic fungal infections.

LYMPHOCYTOSIS

Lymphocytosis is an increase in total lymphocyte count so that it is above the normal range. Lymphocyte counts are rather unreliable as diagnostic tools, because they do not necessarily reflect changes in the rate of their recirculation, synthesis, release, and destruction.
Causes of lymphocytosis include

1. Youth (lymphocytosis is a normal finding in young animals).
2. Leukemia (lymphocytic or lymphoblastic), e.g., bovine leukosis.
3. Autoimmune disease (rare).

LYMPHOPENIA

Lymphopenia is a decrease in absolute lymphocyte numbers. It may be caused by

1. Glucocorticoid (endogenous or exogenous excess).

2. Lymphocyte loss, e.g., lymphangectasia (rare).

3. Viral infection—early stages.

4. Impaired lymphopoiesis, e.g., prolonged glucocorticoid therapy, immunodeficiency in Arabian foals.

THROMBOCYTOPENIA

Thrombocytopenia is a decrease in thrombocyte numbers to below the normal range. It may occur as a result of either decreased production or increased consumption.

The cause of decreased production is bone marrow depression caused by

1. Drugs, e.g., phenylbutazone, chronic furazolidone poisoning in calves, certain chemotherapeutic agents, estrogens, and chemical toxins (e.g., in trichloroethylene-extracted soybean meal).

2. Infectious agents, e.g., *Ehrlichia equi* and African swine fever virus.

3. Immune disease.

4. Ionizing radiation.

5. Toxic plants (e.g., bracken fern).

6. Idiopathy.

The causes of increased consumption are as follows:

1. Hemorrhage.

2. Thrombus formation secondary to vascular damage, localized or disseminated.

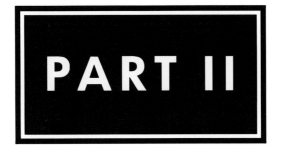

MISCELLANEOUS

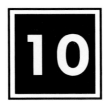

Sudden Death

"Conscientious and careful physicians allocate causes of disease to natural laws, while the ablest men of science go back to medicine for their first principles."

Aristotle

HORSES

Cardiovascular System

Vessel Rupture

Bronchial Artery. Exercise-induced pulmonary hemorrhage.
Parasite-Induced Aneurysms
Aortic Ring Rupture. Aged stallions.
Pulmonary Artery
Coronary Vein
Middle Uterine Artery. Pregnant mares.
Hepatic Portal Vein
Internal Iliac Artery

Occlusive Lesions

Verminous Arteritis. Coronary artery embolism.
Pulmonary Thromboembolism

Diseases of the Heart Valves

Rupture of Mitral Chordae Tendineae

Diseases of the Myocardium

Monensin Poisoning
Yew Poisoning. Taxine causes severe bradycardia.

Arrhythmias. E.g., ventricular fibrillation.

Gastrointestinal System

Gastric or Intestinal Rupture

Ulceration
Distension
Ischemia
Infarction

Intraluminal Obstructions

Enteroliths
Fecoliths
Phytobezoar
Foreign Bodies
Neoplasia

Extraluminal Obstructions

Volvulus
Strangulating Lipoma
Herniation. Inguinal, scrotal, or ventral.

Peracute Enterocolitis

Salmonellosis
Clostridiosis
Blister Beetle Toxicity
Heavy Metal Toxicity

Respiratory System

Exercise-Induced Pulmonary Hemorrhage

Common disease, but rarely fatal.

Neurologic System

Trauma

Fractures of the base of the skull

Leukoencephalomalacia

Moldy Corn Poisoning (Fusarium moniliforme)

Cerebrovascular Accident

  Rare

Infectious Diseases

Septicemia. Especially neonates.
Clostridial Colitis
Clostridial Myositis
Salmonellosis
Anthrax
Tyzzer's Disease. Affects neonates.

Toxins

Heavy Metals

Lead
Arsenic

Molds

  Especially moldy corn

Plants

Yew
Water Dropwort
Poison and Water Hemlock
Black Nightshade
Choke Cherry
Blue Green Algae

Blister Beetle Toxicity

Cantharidin

Drugs, Insect Bites, and Snake Bites

Acute anaphylaxis or localized swelling result.

Trauma

Falling Over Backward. Resultant damage to brainstem.
Fractures of Cervical Vertebrae. Collision with fixed objects, e.g.,
  fences and walls.

Impalement Injuries. Leading to pneumothorax, diaphragmatic hernia, or vessel rupture.

Miscellaneous

Electrocution

Lightning
Fallen Power Lines

Iatrogenic Causes

Intracarotid Injections
Accidental Administration of Water or Medication into the Lungs

Malice

Gunshot Wounds
Insulin Overdose
Potassium Chloride Overdose

CATTLE

Cardiovascular System

Vitamin E/Selenium Deficiency
Ionophore Poisoning. Cardiac and skeletal muscle lesions.
Copper Deficiency. Myocardial lesions.
Clostridial Myositis. *Clostridium chauvoei, C. septicum*, etc.
Vessel Rupture
1. **Vena Caval Syndrome.** Thrombosis of posterior vena cava, leading to pulmonary thromboembolism; acute hemorrhage from pulmonary arterial aneurysm (secondary to hypertension), leading to death.
2. **Rupture of Uterine Artery.** Usually associated with parturition.
Acute Cardiac Tamponade. Resulting from coronary artery trauma, e.g., penetrating reticular foreign body.
Acute Anemia. Bacillary hemoglobinuria (*C. novyi* type D), babesiosis, postparturient hemoglobinuria.

Gastrointestinal System

Primary Bloat. Free gas or frothy bloat.
Secondary Bloat. Choke, tetanus, reticular obstruction, acute ruminal acidosis.
Perforating Abomasal Ulcer

Abomasal Torsion or Volvulus
Intestinal Volvulus
Cecal Torsion or Volvulus
Torsion at Root of Mesentery
Strangulated Umbilical or Inguinal Hernia
Peracute Diarrhea. *Escherichia coli* and *Clostridium perfringens* in calves, salmonellosis, heavy metals.
Acute Diffuse Peritonitis

Respiratory System

Acute Pasteurellosis
Acute *Haemophilus somnus* Infection
Vena Caval Thrombosis

Neurologic System

Haemophilus somnus Septicemia
Aujeszky's Disease. Pseudorabies.
Lead Poisoning
Acute Bacterial Meningitis. Calves.
Hypomagnesemia. Calves and adults.

Infectious Diseases

Septicemia. Especially in neonates.
Blackleg. (*Clostridium chauvoei*)
Malignant Edema. (*C. septicum*)
Black Disease. (*C. novyi* type B)
Anthrax. (*Bacillus anthracis*)
Coliform Mastitis
Acute Staphylococcal Mastitis

Toxins

Heavy Metals

Lead
Arsenic
Mercury
Cadmium

Plants

Canary Grass. (*Phalaris* spp.)
Cyanogenetic Glycoside-Containing Plants

Brassica **spp.** Rape and kale.
Nitrate-Containing Plants. Leading to nitrite poisoning.
Water Dropwort
Water Hemlock
Poison Hemlock
Andromedotoxin. Rhododendron and mountain laurel.
Oleander, *Acacea* **spp., and yew**
Blue-Green Algae

Other Chemicals

Urea. As feed additive.
Manure Gases. In slatted floor systems.
Metaldehyde. Slug bait.
Snake Venom

Miscellaneous

Hypocalcemia
Lightning or Other Electrocutions
Trauma
Iatrogenic. E.g., rapid i.v. administration of calcium.

SHEEP AND GOATS

Cardiovascular System

Vitamin E/Selenium Deficiency

May cause cardiac muscle changes.

Vessel Rupture

E.g., uterine artery. Occurs during lambing/kidding.

Acute Anemia

Haemonchosis. Especially in young animals.
Coccidiosis. Especially kids.
Babesiosis
Copper Poisoning

Gastrointestinal System

Primary Bloat. Free gas or frothy bloat.
Secondary Bloat. E.g., choke or obstruction of reticulum or esophagus.

Braxy. (*Clostridium septicum*)
Intestinal Accidents. Rare in small ruminants.
Peracute Enteritis. *C. perfringens* types B, C, and D; salmonellosis (all
ages); *Escherichia coli* (lambs, kids); heavy metals.
Grain Overload

Respiratory System

Acute Pasteurellosis. More common in sheep than goats; *Pasteurella
haemolytica* most common cause.

Neurologic System

Aujeszky's Disease. Animals housed adjacent to pigs.
Hypomagnesemia
Septic Meningitis Secondary to Septicemia. Neonates.

Infectious Diseases

Septicemic Pasteurellosis. Mainly sheep.
Haemophilus agni. Young lambs.
***Clostridium perfringens* types B, C, and D**
Black Disease. (*C. novyi* type B)
Bacillary Hemoglobinuria. (*C. novyi* type D)
Clostridial Myositis
Anthrax
Acute Staphylococcal Mastitis
Aujeszky's Disease (Pseudorabies)

Toxins

Heavy Metals. E.g., lead, arsenic.
Toxic Plants. E.g., yew, rhododendron, cyanogenetic plants, *Acacea*
spp.

Miscellaneous

Trauma
Worrying. By dogs, other predators.

PIGS

Cardiovascular System

Mulberry Heart Disease. Vitamin E/selenium deficiency.
Endocarditis. *Erysipelothrix rhusiopathiae.*

Electrocution. Naked wires, lightning.
Encephalomyocarditis. Picornavirus.
Monensin Poisoning. Cardiac and skeletal muscle lesions.

Gastrointestinal System

Intestinal Hemorrhage. (*Campylobacter sputorum*).
Enterotoxemia. (*Clostridium perfringens* type C)—piglets.
Colibacillosis. (*Escherichia coli* K88)—piglets.
Swine Fever/African Swine Fever
Salmonellosis. Weaned pigs.
Transmissible Gastroenteritis. (coronavirus)—piglets.
Foot and Mouth Disease. Piglets.
Bowel Edema. (*E. coli*, usually postweaning).
Anthrax. An intestinal form is recognized in pigs.
Intestinal Accidents. Strangulated inguinal hernias.
Gastric Ulcers
Whey Bloat or Gastric Torsion. Usually adults.

Respiratory System

Acute Pasteurellosis
Acute Pleuropneumonia. (*Actinobacillus* spp., *Haemophilus pleuropneumoniae*)

Neurologic System

Septic Meningitis. *Streptococcus suis* types 1 and 2, in neonatal and weaned pigs; *Haemophilus parasuis* in young pigs.
Pseudorabies Encephalitis. Primarily young pigs.
Cytomegalovirus Encephalitis
Bowel Edema. *Escherichia coli*—mainly postweaning.
Hypoglycemia. Neonates.
Trauma

Musculoskeletal System

Malignant Hyperthermia/Porcine Stress Syndrome
Vitamin E/Selenium Deficiency
Clostridial Myositis
Monensin Poisoning. Cardiac and skeletal muscle lesions.

Toxins

Heavy Metals. Arsenicals, etc.
Nitrate Poisoning. Methemoglobinemia.

Gassing with Slurry Fumes. Hydrogen sulfide, sulfur dioxide.
Carbon Monoxide. Gas heaters.

Miscellaneous

Crushing. Piglets.
Cannibalism. Piglets.
Fighting. Often follows mixing of litters; deaths may occur.
Heat Stroke
Navel Bleeding. Isolated occurrence.
Thrombocytopenic Purpura. Sporadic.
Prolapse of Uterus
Septic Metritis/Mastitis

NEW WORLD CAMELIDS

The causes of sudden death in New World Camelids are poorly documented. However, the following conditions have been implicated in cases of sudden death in New World Camelids.

Septicemia. Especially neonates.
Acute Enteritis. E.g., salmonellosis.
Clostridial Myositis
Encephalomyocarditis. Picornavirus.
Trauma
Vitamin E/Selenium Deficiency. Cardiac form.
Gastric Ulcers. Peritonitis.
Intestinal Accidents
Congenital Cardiac Disease. Common.
Heavy Metals
Toxic Plants. Yew, poison hemlock, oleander, rhododendron, mountain laurel.

DIAGNOSTIC PROCEDURES IN THE INVESTIGATION OF SUDDEN DEATH

1. A complete history of the animal(s) and, if applicable, of the herd is essential. All items submitted for analysis should be appropriately labeled.

2. The environment should be examined for potentially harmful or toxic agents.

3. Before conducting a necropsy, the carcass and the area around it should be closely examined. Necrospy or removal of the animal

from the premises is not advised if there is reason to suspect a reportable disease (e.g., anthrax).

4. If possible, the whole carcass should be submitted for necropsy, preferably fresh or chilled, but not frozen. Tissues and other samples should be chilled; formalinized tissue specimens should also be submitted.

5. If poisoning is suspected, samples of whole blood, urine, gastrointestinal contents, liver, and kidney should be collected. Other tissues that might also be useful include hair, hoof, fat, and bone.

6. Samples of feed, water, and other materials such as weeds or chemicals to which the animal had access should also be included.

7. If infectious disease is suspected, appropriate samples should be submitted for culture and/or identification.

8. Clean glass or plastic containers, preferably wide necked, are ideal for specimen submission. Care should be taken to avoid contamination with debris.

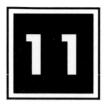

Chronic Weight Loss, Poor Athletic Performance in Horses, and Poor Production in Pigs

CHRONIC WEIGHT LOSS

Weight loss may occur for many reasons. In general, the causes are starvation; inability to prehend, chew, or swallow; failure of the mechanisms of digestion, absorption, and assimilation; and systemic disease, e.g., renal or hepatic failure.

Horses

DIETARY ABNORMALITIES. Inadequate quality or quantity of feed.
DYSPHAGIA
Poor Dentition. Occurs especially in aged horses.
Stomatitis and Glossitis. Caused by ingestion of caustic substances or trauma from the bit or foreign bodies.
Neurologic Disease. Peripheral or central damage to cranial nerves 5, 7, 9, 10, or 12, e.g., protozoal myelitis, trauma, guttural pouch mycosis, or lead poisoning.
Trauma. Fracture of mandible or hyoid apparatus, or trauma to soft tissue.
DIGESTIVE AND ABSORPTIVE ABNORMALITIES
Chronic Gastritis/Gastric Ulceration. May be accompanied by anemia or chronic colic. Associated with prolonged administration of nonsteroidal antiinflammatory drugs or bot infection.
Infiltrative Bowel Disease. Includes lymphosarcoma, granulomatous enteritis, lymphocytic-plasmacytic enteritis, eosinophilic gastroenteritis, basophilic enteritis, and intestinal tuberculosis.
Parasitism. (*Parascaris equorum* in foals and yearlings. Heavy *Strongylus* spp. infections in adults.) Diarrhea due to cyathostomiasis in late winter/early spring. Heavy ectoparasite burden.
Phenylbutazone Toxicity. Gastrointestinal, renal, and bone marrow abnormalities are encountered. Hypoproteinemia is a common finding, caused by extensive colonic ulceration.
Chronic Diarrhea. Many potential causes, e.g., infiltrative disease and chronic parasitism. Many causes are idiopathic.
Liver Disease. Includes chronic hepatitis and cirrhosis (due to pyrrolizidine alkaloid ingestion).
Neoplasia. Lymphosarcoma, mainly in young horses. Gastric squamous cell carcinoma in older horses.
Miscellaneous. Adhesions of abdominal viscera.
CHRONIC RESPIRATORY DISEASE. Includes pneumonia with or without pleuritis; pulmonary abscessation.
RENAL DISEASE. Includes chronic renal failure; protein-losing nephropathies, e.g., glomerulonephritis (equine infectious anemia, purpura hemorrhagica) and amyloidosis; abscessation; and neoplasia.
INFECTIOUS DISEASE. Includes equine infectious anemia, bastard

strangles, systemic fungal infections, and chronic enteric salmonellosis.

HYPERADRENOCORTICISM. Common in older horses.

If a detailed physical examination fails to elucidate a cause for the chronic weight loss, some of the following tests may be indicated.

- Complete blood count
- Serum chemistry profile
- Fecal flotation
- Urinalysis
- Examination of abdominal viscera per rectum
- Agar gel immunodiffusion (AGID) test for equine infectious anemia
- Abdominal paracentesis
- Diagnostic imaging (thorax particularly)
- Thoracocentesis
- Gastroscopy
- Absorption tests (xylose/glucose)
- Liver biopsy
- Rectal mucosal biopsy
- Exploratory laparotomy

Cattle

DIETARY ABNORMALITIES. Inadequate quality or quantity of feed. Trace element deficiency, e.g., copper, cobalt.

DYSPHAGIA

Poor Dentition. Associated with fibrous diets, trauma, and fluorosis.

Stomatitis. Caused by foreign bodies, irritant or caustic substances, and infectious agents, e.g., viral stomatitis, mucosal disease, malignant catarrhal fever, and oral necrobacillosis.

Glossitis. Caused by foreign bodies, infectious agents, e.g., *Actinobacillus lignieresi* (wooden tongue), and ulcerative glossitis (mucosal disease and foot and mouth disease).

Neurologic Disease. Peripheral or central, damage to cranial nerves 5, 7, 9, 10, and 12.

Trauma. Fracture of mandible or hyoid apparatus.

Miscellaneous. Lumpy jaw *(Actinomyces bovis)*, in which dental loss or malocclusion has occurred.

DIGESTIVE AND ABSORPTIVE ABNORMALITIES

Chronic Reticuloperitonitis. May be associated with a foreign body.

Rumenitis. Usually a sequel to grain overload.

Chronic Bloat. Can be caused by mechanical obstruction of cardia with foreign body, ileus or vagus nerve damage, neoplasia, actinobacillosis, or actinomycosis of reticular wall.

Vagal Indigestion. Leads to chronic abdominal distension. Results in inappetence and weight loss.

Lymphosarcoma. Abomasal wall is commonly involved.

Abdominal Abscessation. May occur at any site; commonly involves the liver.

Abomasal Displacement. Uncorrected displacement may lead to weight loss.

Abomasal Ulceration. Common. Associated especially with high-producing cows.

Infiltrative Bowel Disease. Includes Johne's disease (*Mycobacterium johnei*), intestinal tuberculosis, and neoplasia.

Parasitism. Includes ostertagiasis types 1 and 2 and liver fluke (*Fasciola* spp.) infection.

Chronic Diarrhea. Caused by chronic mucosal disease, Johne's disease (*Mycobacterium johnei*), chronic salmonellosis, hepatic fibrosis (pyrrolizidine alkaloids), or copper deficiency/molybdenosis.

Liver Disease. Caused by hepatic lipidosis, pyrrolizidine alkaloid-induced fibrosis, hepatic abscessation, or vena caval thrombosis.

RENAL DISEASE. Includes pyelonephritis (*Corynebacterium renale* and *Escherichia coli*), renal failure, and renal amyloidosis.

NEOPLASIA. E.g., bovine leukosis; thymoma in calves.

RESPIRATORY DISEASE. Includes chronic pneumonia, vena caval syndrome, chronic pasteurellosis, and lungworm (*Dictyocaulus viviparus*) infection.

MUSCULOSKELETAL DISEASE. Includes laminitis, foot abscessation, septic pedal arthritis, vitamin E/selenium deficiency, and sarcocystosis.

MASTITIS. Chronic abscessation with *Staphylococcus aureus* or *Actinomyces pyogenes*.

BLINDNESS. Variety of causes, e.g., severe keratitis due to *Moraxella bovis*. Central causes include congenital hydrocephalus and pituitary abscessation.

CARDIOVASCULAR DISEASE

Endocarditis. Valvular disease; *Actinomyces pyogenes* and *Escherichia coli* are frequently isolated.

Pericarditis. Septic effusion results from pericardial penetration by wire in reticulum. Causes cardiac tamponade.

ANEMIA

Chronic Hemorrhage. Caused by abomasal ulcers or parasitism (e.g., lice infestation).

Bone Marrow Depression. E.g., bracken poisoning.

Nutritional Deficiency. Includes copper or cobalt deficiency, iron deficiency in calves, poor nutrition in general.

BEHAVIORAL ABNORMALITIES. Include increased sexual activity and bullying.

Small Ruminants

DIETARY ABNORMALITIES. Inadequate quantity or quality of feed, especially inadequate trough space. Trace element deficiency, especially cobalt or copper.

DYSPHAGIA

Poor Dentition. Occurs especially in older animals on fibrous feeds or root crops.

Stomatitis. Caused by foreign bodies, caustic substances, dental points, chronic bluetongue infection (orbivirus), and orf (parapox virus).

Glossitis. Caused by foreign bodies. Relatively uncommon in small ruminants.

TRAUMA. Includes fracture of mandible or teeth and damage to soft tissue structures of mouth and pharynx.

DIGESTIVE AND ABSORPTIVE ABNORMALITIES

Rumenitis. May be sequel to grain overload.

Infiltrative Bowel Disease. Johne's disease (*Mycobacterium johnei*), usually not associated with diarrhea.

Parasitism. Usually caused by HOT (*Haemonchus contortus*, *Ostertagia* spp., and *Trichostrongylus* spp.) complex. Common. Esophagostomiasis or fascioliasis may be involved.

Chronic Diarrhea. Caused by parasitism (e.g., *Ostertagia* spp.), chronic coccidiosis, cobalt deficiency, or chronic salmonellosis.

Abomasal Emptying Defect. Occurs in sheep only, Suffolk breed primarily. Abdominal enlargement may be evident. Rumen chloride is increased.

LIVER DISEASE. Caused by liver abscessation (e.g., *Corynebacterium pseudotuberculosis*) or liver fluke (*Fasciola* spp.) infection.

RENAL DISEASE. Chronic renal failure due to ingestion of toxic plants (e.g., oak or oxalate-containing plants). An inherited membranous glomerulonephritis occurs in Finnish Landrace sheep.

INTERNAL ABSCESSATION. Thoracic or abdominal abscessation, usually caused by *Corynebacterium pseudotuberculosis*.

RESPIRATORY DISEASE. Includes chronic *Pasteurella* pneumonia, ovine progressive pneumonia (maedi), pulmonary adenomatosis (sheep only), caprine arthritis and encephalitis (pulmonary form), lung abscesses (e.g., caseous lymphadenitis), parasites (e.g., *Dictyocaulus filaria* and *Protostrongylus* spp.), and enzootic pneumonia.

MUSCULOSKELETAL DISEASE. Includes caprine arthritis and encephalitis in adult goats, foot rot, and other lamenesses.

MASTITIS. Chronic mastitis with mammary abscessation.

ANEMIA. Caused by parasitism, e.g., HOT complex (see Digestive and Absorptive Abnormalities) and coccidiosis; cobalt or copper deficiency; poor nutrition; or chronic systemic disease.

BEHAVIORAL ABNORMALITIES. Include scrapie in adult sheep and goats, blindness, increased sexual activity (especially males), and bullying.

ECTOPARASITISM. Includes lice, keds, and mange (especially *Psoroptes ovis*).

POOR ATHLETIC PERFORMANCE IN HORSES

Poor athletic performance in horses usually refers to either a decreased level of performance or failure to achieve an expected level of performance.

Musculoskeletal Disease

DEGENERATIVE JOINT DISEASE. Most common in fetlocks, hocks, and carpi. Usually a sequel to chronic, low-grade, traumatically induced arthritis or osteochondrosis dissecans.

ISCHEMIC BONE DISEASE. E.g., navicular disease. Usually occurs in older horses.

CHRONIC BONE STRESS. Includes sesamoiditis, splints, and bucked shins.

DESMITIS. Inflammation of ligamentous structures, e.g., suspensory ligament.

TENOSYNOVITIS AND TENDINITIS. E.g., inflammation of the superifical/deep flexor tendon sheath or tendon strain.

MUSCLE TEARS. Localized damage. May be difficult to locate on physical examination.

RHABDOMYOLYSIS. May occur during or after heavy exercise, endurance rides, etc.

Musculoskeletal diseases are the most common cause of poor athletic performance in horses. For more information on musculoskeletal diseases, see Chapter 6.

Respiratory Disease

UPPER AIRWAY DISEASE. Includes left (rarely right) recurrent laryngeal neuropathy, epiglottic entrapment, dorsal displacement of soft palate, ethmoidal hematoma, and nasal septum deviation.

LOWER AIRWAY DISEASE. Includes exercise-induced pulmonary hemorrhage, pneumonia, chronic pleuritis, pulmonary abscess, lungworms, and small airway disease.

Cardiac Disease

ARRHYTHMIAS. E.g., atrial fibrillation.

CONGENITAL CARDIAC DEFECTS. E.g., ventricular septal defect.

VALVULAR DISEASE. Acquired or congenital. Includes mitral valve insufficiency, aortic stenosis, and aortic valve insufficiency.

MYOCARDITIS. Associated with viral disease, e.g., influenza.

Miscellaneous

ANEMIA

ENDOCRINE. E.g., hyperadrenocorticism, hypoadrenocorticism, and thyroid disease.

NEUROLOGIC. Cervical vertebral malformation, degenerative myelopathy, or protozoal myelitis.

GENETIC. Animal is physiologically unable to perform as expected.

INADEQUATE TRAINING/CONDITIONING

INADEQUATE DIET

POOR PRODUCTION IN PIGS

The problem of poor production in pigs is best approached on an age/group basis and in terms of a herd or group problem, because many of the disease states are management related and thus affect many or all of the animals.

Production Targets

Production targets are listed in Table 11–1. These targets apply to intensive, well-managed swine facilities with controlled environments.

TABLE 11–1. PIG PRODUCTION TARGETS

Production Parameters	Production Target
1. Number of piglets born alive/litter	10–11
2. Number of piglets weaned/litter	9–10
3. Mortality up to weaning (overlying 4%, starvation 2%, congenital deformities 1%, enteritis 1%, other 2%)	<10%
4. Weight at birth	1.2–1.5 kg
5. Weight at weaning:	
21 days	5–6 kg
35 days	10 kg
6. Number of litters/sow/year	2.2–2.4
7. Number of piglets/sow/year	20–24
8. Weaning to service interval	6–10 days
9. Return to service	<10%
10. Days to slaughter	(60–65 kg) 125 days

Birth to Weaning Piglets

ENVIRONMENTAL FACTORS. Include low temperature, especially in a wet environment, and poor ventilation. Ideal temperature is 30° C (86° F).

MATERNAL FACTORS. Include agalactia, due to mastitis, hormonal imbalance, failure of milk let-down, ergotism, or obesity; poor mothering (especially gilts); or inadequate number of functioning teats.

DIARRHEA. (*Escherichia coli* and *Clostridium perfringens* type C) Chronic diarrhea leading to emaciation. Recovered cases of transmissible gastroenteritis.

NUTRITIONAL FACTORS. Include iron deficiency, which usually manifests at 3–4 weeks of age as anemia with tachypnea and poor growth rate. Also includes inadequate food intake, excessive number in litter, and low environmental temperature.

RESPIRATORY DISEASE. *Bordetella bronchiseptica* pneumonia in young pigs.

MUSCULOSKELETAL DISEASE

Neonatal Polyarthritis. (*Streptococcus suis* type I or *Actinobacillus suis*) Occurs at 0–2 weeks.

Other Polyarthritides. Include Glasser's disease (*Haemophilus suis*) and polyserositis (*Mycoplasma hyorhinis*).

Postweaning and Fattening Pigs

ENVIRONMENTAL FACTORS

Hypothermia. As piglets age, the optimum temperature for growth decreases.

Poor Ventilation

Immaturity at Weaning. If the pig is weaned earlier than 21 days, the immature intestine may be unable to cope with the change from a liquid to a solid diet.

Overcrowding

GASTROINTESTINAL DISEASE

Postweaning Diarrhea. (*Escherichia coli*)

Swine Dysentery. (*Treponema hyodysenteriae*)

Intestinal Spirochaetosis. (*Treponema* spp.)

Chronic Salmonellosis. (*Salmonella* spp.)

Transmissible Gastroenteritis. (coronavirus)

Porcine Intestinal Adenomatosis. (*Campylobacter sputorum*)

Porcine Epidemic Diarrhea. (etiology not fully described)

Parasitism. (*Esophagostomum* spp. and *Ascaris suum*)

Rectal Stricture. Secondary to rectal prolapse.

RESPIRATORY DISEASE

Atrophic Rhinitis. (*Bordetella bronchiseptica* and *Pasteurella multocida*) (synergistic infection).

Enzootic Pneumonia. (*Mycoplasma hyopneumoniae, Actinobacillus pleuropneumoniae, Pasteurella multocida*, and other pathogens).

Other Chronic Pneumonias. (*Actinobacillus pleuropneumoniae* and *Pasteurella multocida*).

Parasitism. (*Ascaris suum* and *Metastrongylus* spp.)

MUSCULOSKELETAL DISEASE

Arthritis. *Erysipelothrix rhusiopathiae, Mycoplasma hyosynoviae, M. hyorhinis, Streptococcus suis* type II.

Trauma. Can be caused by hard, rough floors.

NEUROLOGIC DISEASE. Spinal abscesses associated with tail biting; hindlimb paralysis is a feature.

NUTRITIONAL FACTORS. Iron deficiency may present postweaning. Failure to balance food ration appropriately may cause herdwide reduction in performance.

MYCOTOXINS. Include ochratoxin, vomitoxin, aflatoxin, ergot, and mycotoxic nephropathy.

MISCELLANEOUS

Behavioral Abnormalities. Include tail biting and bullying.

Weakness. E.g., warfarin poisoning.

Defective Watering Equipment. If water intake varies, pigs may become dehydrated.

Adult Pigs

Many of the causes of weight loss or poor performance in adult pigs are similar to those in postweaning and fattening pigs. However, the following conditions are more common in adults.

FLOORING. Hard or slippery floors may lead to severe foot problems and trauma to bony protuberances, etc.

FOOT PROBLEMS

Foot rot. Poor conditions underfoot, especially wet, dirty flooring, lead to foot abscessation and sole ulceration.

Laminitis. May be seen in sows before or soon after farrowing.

BACK PROBLEMS. Spondylosis usually affects older sows and boars.

CHRONIC MASTITIS. May contribute to weight loss if severe.

PYELONEPHRITIS/CYSTITIS. (*Eubacterium suis*) Signs include bloody urine, fever, and dysuria.

MYCOTOXINS. See Postweaning and Fattening Pigs.

REPRODUCTIVE FAILURE. Consultation of detailed texts on the subject of reproduction is advised.

NUTRITIONAL FACTORS. Failure to feed a balanced ration may lead to poor performance due to weight loss or excessive weight gain.

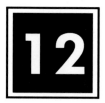

Fluid and Electrolyte Therapy

FLUID HOMEOSTASIS

Distribution of Body Fluids

Body Fluid Compartments

The body contains three fluid compartments—intracellular, interstitial, and intravascular. The interstitial and intravascular fluid, which together constitute the extracellular fluid (ECF), comprise approximately 40% of body fluid. The intracellular fluid (ICF) comprises approximately 60% of body fluid.

Figure 12–1 shows the relative volumes of these compartments in the average adult horse.

In the adult horse, approximately 60% of total body weight

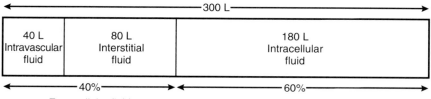

FIGURE 12–1. The relative volumes of fluid in the 500-kg horse's compartments.

consists of water. Thus, a 500-kg adult contains 300 kg (300 L) of water. In the neonate, a greater proportion (approximately 70%) of the total body weight is made up of water.

Fluid Shifts and Equilibration

Fluid movement between the intravascular and extravascular compartments is governed by Starling's equation:

$$\text{Net capillary filtration} = K[(P_{cap} - P_{int}) - \sigma(\pi_{cap} - \pi_{int})]$$

where

K	=	filtration coefficient
P_{cap}	=	capillary hydrostatic pressure (mm Hg)
P_{int}	=	interstitial hydrostatic pressure (mm Hg)
σ	=	oncotic reflection coefficient
π_{cap}	=	capillary oncotic pressure
π_{int}	=	interstitial oncotic pressure

For example, in congestive heart failure, capillary hydrostatic pressure (P_{cap}) may be sufficiently increased to cause interstitial edema. In hypoalbuminemia, the reduced capillary oncotic pressure (π_{cap}) may contribute to interstitial edema.

Clinical Assessment of Hydration Status

Changes in hydration status affect all three fluid compartments, but changes in the intravascular space are manifested acutely, whereas changes in intracellular and interstitial fluid develop more slowly. Therefore, the clinical methods used to evaluate hydration status are focused on the intravascular space and include measurements of heart and pulse rate, pulse quality, arterial pressure, urine output, and rectal temperature. Interstitial fluid content may be estimated by changes in skin turgor, dryness of mucous membranes, and thirst. Intracellular fluid changes are difficult to evaluate; however, changes in mentation may occur with abnormalities of ICF volume.

Clinical Signs of Dehydration

MILD DEHYDRATION (1–5%). Generally undetectable.

MODERATE DEHYDRATION (5–8%). Slight increase in capillary refill time. Moderate depression may be present. Eye is noticeably sunken. Skin is moderately inelastic. Heart rate possibly increased.

MARKED DEHYDRATION (8–12%). Signs of shock; pulse is weak and rapid, eye markedly sunken, extremities cold, tachycardia and depression present.

SEVERE DEHYDRATION (12–15%). Animal is recumbent; worsening status as described under marked dehydration. Death imminent.

Volume Replacement

Sources of fluid loss in the normal animal include urine, feces, and insensible losses via respiration and sweating.

Calculating Fluid Requirements

Maintenance requirements are usually calculated on the basis of body weight; however, because this relationship is not linear, a more accurate approach is to calculate the requirements based on the body surface area, which is determined according to the following formula:

$$\text{Surface area (m}^2) = 0.1 \times \text{body weight (kg)}^{0.66}$$

Hence, the surface area of a 50-kg foal is as follows:

$$\text{Surface area (m}^2) = 0.1 \times 50 \text{ kg}^{0.66}$$
$$= 1.32 \text{ m}^2$$

The maintenance requirement is 2 L/m²/day, so for this 50-kg patient:

$$\text{Fluid requirement} = 1.32 \text{ m}^2 \times 2 \text{ L/m}^2 = 2.64 \text{ L, or 53 ml/kg/day}$$

Using the same formula, the surface area for a 450-kg cow is

$$\text{Surface area} = 0.1 \times 450 \text{ kg}^{0.66}$$
$$= 5.64 \text{ m}^2$$

$$\text{Fluid requirement} = 5.64 \text{ m}^2 \times 2 \text{ L/m}^2 = 11.3 \text{ L or 25 ml/kg/day}$$

If the fluid requirement had been calculated based on body weight, the fluid dosage would have been 450 kg × 50 ml/kg = 22.5 L, which is twice the amount calculated based on surface area.

Table 12–1 shows examples of daily water requirements based on

TABLE 12–1. EXAMPLES OF DAILY WATER REQUIREMENTS BASED ON SURFACE AREA

Kg	SA (m²)	Total Fluid Required (L)	ml/kg/24 h
1	0.1	0.2	200
5	0.29	0.58	116
10	0.46	0.91	92
20	0.72	1.44	72
50	1.32	2.64	53
100	2.1	4.2	42
250	3.83	7.65	31
450	5.64	11.28	25
500	6.04	12.1	24
800	8.24	16.5	21
1000	9.55	19.1	19

surface area. While there is a 100-fold increase in body weight from 10 kg to 1000 kg, there is only a 20-fold increase in surface area. This demonstrates that the relationship between body weight and maintenance fluid requirement is nonlinear.

EXAMPLE: The patient is a 2-day-old (45-kg) calf, depressed and recumbent, with watery diarrhea, hypothermia, tachycardia, weak pulse, increased capillary refill time, cold extremities, sunken eyes, and decreased skin turgor. It is estimated to be 10–12% dehydrated, with a packed cell volume of 52%. Provisional diagnosis is circulatory collapse, secondary to enterotoxigenic *Escherichia coli*–induced diarrhea. The fluid lost will contain significant amounts of Na^+, K^+, Cl^- and HCO_3^-.

Calculation of the Fluid Requirements. The calf is 10% dehydrated, i.e., has lost 10% of its total body water; because total body water in neonates is 70% of body weight, it follows that water loss is 7% of body weight (10% of 70 = 7%). (For simplicity, the percentage of dehydration is usually calculated based on body weight). In the present example this would mean a replacement requirement of 4.5 L (which somewhat overestimates the fluid requirement).

Existing deficit (7% of body weight)	3.15 L
Ongoing losses (approx.)	3.00 L
Maintenance requirement @ 50 ml/kg	2.25 L
Total requirement for 24 hours	8.40 L

Therapy. A balanced electrolyte solution such as lactated Ringer's is suitable. An initial resuscitating dose of 90 ml/kg, given at a rate of up to 6 ml/kg/min, can be tolerated in most instances. However, complications, particularly pulmonary edema, may occur at this infusion rate. In practice, it is difficult to achieve such high infusion rates with a single i.v. catheter. The remaining 3–5 L may be given at a constant rate over the next 24 h, either intravenously, or both intravenously and orally, depending on the response to therapy. If diarrhea persists, supplementation of K^+ may be required.

Hypoglycemia is a common finding in sick neonates, and blood glucose concentrations can be measured under field conditions using a portable meter. One could assume that all comatose or weak neonates are hypoglycemic and should therefore receive dextrose. Administration of 1 L of a 5% solution in association with initial resuscitating fluids should be sufficient to correct the imbalance in the short term.

Routes of Fluid Administration

ORAL. The oral route provides a safe, convenient, practical, and economical means of delivering fluids, electrolytes, and nutrients. Various oral preparations are available, containing electrolytes, glucose, glycine, and other amino acids. Both commercial products and homemade solutions are used. The limitations to the use of oral fluids include severe dehydration, ileus, or intestinal obstruction. Whole milk is the most practical choice for neonates, since it supplies a source of water and energy. Anorexic or dysphagic animals will need to have the fluids delivered by stomach tube.

SUBCUTANEOUS. Crystalloid solutions may be given by the subcutaneous route to maintain hydration but they are poorly absorbed when the peripheral circulation is impaired. Their usefulness is generally confined to smaller animals, such as lambs. Hypertonic solutions should not be used subcutaneously.

INTRAPERITONEAL. Strict asepsis is crucial when administering intraperitoneal fluids; occasionally, whole blood is administered by this route, such as when immunoglobulin supplementation is required in neonates. In lambs and kids, intraperitoneal glucose (20% solution, 10 ml/kg) is administered for the treatment of hypoglycemia.

INTRAVENOUS. This route is indicated when rapid expansion of intravascular volume is required. In addition to the commonly used crystalloid solutions, colloids such as modified gelatins and synthetic starch solutions are available for intravenous use.

Types of Fluids

COLLOIDS
Blood Derivatives. Plasma is the only blood derivative commonly used in veterinary medicine. Concentrated albumin has been used in human medicine but is too expensive for use in large animals. The expected half-life of transfused plasma proteins is 5–10 days.

Dextran Solutions. Dextrans are polysaccharide molecules produced by the actions of the bacterium *Leuconostoc mesenteroides* on sucrose. Low molecular weight dextrans (40,000 daltons) are safer than the higher molecular weight dextrans (70,000 daltons), which tend to interfere with hemostasis. One gram of dextran retains 20 ml of water in the intravascular space. Dosage for Dextran 40 should not exceed 20 ml/kg over a 24-h period.

HYPERTONIC SALINE SOLUTIONS. When rapid expansion of the blood volume is required, such as in hemorrhage or circulatory shock secondary to endotoxemia, intravascular volume can be expanded by infusion of hypertonic saline solutions such as 7.5% NaCl. The increase in intravascular osmolality causes fluid to move from the interstitial and intracellular spaces to the intravascular space.

Only small volumes are required (4 to 5 ml/kg for 7.5% NaCl), and the solution has a positive inotropic effect.

Following initial resuscitation of the patient with 7.5% NaCl, volume expansion should continue with a balanced electrolyte solution, such as lactated Ringer's. The addition of 5% dextrose in water will facilitate intracellular rehydration.

CRYSTALLOIDS. Balanced electrolyte solutions such as lactated Ringer's and Hartmann's solutions are appropriate for replacing lost fluid volume in most situations, because their ionic composition is similar to plasma's. Normal saline (0.9% NaCl) is not appropriate in most situations because of its high chloride content (Na^+ 154 mmol/L, Cl^- 154 mmol/L). Long-term use of normal saline would cause hyperchloremia, hypokalemia, and metabolic acidosis.

Aims of Fluid Therapy

1. Replace existing deficits. The composition of the fluid lost in most disease conditions is similar, with the exception of conditions involving pyloric obstruction and/or vomiting.
2. Replace ongoing losses.
3. Provide maintenance requirements.

ELECTROLYTE DERANGEMENTS

Sodium Imbalances

Sodium (Na^+) is the most plentiful electrolyte in the ECF, where its concentration is 135–145 mmol/L. In ICF its concentration is approximately 15 mmol/L. Sodium has an important role in regulating ECF volume; it has been called the "osmotic skeleton" of the ECF. Changes in ECF sodium concentration are usually accompanied by changes in water content.

Hyponatremia

Hyponatremia refers to a serum sodium concentration below the normal range (<135 mmol/L). It is due to a relative excess of water and may result from an excessive loss of sodium or gain of water. Hyponatremia may coexist with a water deficit or excess.

EXAMPLES OF HYPONATREMIC STATES

Hyponatremia with ECF Excess. In cardiac failure, a total body increase in sodium and water may develop; however, the total body water is increased to a greater degree.

Hyponatremia with ECF Deficit. In this condition, deficits exist in total body sodium and water, with the sodium deficit being relatively greater. In large animals this condition is usually a sequel to diarrhea, resulting in "hypotonic dehydration."

Hyponatremia with Normal ECF Volume. A low serum sodium concentration with normovolemia may occur in association with excessive antidiuretic hormone activity.

CLINICAL SIGNS OF HYPONATREMIA. The clinical signs depend on the magnitude, rate of onset, and cause of the hyponatremia. Most signs are associated with neurologic abnormalities such as depression, weakness, muscle twitching, and convulsions and are related to cellular swelling. Neurologic changes are more severe in acute hyponatremia, as may occur in acute water overloading. Cerebral swelling is less severe if the hyponatremia develops more slowly.

T R E A T M E N T: In large animals, hyponatremia usually results from diarrhea (hypotonic dehydration), and therefore treatment involves sodium administration accompanied by ECF expansion. If the patient is mildly affected, electrolyte solutions may be administered orally. In most situations, hyponatremia is treated by volume expansion with intravenous polyionic solutions. Lactated Ringer's solution or 0.9% NaCl is suitable in most instances.

In cases of extreme hyponatremia (<125 mmol/L), solutions of hypertonic saline may be infused. However, they should be administered judiciously, with the following considerations:

1. They should *not* be infused if the patient is volume depleted, or intracellular dehydration could result.

2. The aim of therapy is to increase the serum sodium concentration enough to alleviate neurologic signs, *not* to rapidly restore the serum sodium to normal.

3. Only small volumes of hypertonic saline are required; e.g., the serum concentration can be increased 10 mmol/L by the infusion of 6 ml/kg of 5% NaCl, slowly i.v.

EXAMPLE: For a 50-kg calf:

$$6 \text{ ml/kg} \times 50 \text{ kg} = 300 \text{ ml NaCl (5\%)}$$

Hypernatremia

Hypernatremia refers to a serum sodium concentration above the normal range (>145 mmol/L). It can result from conditions causing a loss of water relative to sodium or an excess of sodium relative to water.

EXAMPLES OF HYPERNATREMIC STATES

Hypernatremia Associated with ECF Deficit. This condition is most frequently seen with watery diarrhea, but it can occur in water deprivation, heatstroke, and diabetes insipidus. It results in "hypertonic dehydration."

Hypernatremia Associated with ECF Excess. This condition may result from the excessive administration of hypertonic sodium solutions (e.g., 7.5% NaCl or sodium bicarbonate). It has occurred in calves following tube feeding of electrolyte solutions in association with inadequate water supplementation.

CLINICAL SIGNS OF HYPERNATREMIA. As in hyponatremia, the signs are associated with neurologic abnormalities, including altered mentation, ataxia, and seizures. Hypernatremia results in intracellular dehydration.

T R E A T M E N T: The aim of treatment is to reduce the serum sodium gradually to avoid causing cerebral edema.

Acute hypernatremia is treated by the administration of hypotonic polyionic solutions (e.g., half-strength lactated Ringer's).

In chronic hypernatremia, the existing high intracellular osmotic pressure may lead to cellular swelling if hypotonic solutions are administered. In general, it is probably safe to reduce the serum Na^+ by 10–15 mmol/L over an 8-h period. Isotonic fluids may be infused to expand the ECF and cause a gradual reduction in serum Na^+.

The free water deficit may be calculated using the following equation:

$$\text{Free water deficit (L)} = 0.6 \times \text{body weight (kg)} \times \frac{(\text{actual } Na^+ - 140)}{140}$$

EXAMPLE: For a 50-kg foal, with diarrhea, depression, dehydration, and a serum Na^+ of 178 mmol/L:

$$\text{Free water deficit (L)} = 0.6 \times 50 \text{ kg} \times \frac{(178 \text{ mmol/L} - 140)}{140}$$

$$= 8.1 \text{ L}$$

Potassium Imbalances

Potassium (K^+) is the major intracellular electrolyte, and the ICF accounts for 98% of the body's potassium. The 2% in the ECF has an important role in neuromuscular function, and deviations from normal serum concentrations produce alterations in myocardial irritability. Serum potassium concentration is affected by alterations in acid–base balance. A decrease in pH of 0.1 unit causes an increase in K^+ of 0.3 to 0.7 mmol/L, depending on total body potassium balance.

Hypokalemia

Hypokalemia refers to a serum potassium below the normal range (<3.5 mmol/L). It is usually indicative of a deficit in total body potassium.

Gastrointestinal losses, especially diarrhea, are the most common cause of potassium depletion. Diarrheal fluid may contain 20–30 mmol/L of potassium. Renal losses may occur with long-term diuretic use. Potassium depletion occurs during prolonged periods of anorexia, because a daily intake must be maintained.

T R E A T M E N T: Mild deficiencies can be treated by oral supplementation with KCl. One gram of KCl contains 13 mmol of K^+.

(1 level tablespoon of KCl weighs 14 g.) Supplementation may need to be continued for up to 5 days.

EXAMPLE: A 50-kg calf has a history of diarrhea of 3 days' duration. The diarrhea has resolved, but the serum K^+ is 2.5 mmol/L. The calf may be given orally approximately 170 mmol of KCl (1 tablespoon) daily for 5 days, in conjunction with a normal intake of milk. Administration with food reduces gastrointestinal irritation.

If potassium depletion is severe, intravenous supplementation with K^+ is necessary. With serum K^+ of <2.5 mmol/L, 2.5–3.0 mmol/L, or 3.0–3.5 mmol/L, the concentration of K^+ in the *maintenance* fluids should be increased to 80, 60, and 40 mmol/L, respectively. With these high concentrations of K^+, daily monitoring of serum K^+ is advised. In the absence of monitoring of serum K^+, it is generally safe to administer up to 0.5 mmol of K^+/kg/h in animals up to 50 kg, and empirically up to 0.25 mmol/kg/h in larger animals.

Before administering high-potassium solutions, it is important to ensure that renal function is adequate.

Also, observe the following precautions when administering intravenous KCl:

1. Never infuse KCl solutions directly from ampules without adequately diluting them.

2. To ensure adequate mixing of KCl with infusion solutions, invert and agitate the container several times.

3. Avoid subcutaneous administration, since concentrations >10 mmol/L are irritating.

Hyperkalemia

Hyperkalemia refers to a potassium concentration above the normal range (>5.5 mmol/L). The condition rarely occurs in animals with adequate urine output.

Causes include decreased renal perfusion, e.g., severe dehydration; acute renal failure; renal disease, e.g., ruptured bladder or urethra; metabolic acidosis; iatrogenic causes, e.g., rapid intravenous infusion of potassium-containing solutions; and, rarely, adrenal insufficiency (reduced aldosterone concentration).

CLINICAL SIGNS. The most important clinical effects of hyperkalemia are on the myocardium. Changes in the electrocardiogram (ECG) are generally present when the serum K^+ concentration exceeds 8 mmol/L. These changes include tall T waves, a prolonged P-R interval, and a decrease in amplitude, followed by disappearance of P waves and a widening of QRS complexes, progressing to ventricular arrhythmias and cardiac arrest.

T R E A T M E N T:

1. Provide volume expansion with K^+-free fluids, e.g., 0.9% NaCl.
2. Correct underlying abnormalities, e.g., metabolic acidosis.
3. In severe cases, insulin therapy may be indicated. Insulin is administered in a solution containing 5% dextrose and 0.45% NaCl, at a dose rate of 0.5 I.U. of insulin/g dextrose. Administration of 20 ml of the solution/kg/h is recommended, with hourly checks of glucose and K^+; the dosage should be decreased in accordance with the response to therapy and to avoid volume overload.
4. In severe cases, such as renal failure or ruptured urinary bladder (presurgically), peritoneal dialysis should be considered. In large animal practice this is usually feasible only in neonates.
5. If serious cardiac arrhythmias are occurring, administration of calcium may be necessary. Calcium gluconate (10% solution) at a dose rate of 1–2 ml/10 kg, should be infused over 3–5 min. ECG monitoring is recommended during the infusion. The infusion should be stopped if bradycardia occurs.

The myocardial protective effects of calcium are transient, and efforts to reduce the serum K^+ concentration should be continued.
6. Ion-exchange resins, which cause sodium to be exchanged for potassium in the intestine, may be given as a retention enema. Preparations marketed for humans may be suitable for neonatal animals.

Sodium Bicarbonate

The bicarbonate deficit in the ECF can be calculated according to the following equation:

$$HCO_3^- \text{ deficit (mmol/L)} = \text{plasma } HCO_3^- \text{ deficit} \times \text{body weight (kg)} \times 0.3 \text{ (0.4 in neonates)}$$

This dosage, or part thereof, should be given slowly, in association with volume expansion, to allow equilibration between the intravascular and interstitial fluid spaces.

EXAMPLE: For a 50-kg calf with severe depression and dehydration subsequent to *E. coli*–induced diarrhea: analysis of venous blood indicates a pH of 6.95 and HCO_3^- of 8 mmol/L.

Plasma HCO_3^- deficit (mmol/L) = Normal − actual

$$= 24 \text{ mmol/L} - 8 \text{ mmol/L}$$
$$= 16 \text{ mmol/L}$$

ECF deficit
$$= 16 \text{ mmol/L} \times 50 \text{ kg} \times 0.4$$
$$= 320 \text{ mmol/L}$$

It is recommended that one quarter of the calculated dose (80 mmol) of NaHCO$_3$ be administered over a 1-h period in conjunction with volume expansion, the remainder being administered over the following 12–24 h. In many cases, volume expansion alone will improve renal and tissue perfusion sufficiently to remove the need for NaHCO$_3$. The overzealous administration of sodium bicarbonate is discouraged, as fatal complications may arise, especially in the dehydrated animal.

Calcium Imbalances

Calcium has an important role in neuromuscular function and is involved in the initiation and propagation of nerve impulses, as well as being an important component of bone and teeth. In plasma, approximately half of the calcium is unbound (ionized), while the remainder is bound to albumin, with a small amount chelated. The ionized calcium is the biologically important fraction, and measurement of this form is of more value clinically than knowledge of the total plasma calcium.

Normal plasma calcium (total) concentration is 2–2.70 mmol/L (8.13–10.98 mg/dl) in cattle; 2.80–3.40 mmol/L (11.38–13.80 mg/dl) in horses.

Hypocalcemia

Parturient paresis of dairy cattle, "milk fever," is the most common clinical manifestation of hypocalcemia. It occurs commonly in high-producing dairy cows soon after calving.

CLINICAL SIGNS. Three stages of the disease are recognized. In stage 1, the cow is able to stand but appears agitated. She has mild ataxia with muscle twitching, and occasionally she exhibits bellowing.

In stage 2, the cow is down but has sufficient muscle tone to remain in sternal recumbency and usually has the neck flexed with the head resting on the flank.

In stage 3, the cow is in lateral recumbency, with cold extremities and tachycardia. The animal is in urgent need of treatment.

Hypocalcemia occurs in pregnant ewes in late pregnancy, and mares may develop the condition in early lactation or immediately after weaning (1–2 days). On rare occasions it is associated with transport (transit tetany).

T R E A T M E N T: Calcium borogluconate is preferred for parenteral infusion. It contains 8.3% calcium. Cows and mares require approximately 12 g of calcium, while sheep require 0.5–1 g.

To obtain a rapid response, the solution should be administered intravenously. In mild cases, subcutaneous administration may be adequate.

Because calcium has a direct action on the myocardium, rapid infusion may cause cardiac arrest. Toxicity can be avoided by slowly infusing the calcium and monitoring the heart rate.

Hypercalcemia

Hypercalcemia is not a common finding in large animals. An increase in plasma albumin, as may occur in dehydration, may cause a mild hypercalcemia but would not result in clinical signs of hypercalcemia.

Clinical diseases giving rise to hypercalcemia include the following:

Renal disease in the horse (in some cases)
Primary hyperparathyroidism, e.g., neoplasia of the parathyroid
Primary pseudohyperparathyroidism, due to production of parathormone by a tumor elsewhere in the body
Hypervitaminosis D due to oversupplementation with vitamin D
Ingestion of plants with a vitamin D_3–like activity, e.g., *Solanum malacoxylon*
Neoplasia that produces osteoclastic factors (rare)

CLINICAL SIGNS. Signs include depression, anorexia, bowel stasis, polydipsia, and polyuria. Soft tissue mineralization results in a stiff gait. Pressure on the flexor tendons and sesamoid ligament may elicit a pain response.

TREATMENT: Removal of the underlying cause may be helpful in animals that are ingesting plants containing vitamin D_3. Treatment is generally not practical for other causes of hypercalcemia, such as malignancy.

Palliative treatment for hypercalcemia includes the following:

Diuresis—0.45% or 0.9% NaCl i.v. (Na^+ inhibits tubular reabsorption of Ca^{++})
Furosemide—promotes diuresis and increases calcium excretion
Corticosteroids—decrease bone turnover and tubular reabsorption of Ca^{++} (for patients with malignancy)
Mithramycin—antibiotic with cytotoxic properties; inhibits bone resorption (toxic side effects are important)
Calcitonin—rapidly decreases serum calcium

Magnesium Imbalances

Most of the magnesium in the body is intracellular. The magnesium concentration in the serum is 0.8–1.2 mmol/L. (1.8–3.0 mg/dl). Approximately two thirds of serum magnesium is in the unbound (ionized) form.

Hypomagnesemia

Clinical hypomagnesemia (grass tetany, grass staggers) is common in adult cows and occurs less frequently in sheep and goats. Hypomagnesemia has been associated with sudden death in bucket-fed calves. The classic form of the disease occurs in in-wintered lactating dairy cows following turnout to lush pasture in springtime.

CLINICAL SIGNS. Magnesium is necessary for the release of acetylcholine at myoneural junctions. Hypomagnesemia predisposes to cardiac arrythmias, and ECG changes include prolongation of P-R and Q-T intervals.

In the acute form of the disease, cows become hyperesthetic and may gallop around wildly and bellow. Ataxia and recumbency may follow, with nystagmus and frothing at the mouth. Death usually follows rapidly if treatment is not given.

In the subacute form, clinical signs develop over a few days. The cow develops an anxious facial expression with muscle tremors, ataxia, and an exaggerated response to noise.

T R E A T M E N T: Most cases of hypomagnesemia respond well to the intravenous infusion of a calcium and magnesium mixture. Magnesium sulfate ($MgSO_4$), 150–250 ml of a 20% solution, can be added to calcium borogluconate and injected *slowly* i.v.

A more sustained increase in the serum magnesium concentration can be achieved with the subcutaneous injection of 200 ml of a 20% solution of $MgSO_4$. The dosage for sheep and goats is approximately 20 ml of the 20% solution.

Hypermagnesemia

Hypermagnesemia is rare in animals.

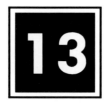

Cardiovascular Shock

Cardiovascular shock is a clinical condition that results from failure of the heart to pump sufficient blood to maintain adequate tissue perfusion.

ETIOLOGIC CLASSIFICATION OF SHOCK

Cardiogenic Shock

Cardiogenic shock is rare in large animals.

Causes

MYOCARDIAL DISEASE. E.g., monensin poisoning, mulberry heart disease, and inherited cardiomyopathy of Holstein cattle.

VALVULAR DISEASE. Ruptured chordae tendineae or valvular endocarditis.

CARDIAC TAMPONADE. E.g., pericardial effusion

ARRHYTHMIAS. E.g., atrial fibrillation, ventricular tachycardia, and heart blocks.

Hypovolemic Shock

Hypovolemic shock is failure to maintain adequate preload (end-diastolic volume).

Causes

Causes include hemorrhage and fluid loss, e.g., from diarrhea or burns (plasma loss).

Septic or Endotoxic Shock

Two Phases

The early, *hyperdynamic* phase is associated with a reduced systemic vascular resistance and increased cardiac output.

The later, *hypodynamic* state is characterized by persistent hypotension, decreased cardiac output, increased pulmonary vascular resistance, hypoxemia, and acidemia.

Predisposing Factors

COLOSTRUM. Inadequate ingestion of colostrum by neonates or poor quality of colostrum.
IMMUNOSUPPRESSIVE THERAPY
INDWELLING VASCULAR CATHETERS
NEOPLASIA
HYPOVOLEMIA

Causes

MASTITIS. Coliform or staphylococcal.
SEPTIC METRITIS
SEPTICEMIA. E.g., umbilical infection in neonates or acute *Pasteurella* spp. septicemia in cattle, pigs, or small ruminants.
SEPTIC PERITONITIS/INTESTINAL ACCIDENT

Anaphylactic and Anaphylactoid Shock

Anaphylactic shock involves the release of vasoactive amines (e.g., histamine) from mast cells in response to exposure to an allergen to which the patient has previously been sensitized (immunoglobulin E mediated).

Anaphylactoid shock is similar to anaphylactic shock, without being immune mediated. Anaphylactoid shock usually follows administration of a drug. The net result of vasoactive amine release on the circulatory system is decreased venous return. Bronchial constriction is another significant effect.

Neurogenic Shock

Sympathetic blockade is the most probable cause of neurogenic shock. Examples of sympathetic blockade are high epidural block with local anesthesia and damage to the vasomotor center (e.g., head trauma).

Traumatic Shock

Shock can follow severe trauma (e.g., long bone fracture or muscle trauma). Blood pools in the affected area, causing a decrease in venous return and a subsequent reduction in cardiac output.

Endocrine Shock

Endocrine shock is a consequence of adrenal failure, as in Addison's disease.

CLINICAL SIGNS OF SHOCK

- Hypotension, manifested by weak pulse
- Tachycardia
- Cold extremities
- Depression
- Pallor of mucous membranes and increased capillary refill time
- Fever (early stages of septic shock)

MANAGEMENT OF SHOCK

Starling's Law of the Heart

An insight into the pathophysiology and, consequently, the management of shock can be gained from referring to Frank and Starling's classic "law of the heart."

Frank and Starling stated that the energy of contraction is a function of the length of the resting cardiac muscle fiber. In clinical terms this means that, within limits, the stroke volume is proportional to the left ventricular end-diastolic volume (preload).

Specific Therapies

Preload

The main goal of therapy is to optimize preload. In cardiogenic shock due to myocardial failure or in cardiac tamponade, moderate increases in circulating volume may optimize the cardiac output.

In hypovolemic and septic shock, the optimal cardiac output is achieved by the administration of crystalloids, colloids (plasma or a dextran), or blood, depending on the circumstances.

When crystalloids are used, high doses of up to 90 ml/kg as a bolus may be required in severe cases, delivered at a rate of up to 6 ml/kg/min.

Venous return may be facilitated by positioning the patient appropriately (where practical). Elevating the hindlimbs promotes venous return.

Increasing Myocardial Contractility

If cardiac output remains low despite adequate preload, inotropic agents may be indicated. Their main application in large animals is during general anesthesia to combat the myocardial-depressant effects of anesthetic agents (Table 13–1).

Afterload Reducers

Afterload reducers decrease systemic vascular resistance. Their effects include reduced resistance to forward flow, leading to improved cardiac output and decreased myocardial oxygen consumption. Examples of afterload reducers are hydralazine, nitroprusside, and prazosin.

Correction of Metabolic Abnormalities

In metabolic acidosis (pH < 7.2), the administration of $NaHCO_3$ may be indicated. However, there is no evidence that acidosis affects cardiac contractility, and recent experimental data indicate that $NaHCO_3$ may exacerbate myocardial depression in septic patients.

Where respiratory compromise is present, administration of O_2, and occasionally intubation and ventilatory support, may be required.

Steroids

The use of corticosteroids in the treatment of shock is controversial. Drugs used include methyl prednisolone (30 mg/kg i.v. every 4 h) and dexamethasone (3 mg/kg i.v.).

Nonsteroidal Antiinflammatory Drugs

Flunixin meglumine has been used to attenuate the effects of endotoxin and may be beneficial in the treatment of endotoxic/septic shock, at a dose range of 0.25–1.0 mg/kg every 8–12 h.

TABLE 13–1. AGENTS USED TO INCREASE MYOCARDIAL CONTRACTILITY

Agent	Dosage (μg/kg/min)	Cardiac Output	Heart Rate	Renal Blood Flow
Dopamine	2.5–5.0	+	+	+
	>10.0	+	+	−
Dobutamine	2.0–10.0	+	o	+
Epinephrine	0.05–0.15	+	+	−

Antibiotics

Antibiotics are indicated in septic shock and may be indicated in other forms of shock if bacterial translocation is suspected. Because in the majority of cases septic shock is caused by gram-negative organisms, the appropriate antibiotics must be used. These include

- Aminoglycosides, e.g., gentamicin and amikacin. These are often used in combination with penicillins or other drugs with a good spectrum of activity against gram-positive organisms.
- β-lactam antibiotics, e.g., penicillin; semisynthetic penicillins such as ampicillin, amoxicillin, or ticarcillin, alone or in combination with clavulanic acid; and third-generation cephalosporins such as ceftiofur sodium and moxalactam.
- Chloramphenicol, a broad-spectrum bacteriostatic drug. Note: Chloramphenicol is not for use in food animals.
- Potentiated sulfonamides, e.g., trimethoprim with a sulfonamide drug.

Anaphylactic Shock

Some of the drugs used specifically to treat anaphylactic shock are listed below.

Epinephrine

Epinephrine (5–15 μg/kg) may be administered intramuscularly or diluted and given slowly intravenously (over 5 min). Absorption from subcutaneous sites is reduced in shock states. Effects include vasoconstriction (leading to increased venous return) and bronchodilation.

Antiinflammatory Agents

CORTICOSTEROIDS. E.g., methylprednisolone or dexamethasone.

NONSTEROIDAL ANTIINFLAMMATORY DRUGS. E.g., flunixin meglumine.

BRONCHODILATORS. E.g., aminophylline (1 mg/kg, slowly i.v.), clenbuterol (0.8 μg/kg, i.v.) are indicated if severe bronchoconstriction is present.

ANTIHISTAMINES. E.g., tripelennamine (0.5 mg/kg, i.m.).

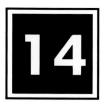

Blood Gases and Acid–Base Balance

Maintenance of the acid–base balance is accomplished by interaction between the extracellular fluid (ECF) and the pulmonary, renal, and gastrointestinal systems.

Disorders of the acid–base balance are accompanied by various clinical abnormalities. These abnormalities have been attributed directly to changes in hydrogen ion concentration [H$^+$]. For convenience, the hydrogen ion concentration is expressed in pH units. A pH unit is equal to the negative logarithm of the hydrogen ion concentration: pH $= -\log[\text{H}^+]$.

The Henderson-Hasselbalch equation states,

$$pH = pKa + \log \frac{[\text{base}]}{[\text{acid}]}$$

where pKa $=$ the pH at which 50% of the solution is ionized.

Because HCO_3^- represents approximately 80% of the buffering capacity of the ECF, the Henderson-Hasselbalch equation is usually written as follows:

$$pH = pKa + \log \frac{[\text{HCO}_3^-]}{[\text{H}_2\text{CO}_3]}$$

This is sufficiently accurate for clinical purposes.

When hydrogen ions combine with bicarbonate, carbonic acid (H_2CO_3) is formed, which dissociates to CO_2 and H_2O.

$$H^+ + HCO_3^- \rightleftharpoons H_2CO_3 \rightleftharpoons CO_2 + H_2O$$

The equilibrium of the reaction is predominantly to the right, and the concentration of CO_2 (dissolved) is more than 1000 times that of H_2CO_3. So the revised Henderson-Hasselbalch equation (p. 263) can be rewritten as follows:

$$pH = pKa + \log \frac{[HCO_3^-]}{[\alpha PCO_2]}$$

where α = solubility of CO_2 at 37° C = 0.03 mmol/L of ECF, HCO_3^- = 24 mmol/L, and pKa = 6.1 for bicarbonate buffer system.

$$pH = pKa + \log \frac{24}{0.03[40]}$$

$$= 6.1 + \log \frac{24}{1.2}$$

$$= 6.1 + \log 20 \; [1.3]$$

$$= 7.4$$

ACIDEMIA, ALKALEMIA, AND COMPENSATORY MECHANISMS

When blood pH decreases below the normal range of 7.35–7.45, *acidemia* results. When blood pH increases above that range, *alkalemia* results.

Respiratory acidosis, respiratory alkalosis, metabolic acidosis, and metabolic alkalosis describe the conditions that give rise to acidemia and alkalemia.

The body attempts to maintain a pH close to the normal range in the presence of fluctuations of $[H^+]$. This is achieved by maintaining the ratio of $[HCO_3^-]$ to $[CO_2]$ close to the normal ratio of 20:1.

Respiratory Acidosis

In respiratory acidosis (alveolar hypoventilation), the accumulation of CO_2 decreases the pH. If this condition persists, the kidney conserves HCO_3^-. The resulting increase in $[HCO_3^-]$ tends to restore the $[HCO_3^-]:[CO_2]$ ratio toward normal, but this is never complete. The plasma bicarbonate concentration reflects the degree of renal compensation.

Respiratory Alkalosis

In respiratory alkalosis (alveolar hyperventilation), the increase in pH is secondary to the reduction of CO_2. Renal compensation is achieved by increased excretion of bicarbonate. The plasma bicarbonate is thus less than normal.

Metabolic Acidosis

In metabolic acidosis, a primary decrease in $[HCO_3^-]$ occurs. This may be the result of poor tissue perfusion or excessive gastrointestinal or renal HCO_3^- loss. Respiratory compensation occurs by increased ventilation and reduction of the CO_2. Complete compensation can be predicted by the equation $PaCO_2 = 1.5\ [HCO_3^-] + 8\ (\pm 2)$.

Metabolic Alkalosis

In metabolic alkalosis, an increase in plasma $[HCO_3^-]$ occurs. It may occur after marked chloride loss, e.g., abomasal sequestration of HCl. Respiratory compensation (CO_2 retention) is usually minimal. Complete compensation can be predicted by the equation $PaCO_2 = 0.7\ [HCO_3^-] + 20(\pm 2)$.

Mixed Derangements

Mixed metabolic and respiratory derangements may coexist. Less commonly, acute changes may be superimposed on a chronic condition.

Total CO₂

Total CO_2 (TCO_2) is used as an indirect measure of $[HCO_3^-]$. TCO_2 determines total CO_2 in plasma; this CO_2 consists of ionized and un-ionized forms.

      Ionized forms: HCO_3^-, and carbamine compounds
      Un-ionized forms: H_2CO_3 and dissolved CO_2

So $TCO_2 = HCO_3^- + $ dissolved CO_2.

In general, the dissolved CO_2 varies from 0.6 to 1.8 mmol/L. Let's assume a mean value of 1.0 mmol/L. $TCO_2 = (HCO_3^- + 1.0)$. Therefore, $HCO_3^- = (TCO_2 - 1.0)$.

The limitations of TCO_2 measurement are that (1) it estimates only the metabolic component, and (2) in pulmonary disease with CO_2 retention, HCO_3^- will be falsely increased.

Base Excess/Deficit

The base excess/deficit value indicates the number of millimoles of acid or base required to titrate 1 L of blood to a pH of 7.4 at 37° C and a $PaCO_2$ of 40 mm Hg. This takes into account the buffering capacity of HCO_3^- (correct for PCO_2, hemoglobin, phosphates, etc.).

NORMAL ACID–BASE AND ARTERIAL BLOOD GAS VALUES FOR CATTLE AND HORSES

pH	7.35–7.45
PO_2	85–100 mm Hg
PCO_2	35–45 mm Hg
HCO_3^-	24 ± 4 mmol/L
Base excess	0 ± 3 mmol/L

Alveolar Gas Equation

The alveolar partial pressure of O_2 (PAO_2) may be determined by the following simplified equation:

$$PAO_2 = P_IO_2 - \frac{PaCO_2}{R}$$

where P_IO_2 = inspired oxygen concentration and R = the respiratory quotient. At sea level (760 mm Hg), the oxygen in the inspired air is 20.9%, and $PaCO_2$ = 40 mm Hg. At body temperature (37° C), the water vapor pressure in the airway is 47 mm Hg and R = 0.8. Therefore, solving for the above equation:

$$PAO_2 = [20.9\% \, (760 - 47)] - \frac{40}{0.8}$$
$$= (.209 \times 713) - 50$$
$$= 150 - 50$$
$$\approx 100 \text{ mm Hg}$$

If lung function were ideal, the arterial $O_2(PaO_2)$ would equal the PAO_2. However, because of a minor ventilation–perfusion mismatch, there is usually a disparity of ≤ 10 mm Hg in the normal lung. This is described as the alveolar–arterial oxygen difference and is written as $(A - a)PO_2$.

Oxygen Transport

O_2 transport to the tissues is affected by a number of mechanisms, which can be described by the following equation:

O_2 transport (L/min) = cardiac output (L/min) × hemoglobin (g/L) × % saturation of hemoglobin × 1.34

(1.34 = the number of milliliters of O_2 carried by each gram of hemoglobin)

Conditions (e.g., hypovolemia, anemia, and cardiac disease) that affect any of these parameters will impair O_2 transport.

INFLUENCE OF CHANGES IN HCO_3^- AND CO_2 ON pH

CO_2

Normal arterial value is approximately 40 mm Hg.

$$\uparrow PaCO_2 \text{ by 20 mm Hg} = \downarrow pH \text{ of } 0.1$$
$$\downarrow PaCO_2 \text{ by 10 mm Hg} = \uparrow pH \text{ of } 0.1$$

HCO_3^-

Normal value is approximately 24 mmol/L.

$$\uparrow \text{ or } \downarrow [HCO_3^-] \text{ by 10 mmol/L} = \uparrow \text{ or } \downarrow pH \text{ by } 0.15$$

Acute Respiratory Acidosis/Alkalosis

$$\uparrow PaCO_2 \text{ by 10 mm Hg} \rightarrow \uparrow [HCO_3^-] \text{ by 1 mmol/L}$$
$$\downarrow PaCO_2 \text{ by 10 mm Hg} \rightarrow \downarrow [HCO_3^-] \text{ by 2 mmol/L}$$

Chronic Respiratory Acidosis/Alkalosis

$$\uparrow PaCO_2 \text{ by 10 mm Hg} \rightarrow \uparrow [HCO_3^-] \text{ by 4 mmol/L}$$
$$\downarrow PaCO_2 \text{ by 10 mm Hg} \rightarrow \downarrow [HCO_3^-] \text{ by 5 mmol/L}$$

INTERPRETATION OF BLOOD GASES

$PaCO_2$ Evaluation

The following information may be deduced from the $PaCO_2$:

a. The adequacy of alveolar ventilation ($\dot{V}_A$) is assessed according to

$$PaCO_2 \text{ is proportional to } \frac{1}{\dot{V}_A}$$

b. The $PaCO_2$ allows estimation of PAO_2 according to the alveolar gas equation:

$$PAO_2 = P_IO_2 - \frac{PaCO_2}{R}$$

where R = respiratory quotient (0.8).

   c. $PaCO_2$ aids in evaluating the contribution of respiration to the acid–base balance.

PaO_2 Evaluation

The PaO_2 may be used to determine the efficiency of gas exchange in the lung. The $(A - a)PO_2$ may be calculated according to $PAO_2 = P_IO_2 - PaCO_2/R$.

pH Evaluation

Relate this to $PaCO_2$, because breathing is the main mechanism that influences acid–base status in the short term. Decide what the implications are regarding respiratory and metabolic changes in $[H^+]$. The interpretation of these changes requires the identification of the primary abnormality. This is sometimes a clinical decision.

Examples

In the following examples it is assumed that hemoglobin concentration is within the normal range.

EXAMPLE 1: A 2-day-old, 45-kg calf has severe watery diarrhea of 12 hours' duration and estimated 8–12% dehydration. Blood gas is as follows:

$$\begin{aligned} \text{pH} &= 7.15 \\ PaCO_2 &= 30 \text{ mm Hg} \\ HCO_3^- &= 8 \text{ mmol/L} \end{aligned}$$

What is the acid–base status?

1. The $PaCO_2$ indicates moderate hyperventilation.

    The predicted $PaCO_2$ = 1.5 × $[HCO_3^-]$ + 8 (± 2)
                       = 1.5 × 8 + 8 (± 2)
                       = 20 (± 2)

2. The pH of 7.15 indicates severe acidemia. Because the bicarbonate is altered in the direction of the pH, the primary abnormality is metabolic.

DIAGNOSIS. This is an example of a partially compensated metabolic acidosis. The disease process is typical of enterotoxigenic *Escherichia* coli–induced diarrhea with subsequent dehydration.

T R E A T M E N T: Institute intravenous volume replacement. A balanced electrolyte solution such as lactated Ringer's solution is the most important aspect of treatment.

Administer $NaHCO_3$ at the appropriate dosage, e.g., 1–2 mmol/kg, in association with volume replacement.

Provide nursing care.

Because the calf may also be hypoglycemic, in the absence of a blood glucose determination, 1 L of 5% dextrose should be infused intravenously.

EXAMPLE 2: A 12-h-old, 40-kg foal is depressed, recumbent, and hypothermic, with tachycardia, increased capillary refill time, and weak pulse. Arterial gas analysis reveals the following:

$$\begin{aligned}
\text{pH} &= 7.1 \\
\text{PaCO}_2 &= 70 \text{ mm Hg} \\
\text{HCO}_3^- &= 13 \text{ mmol/L} \\
\text{PaO}_2 &= 46 \text{ mm Hg}
\end{aligned}$$

What is the blood gas and acid–base status?

1. The $PaCO_2$ indicates:
   a. Alveolar hypoventilation.

   $$\begin{aligned}
   \text{Expected PaCO}_2 &= (1.5 \times 13) + 8 \\
   &= 27 \text{ mm Hg}
   \end{aligned}$$

   b. $PAO_2 = P_1O_2 - \dfrac{PaCO_2}{0.8}$

   $$\begin{aligned}
   &= 20.9 \,(760 - 47) - \frac{70}{0.8} \\
   &= 150 - 87.5 \\
   &= 62.5
   \end{aligned}$$

   The increase in $PaCO_2$ (and hence $PACO_2$) is responsible for the decrease in PAO_2.
2. The PaO_2 of 46 indicates hypoxemia.
3. The pH of 7.1 indicates marked acidemia; increased $PaCO_2$ and decreased $[HCO_3^-]$ indicate a mixed metabolic and respiratory acidosis.

DIAGNOSIS. This is an example of a combined respiratory and metabolic acidosis. The foal's condition is typical of neonatal septicemia.

TREATMENT: Volume replacement, e.g., with balanced electrolyte solutions.

Is $NaHCO_3$ administration necessary? Volume replacement may improve the pH independent of the administration of $NaHCO_3$. The metabolic component is not excessive (if the $PaCO_2$ is normal, the expected pH is 7.25). In fact, $NaHCO_3$ could aggravate the increase in $PaCO_2$ and increase respiratory work.

Is ventilatory assistance necessary? The PaO_2 of 47 indicates hypoxemia, and in view of the low cardiac output there is probably marked tissue hypoxia. Thus O_2 therapy, either by nasal insufflation or in association with mechanical ventilation, is indicated while volume status is being restored.

Blood gas analysis should be repeated after initial stabilization. If no improvement in respiratory status is noted, mechanical ventilation is indicated.

The foal is probably hypoglycemic, and administration of dextrose should be part of the fluid therapy.

EXAMPLE 3: An aged, 500-kg horse with a history of small airway disease (chronic obstructive pulmonary disease) is presented with an acute attack of respiratory distress. Signs include tachypnea, increased work of breathing, and tachycardia. An arterial blood gas analysis reveals the following:

Sample A (Pretreatment):

$$pH = 7.4$$
$$PaCO_2 = 43 \text{ mm Hg}$$
$$PaO_2 = 66 \text{ mm Hg}$$
$$HCO_3^- = 25 \text{ mmol/L}$$

DIAGNOSIS: The PaO_2 of 66 mm Hg is much less than normal, indicating a derangement of oxygen transport across the lung.

T R E A T M E N T: Treatment consists of 10 mg of atropine administered intravenously and 500 mg of aminophylline administered by slow intravenous injection.

Twenty minutes later the horse appears to be breathing more easily. A blood gas sample at this stage reveals the following:

Sample B (Post-treatment):

$$pH = 7.38$$
$$PaCO_2 = 34 \text{ mm Hg}$$
$$PaO_2 = 59 \text{ mm Hg}$$
$$HCO_3^- = 22 \text{ mmol/L}$$

Has the respiratory function improved?

1. The $PaCO_2$ has decreased, indicating an increase in alveolar ventilation. It also implies that alveolar PO_2 (PAO_2) is increased:

Sample A:

$$PAO_2 = 20.9\% \ (760 - 47) - 43/0.8$$
$$= 150 - 54$$
$$= 96$$

Sample B:

$$PAO_2 = 150 - 34/0.8$$
$$= 150 - 42$$
$$= 108$$

2. The PaO_2 has decreased by 7 mm Hg. Although small, this is a significant finding, as demonstrated by the increase in the $(A-a)PO_2$.

Sample A:

$$(A-a)PO_2 \rightarrow 96 - 66 = 30 \text{ mm Hg}$$

Sample B:

$$(A-a)PO_2 \rightarrow 108 - 59 = 49 \text{ mm Hg}$$

COMMENT: The increasing $(A-a)$ gradient indicates a deterioration of oxygen transfer in the lung. This effect is probably secondary to aminophylline administration, which in addition to its bronchodilatory effects, increases blood flow to previously hypoxic areas of the lung. It does this by increasing cardiac output and causing pulmonary vasodilation. This reduces the ventilation/perfusion ratio in affected areas of the lung.

EXAMPLE 4: A 5-year-old cow, 2 weeks post partum, has inappetence, decreased milk production, decreased ruminal movements, and 15-inch-diameter ping in the left paralumbar fossa. The diagnosis is displacement of the abomasum to left side. Arterial blood gas findings are as follows:

$$pH = 7.60$$
$$PaCO_2 = 49 \text{ mm Hg}$$
$$PaO_2 = 89 \text{ mm Hg}$$
$$HCO_3^- = 45 \text{ mmol/L}$$

What is the acid–base status?

1. The $PaCO_2$ indicates alveolar hypoventilation.
2. The pH indicates alkalemia of metabolic origin because the $[HCO_3^-]$ is changed in the same direction as the pH.

$$\text{Predicted } PaCO_2 = 0.7 \ (HCO_3^-) + 20 \ (\pm 2)$$
$$= 0.7 \ (45) + 20 \ (\pm 2)$$
$$= 31 + 20$$
$$= 51 \ (\pm 2)$$

3. The increased $[HCO_3^-]$ arises secondary to sequestration of Cl^- and H^+ in the abomasum, with renal conservation of Na^+ and HCO_3^-.

DIAGNOSIS: This represents a compensated metabolic alkalosis and not a respiratory acidosis. If we consider that the normal response to a metabolic alkalosis is hypoventilation, then this is an example of compensatory hypoventilation.

TREATMENT:
1. Correct the displacement (surgically).
2. Correct volume deficit.
3. Correct Cl^- and K^+ deficits.
4. Administer acidifying solution, typically 0.9% NaCl with KCl added.

PARADOXICAL ACIDURIA

In the normal animal, when Na^+ is conserved in the distal tubule, either it is exchanged for a positive ion (H^+ or K^+) or a negative ion (HCO_3^- or Cl^-) is resorbed concurrently.

In conditions such as chronic abomasal displacement, Cl^- and H^+ are lost from the ECF due to intestinal pooling. The accompanying dehydration leads to a reduction in circulating blood volume, and glomerular filtration is less than adequate. The release of aldosterone is stimulated, leading to K^+ excretion and Na^+ retention. The reduced glomerular filtration results in a maximum resorption of Na^+ in the proximal tubule, and the lack of Na^+ in the loop and distal tubule affects ion regulation. This leads to inappropriate retention of HCO_3^- and continued K^+ excretion.

Eventually a state of potassium depletion is reached and H^+ excretion is promoted, despite the alkalemia.

TREATMENT:
1. Restore circulating volume. This is of primary importance.
2. Provide K^+ supplementation.
3. Supply acidifying solution, e.g., 0.9% NaCl with KCl added.
4. Correct the underlying problem.

Antimicrobial Drugs

"Stimulate the phagocytes. Drugs are a delusion."
G. B. Shaw

Antibiotics are commonly used in large animal practice; however, the indications for their use are not always well defined.

CHOICE OF DRUG

Ideally the choice of antibiotic should be based on a rational assessment of the probable infecting organism(s), the sensitivity pattern of the bacterium, and the location of the infection (e.g. lung, central nervous system). In the clinical setting, however, one's choice of antibiotics is often based on an educated guess.

Broad-spectrum antibiotics or combinations of narrow-spectrum antibiotics are indicated when the animal is seriously ill, and when the sensitivity pattern is unknown. Narrow-spectrum drugs are preferred because of their greater specificity, and they exert a less deleterious effect on the normal body flora.

GENERAL PRINCIPLES OF DRUG ADMINISTRATION

In order to achieve adequate tissue concentrations of the drug, several factors should be considered.

AGE OF ANIMAL. Higher doses of drug and a reduced frequency of administration are generally recommended for neonates, because of a greater volume of drug distribution and immature metabolic mechanisms, which lead to decreased drug clearance.

DEGREE OF HYDRATION. Dehydration, by decreasing renal clearance, will decrease the required frequency of administration. To adhere to the standard dosing interval in a situation of dehydration is to court toxicity (e.g., renal toxicity with aminoglycosides).

ROUTE OF ADMINISTRATION. Some drugs (e.g., aminoglycosides) are poorly absorbed from the gastrointestinal tract and thus fail to exert systemic effects. Ruminal bacteria may deactivate drugs administered orally.

ANTIBACTERIAL DRUGS

β-Lactam Antibiotics

Table 15–1 lists the route of administration and spectrum of activity for the β-lactam antibiotics.

Mechanism of Action

The β-lactam antibiotics act by inhibiting transpeptidation during bacterial cell wall synthesis, leading to weak cell walls and lysis of the organism. Efficacy of the β-lactam antibiotics is determined by their ability to penetrate the outer layer of the bacterium and bind to certain intracellular proteins, and by their susceptibility to β-lactamases. An important aspect of β-lactam antibiotic therapy is the maintenance of serum concentrations greater than the minimum inhibitory concentration. The antibacterial action of these drugs is time dependent.

Types of β-Lactam Antibiotics

PENICILLINS. Members of this group in common use include benzyl penicillin (penicillin G), ampicillin, amoxicillin, cloxacillin, and ticarcillin.

CEPHALOSPORINS. These drugs are not commonly used in large animals because of their high cost. Two exceptions are ceftiofur sodium, a third-generation cephalosporin, and cephaloridine, a first-generation cephalosporin.

Toxicity

In general, β-lactam antibiotics have low toxicity.

TABLE 15–1. THE β-LACTAM ANTIBIOTICS

Drug	Route of Administration*	Spectrum of Activity	Comments
Penicillins			
Benzyl penicillin (penicillin G)	i.v., i.m., s.c., i.my.	Gram-positive organisms, anaerobes, except *Bacillis fragilis*	Penetrates poorly into central nervous system; inactivated by β-lactamase
Penicillin V	p.o.	Gram-positive organisms	Very high oral doses required to attain effective serum concentrations
Ampicillin	i.v., i.m., i.my., s.c., p.o.	Gram-positive, some gram-negative organisms	Inactivated by β-lactamase; oral route useful in foals; low serum concentrations with i.m. administation
Amoxicillin	i.v., i.m., p.o.	Gram-positive, some gram-negative organisms	Used orally in foals; otherwise rarely used in horses or other large animals
Ticarcillin	i.v., i.u., i.m.	Broad spectrum, especially *Pseudomonas* spp.	Susceptible to β-lactamase, synergistic with aminoglycosides
Ticarcillin and clavulanic acid	i.v., i.u.	Broad spectrum, especially *Pseudomonas* spp.	Addition of clavulanic acid overcomes β-lactamase activity
Cloxacillin	i.my.	Gram-positive organisms, especially β-lactamase-producing bacteria	Very effective in *Staphylococcus aureus* mastitis
Cephalosporins			
Cephapirin	i.m., i.my.	Gram-positive organisms; anaerobes, except *B. fragilis*	Most commonly used as lactating and dry cow intramammary infusions
Ceftiofur	i.m.	Gram-positive, gram-negative organisms	Approved for use only in beef and dairy cattle

*i.v. = intravenous, i.m. = intramuscular, s.c. = subcutaneous, p.o. = per os, i.my. = intramammary, i.u. = intrauterine.

Aminoglycosides

Table 15–2 lists the route of administration and spectrum of activity for the aminoglycosides.

Mechanism of Action

Members of this group act by inhibiting protein synthesis at the ribosomal level. To achieve maximum bactericidal effect, aminoglycosides should be administered to achieve high serum concentrations. The antibacterial effect of these drugs is concentration dependent, and it is not necessary or desirable to maintain serum concentrations greater than the minimum inhibitory concentration for prolonged periods.

Toxicity

Toxicity is related to serum trough concentration, rather than to peak concentration.

NEPHROTOXICITY. Nephrotoxicity is a complication of prolonged therapy. Occurrence is related to age, duration of therapy, frequency of administration, hydration status, and the particular drug used.

OTOTOXICITY. Damage to the auditory and vestibular neural tissue may occur.

NEUROMUSCULAR BLOCKADE. Aminoglycosides should be used with caution in anesthetized patients, and they probably should not be used in association with neuromuscular blocking agents.

Resistance

Resistance to aminoglycosides is mediated by bacterial enzymes. Amikacin appears to be more resistant to enzymatic degradation than other aminoglycosides (e.g., gentamicin and streptomycin).

Tetracyclines

Table 15–3 lists the route of administration and spectrum of activity for the tetracyclines.

Mechanism of Action

The tetracyclines interfere with protein synthesis at the ribosomal level.

Toxicity

GASTROINTESTINAL. Diarrhea occurs due to changes in intestinal microflora. Mainly a problem in horses. The real incidence is unknown but appears to be low.

TABLE 15–2. THE AMINOGLYCOSIDES

Drug	Route of Administration*	Spectrum of Activity	Comments
Streptomycin	i.m., i.my.	Gram-negative, *Leptospira* spp.	Not very effective in horses; resistance common
Neomycin	Topical, p.o., i.my., Op.	Gram-negative organisms	Commonly used for mastitis, for ophthalmic infections, and as topical ointments; very nephrotoxic if administered parenterally
Gentamicin	i.m., i.v., Op., i.u.	Gram-negative organisms, especially *Pseudomonas* spp.; some gram-positive effect	Commonly used in equine practice for systemic infections, septicemia; also effective for endometritis; do not mix with other drugs in same container
Amikacin	i.m., i.v., Op.	Gram-negative organisms primarily; some gram-positive effect	Widest spectrum activity of aminoglycosides in current use; often efficacious against organisms resistant to other aminoglycosides (especially *Pseudomonas*)
Tobramycin	Op.	Gram-negative organisms, especially *Pseudomonas* spp.; some gram-positive effect	Frequently useful for treatment of gentamicin-resistant strains of *Pseudomonas*; generally too expensive for systemic administration

*Op. = ophthalmic ointment or solution. The rest of the abbreviations are defined in Table 15–1.

TABLE 15–3. THE TETRACYCLINES

Drug	Route of Administration*	Spectrum of Activity	Comments
Chlortetracycline	p.o., i.my., i.u.	Gram-positive organisms; gram-negative organisms; rickettsiae; *Mycoplasma* spp.	Not in common use
Oxytetracycline	i.m., i.v.	Gram-positive organisms; gram-negative organisms; rickettsiae; *Mycoplasma* spp.	Achieves high concentrations in body tissues; irritant if administered i.m. or perivascularly (especially in horses); long-acting depot preparation available
Tetracycline	i.m., i.v.	See Chlortetracycline and Oxytetracycline	See Chlortetracycline and Oxytetracycline
Doxycycline, minocycline	i.v.	Wider spectrum of activity against gram-positive organisms, gram-negative organisms, rickettsiae, anaerobes	Expensive

*Abbreviations are defined in Table 15–1.

RENAL. Renal tubular necrosis can occur, especially in the presence of endotoxemia or dehydration.

OTHER. Rapid intravenous administration of tetracycline solutions can cause hypotension and syncope. Chelation of calcium by tetracycline may be responsible for these signs.

Sulfonamides and Potentiated Sulfonamides

Table 15–4 lists the route of administration and spectrum of activity for the sulfonamides and potentiated sulfonamides.

Mechanism of Action

Sulfonamides, trimethoprim, and pyrimethamine act by inhibiting folic acid synthesis. Pyrimethamine and trimethoprim inhibit tetrahydrofolate reductase. Whereas trimethoprim has high affinity for the bacterial enzyme, pyrimethamine is more effective in inhibiting protozoal tetrahydrofolate reductase. Sulfonamides and trimethoprim are often combined (potentiated sulfonamides), resulting in bactericidal activity. Either agent used alone is bacteriostatic.

Toxicity

Renal tubular toxicity may occur. It is predisposed to by volume depletion and acid urine.

Macrolides

Table 15–5 lists the route of administration and spectrum of activity for the macrolides.

Mechanism of Action

Macrolides inhibit RNA-dependent protein synthesis in the bacterial cell.

Toxicity

Macrolides must *not* be given orally to ruminants; these agents have been associated with diarrhea in this species. Mild diarrhea is a common side effect of erythromycin therapy in foals. The gastrointestinal effects of erythromycin (diarrhea) are probably related to its action at motilin receptors.

In pigs, rectal edema, erythema of skin, and diarrhea occur, especially with tylosin.

Text continued on page 285

TABLE 15–4. THE SULFONAMIDES AND POTENTIATED SULFONAMIDES

Drug	Route of Administration*	Spectrum of Activity	Comments
Gut Acting			
Sulfaguanidine	p.o.	Gram-positive, some gram-negative organisms	Poorly absorbed from gastrointestinal tract; used historically for treatment of diarrhea in farm animals
Phthalylsulfathiazole	p.o.		
Sulfathiazole	p.o.		
Other Sulfonamides			
Sulfamethazine (sulfadimidine)	i.v., p.o.	Gram-positive, some gram-negative organisms	Useful for treatment of systemic and urinary tract infections; irritant if administered perivascularly or intraperitoneally; rapidly absorbed from gut, rapidly excreted
Sulfamerazine	p.o., i.v.	Gram-positive organisms, some gram-negative organisms	Similar to sulfadimidine
Sulfamethoxazole	p.o., i.v.		
Sulfadiazine	p.o., i.v.		
Potentiated Sulfonamides[a]			
Trimethoprim and			
Sulfadiazine	p.o., s.c., i.v.	Gram-positive organisms, gram-negative organisms, ineffective against *Leptospira, Pseudomonas, Bacteroides,* and *Erysipelothrix* spp; effective against *Toxoplasma gondii,* other protozoa	Combinations are bactericidal; all sulfonamides are potentially nephrotoxic; combinations penetrate into central nervous system to achieve therapeutic concentrations
Sulfadoxine	p.o., i.v., i.m.		
Sulfamethoxazole	p.o.		

*Abbreviations are defined in Table 15–1.
[a]Combinations of trimethoprim and a sulfonamide, usually in a ratio of 1:5.

TABLE 15–5. THE MACROLIDES

Drug	Route of Administration*	Spectrum of Activity	Comments
Erythromycin	p.o., i.m., i.v.	Gram-positive organisms, esp. *Staphylococcus*, *Streptococcus*, *Clostridium*, *Mycoplasma*, and *Leptospira* spp.	Low toxicity, cholestasis and hepatotoxicity can occur; erythromycin and rifampin are used in combination for *Rhodococcus equi* infection in foals; a long-acting intramuscular preparation has recently been developed
Tilmicosin	s.c.	*Pasteurella* spp., *Haemophilus somnus*, *Staphylococcus* spp., *Actinomyces pyogenes*, *Clostridium* spp., *Mycoplasma* spp.	Marketed for treating shipping fever in cattle; 28-day meat withdrawal required; claimed to achieve effective tissue concentrations for prolonged period, hence a 72-h dosing interval
Tylosin	i.m.	Similar to erythromycin; very effective for *Mycoplasma* spp. infections, gram-positive organisms and some gram-negative organisms	Can cause pruritus and rectal edema in pigs; the drug is primarily used in pigs, but may be used to treat pneumonias in cattle

*Abbreviations are defined in Table 15–1.

TABLE 15–6. MISCELLANEOUS ANTIMICROBIAL DRUGS

Drug	Route of Administration*	Spectrum of Activity	Comments
Antibacterial Agents			
Bacitracin	p.o., topical	Gram-positive organisms, little activity against gram-negative organisms	Very toxic if given parenterally; most commonly used as a component of triple-antibiotic ophthalmic ointments; oral form used as growth promoter for swine
Chloramphenicol	p.o., i.m., i.v.	Broad spectrum; aerobic and anaerobic bacteria; especially useful for salmonellosis, other gram-negative infections	Enters cerebrospinal fluid even when meningitis is not present; penetrates most tissues (e.g., pleurae, mammary glands); banned for use in food animals in some countries
Lincomycin, clindamycin	i.m., i.v.	Gram-positive organisms, similar to erythromycin; effective against anaerobes	Must not be given orally to ruminants; has caused severe depression, diarrhea, death
Polymixin	p.o., i.my., topical	Gram-negative organisms; binds endotoxin	Used as a component of intramammary preparations and oral antidiarrheal boluses; high risk of nephrotoxicity if administered systemically
Nitrofurazone	p.o., topical	Gram-positive organisms, gram-negative organisms	Used orally for salmonellosis in food animals; has antiprotozoal activity; used topically for wound infections; nephrotoxic if administered systemically
Furazolidone	p.o.	Gram-positive organisms, gram-negative organisms, some protozoa	Poorly absorbed when given orally; used for treatment of enteric diseases such as salmonellosis
Rifampicin	p.o.	Gram-positive organisms, bacteria, chlamydia, some antiviral effects	Resistance develops quickly, therefore usually used in combination (e.g., with erythromycin for *Rhodococcus equi* pneumonia)

Arsanilic acid, sodium arsanilate	p.o.	Some gram-negative organisms	Used for prevention of scours in pigs, especially swine dysentery
Metronidazole	p.o., i.v.	Anaerobes	Effective for anaerobic infections (e.g., pulmonary abscessation); used topically for irrigation of foot abscesses; rapid i.v. administration may cause collapse
Tiamulin	p.o.	Treponema hyodysenteriae	Used in the treatment of swine dysentery; administered in drinking water; not recommended for use in breeding swine
Antifungal Agents			
Griseofulvin	p.o.	Dermatophytes	Concentrates in stratum corneum; fungistatic effect; not recommended for use in pregnant animals
Thiabendazole	p.o., topical	Dermatophytes	Useful for topical fungal infections; has been used for mycotic ruminitis in cattle
Miconazole	Op.	Broad spectrum	Used for treatment of mycotic keratitis; expensive
Amphotericin B	Op., parenteral	Broad spectrum	Main use is for treatment of mycotic keratitis; 0.10–0.25% solution
Pimaricin	Op.	Broad spectrum	Can be used as a 5% solution for treatment of mycotic keratitis
Nystatin	Topical, Op.	Dermatophytes; *Aspergillus, Candida* spp.	Poorly absorbed; too toxic for parenteral use

Table continued on following page

TABLE 15–6. MISCELLANEOUS ANTIMICROBIAL DRUGS Continued

Drug	Route of Administration*	Spectrum of Activity	Comments
Antiprotozoal Agents			
Furazolidone	p.o.	Coccidia	Also effective against some bacterial infections
Potentiated sulfonamides	p.o., i.v., s.c.	Coccidia, other protozoa (e.g., Toxoplasma gondii, Sarcocystis spp.)	Antibacterial effects also
Amprolium	p.o.	Coccidia	Used for prevention and treatment of coccidiosis in several species
Monensin, lasalocid, salinomycin	p.o.	Coccidia, T. gondii	Used as growth promoters in ruminants, modifiers of ruminal flora; also have significant antiprotozoal activity
Pyrimethamine	p.o.	Sarcocystis spp., T. gondii	Used in conjunction with potentiated sulfonamides for treatment of equine protozoal myelitis
Amicarbalide	i.m., s.c.	Babesia spp.	Can be given slowly i.v., but usually administered intramuscularly
Quinuronium	s.c.	Babesia spp.	Can occasionally cause sudden onset of hypotension and shock; some preparations contain epinephrine to prevent bradycardia and hypotension
Imidocarb	s.c., i.m.	Babesia, Anaplasma, Ehrlichia spp.	Useful for prevention of disease, if higher doses are used
Diminazene	s.c., i.m.	Babesia spp.	Few side effects; occasionally severe reactions at injection site, especially in horses

*Abbreviations are defined in Table 15–1.

MISCELLANEOUS ANTIMICROBIAL DRUGS

Table 15–6 lists other antibacterial agents, as well as antifungal and antiprotozoal agents.

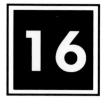

Parasitology

HORSES

Endoparasites

Foals (Up to 6 Months)

THREADWORMS. (*Strongyloides westeri*) Affect younger foals.
Prepatent Period. Approximately 5–7 days.
Pathogenesis. Enteritis, with diarrhea, may result from heavy infestations. Infection is usually by ingestion of mare's milk; percutaneous infection may occur.
T R E A T M E N T: Benzimidazoles (BZD), ivermectin, or pyrantel.

ROUNDWORMS. (*Parascaris equorum*) Affect foals up to 1 year of age.
Pathogenesis. Ingestion, followed by hepatotracheal migration. Coughing, nasal discharge within a few days of infection, poor growth, and diarrhea. Occasionally ileal impaction may result from heavy infections.
T R E A T M E N T: Administer BZD, ivermectin, levamisole, piperazine, pyrantel, or organophosphates.

LARGE STRONGYLES. (*S. vulgaris, S. equinus, S. edentatus*) Affect older foals.

Prepatent Period. S. *vulgaris:* 180–200 days; S. *equinus:* 270 days; S. *edentatus:* 300–320 days.

Pathogenesis. Migrating S. *vulgaris* causes cranial mesenteric arteritis; occasionally other arteries are affected. S. *equinus* migrates through liver and pancreas, and S. *edentatus* migrates through subperitoneal tissues, especially in the right flank. Adult large strongyles are bloodsuckers in the large colon and cecum. Anemia may result from heavy infections. Colic may occur. Only migratory stages are of clinical importance in foals.

T R E A T M E N T: Immature stages: Thiabendazole (TBZ) (440 mg/kg) or fenbendazole (FBZ) (50 mg/kg) for 2 consecutive days, or FBZ (10 mg/kg) for 5 consecutive days, or ivermectin (0.2 mg/kg) once, or oxfendazole (OFZ) (10 mg/kg) once. Adult stages: BZD at standard dosages, febantel (6 mg/kg), pyrantel (6.6 mg/kg), or trichlorfon (40 mg/kg).

SMALL STRONGYLES. (cyathostomes) Over 40 species affect all age groups.

Prepatent Period. 5–14 weeks.

Pathogenesis. Usually moderately pathogenic. Now considered to be more pathogenic than was thought previously. Hypobiotic larvae may exsheath simultaneously from the cecal and colonic mucosae in early spring, causing a marked protein-losing enteropathy, with diarrhea and weight loss.

T R E A T M E N T: Larval stages: As for large strongyles. Adults: As for large strongyles. BZD-resistant cyathostome strains are recognized. These are susceptible to the non-BZD drugs mentioned above and to oxibendazole (OBZ) (10 mg/kg) for adult stages.

TAPEWORMS. (*Anoplocephala perfoliata, A. magna, Paranoplocephala mamillana*) Affect all age groups. Oribatid mites act as intermediate hosts.

Pathogenesis. Adult tapeworms develop 4–6 weeks after ingestion of mites. Parasite colonizes gut in region of ileocecal orifice. Has been incriminated in catarrhal enteritis, ulceration, and intussusception.

T R E A T M E N T: Pyrantel (13.2 mg/kg), mebendazole (MBZ) (15–20 mg/kg), or niclosamide (100–300 mg/kg).

Adult Horses

The foal, weanling, and adult horse have many parasites in common. The following are of clinical significance in the adult horse.

LARGE AND SMALL STRONGYLES. (*Strongyloides vulgaris, S. equinus, S. edentatus*) See Foals.

ROUNDWORMS. (*Parascaris equorum*) Affect horses up to 2 years. Age-related resistance develops.

TAPEWORMS. (*Anoplocephala perfoliata, A. magna, Paranoplocephala mamillana*) See Foals.

PINWORMS. (*Oxyuris equi*) Mainly affect adult horses.

Prepatent Period: 120–150 days.

Pathogenesis: Colonize rectum, colon, and cecum. Pruritus of perineum develops; horses lose tail hairs from constant rubbing.

T R E A T M E N T: Adult stages: BZD, ivermectin (0.2 mg/kg), organophosphates, or febantel (6 mg/kg).

STOMACH WORMS. (*Trichostrongylus axei, Draschia megastoma, Habronema muscae, H. majus*) May affect any age group, but mainly adults. Gastritis and ulceration may result; *D. megastoma* may cause gastric granuloma. The spirurid worms (*Draschia* and *Habronema* spp.) are associated with cutaneous lesions, i.e., "summer sore."

T R E A T M E N T: Administer ivermectin orally (0.2 mg/kg).

BOT-FLY LARVAE. (*Gasterophilus* spp.) Affect all age groups.

Pathogenesis. Life cycle is completed in 1 year. During the summer, the fly deposits eggs on the horse's coat, especially the forelegs and shoulders. Following ingestion, larvae attach to the gastric mucosa. In early spring they are shed, pupate, exsheath, and mate. Lesions vary— mild gastritis to gastric ulceration, rarely perforation.

T R E A T M E N T: Treat in late fall (once all adult flies are dead) to break life cycle. Trichlorfon (40 mg/kg), dichlorvos (20 mg/kg), or ivermectin (0.2 mg/kg).

LUNGWORMS. (*Dictyocaulus arnfieldi*) Affect adult horses in temperate regions.

Prepatent Period. Approximately 4 weeks. Rarely becomes patent in the horse. The donkey is the natural host and is the usual source of infection for the horse.

Pathogenesis. Severe bronchitis and hyperplasia of bronchial epithelium, with coughing.

T R E A T M E N T: Deworm donkeys or remove them from pasture. Effective anthelmintics include ivermectin (0.2 mg/kg) or MBZ (15–20 mg/kg) daily for 5 consecutive days.

Parasites of Skin and Subcutaneous Tissues (All Ages)

WORM NODULE DISEASE. (*Onchocerca cervicalis*) Affects all ages. Transmitted by midges. Adults are found in the ligamentum nuchae and subcutaneous tissue. Microfilariae may be seen in dermal tissues and lymph vessels. *O. cervicalis* has been implicated in cases of periodic ophthalmia.

T R E A T M E N T: Administer ivermectin orally (0.2 mg/kg).

SUMMER SORES. (*Habronema majus, H. muscae, Draschia megastoma*) Affect all age groups; horses in warm climates.
Pathogenesis. These spirurid nematodes are deposited as larvae on open wounds by the housefly or stable fly. Granulomatous reaction ensues (cutaneous habronemiasis, called "summer sores"). Affects distal limbs, occasionally head region, conjunctivae, and prepuce.
T R E A T M E N T: Administer ivermectin orally (0.2 mg/kg).

Ectoparasites

Lice

BITING LOUSE. (*Damalinia equi*) Affects all age groups.
Pathogenesis. Skin irritation, with pruritus and ill-thrift in heavy infestations. Head, mane, tail most frequently affected.
T R E A T M E N T: Ivermectin (0.2 mg/kg) or topical organophosphates or pyrethrins (two treatments 14 days apart) are recommended.

SUCKING LOUSE. (*Haematopinus asini*). Affects all age groups.
Pathogenesis. Similar signs to *D. equi.*
T R E A T M E N T: Topical organophosphates or pyrethrins (two treatments 14 days apart) are recommended. Ivermectin (0.2 mg/kg) may be effective.

Mites

CHORIOPTES EQUI. Fetlocks most frequently affected. Causes irritation and occasionally kicking out with hindlimbs; more common on heavily feathered limbs.
T R E A T M E N T: Topical organophosphate washes (two treatments 2 weeks apart) or ivermectin orally (0.2 mg/kg).

SARCOPTES SCABIEI. Rare. Head, neck, and shoulder are affected initially. Scaling, weeping, and hair loss occur. Reportable disease.
T R E A T M E N T: Ivermectin (0.2 mg/kg), topical organophosphates, or lime sulfur may be used.

PSOROPTES EQUI, P. CUNICULI. Occasionally causes head shaking if ear canal is infested. Mane and tail area and sometimes fetlock may be affected.
T R E A T M E N T: Ivermectin (0.2 mg/kg), topical organophosphates, or lime sulfur may be used.

CHIGGERS. (*Trombicula autumnalis*) Occasionally cause weals, small papules; pruritus develops. Usually self-limiting.

T R E A T M E N T: Topical organophosphates or lime sulfur may be used.

Flies

BITING FLIES. (*Stomoxys calcitrans, Simulium, Haemotobia, Culicoides* spp.) *S. calcitrans*, tabanids, black flies (*Simulium* spp.), and the face fly (*Haematobia*) may cause painful bite wounds. *Culicoides* spp. are associated with hypersensitivity reactions (sweet itch), especially over base of tail.

T R E A T M E N T: Topical fly repellents. Systemic corticosteroids are recommended for severe hypersensitivity to *Culicoides* spp.

Parasite Control

Fecal egg output follows a seasonal pattern. Two peaks in egg numbers occur, one in spring and a second in summer. Corresponding to this are summer/autumn peaks of infective larvae on pasture. Treatment strategies are designed to reduce the degree of pasture contamination, and consequently the worm challenge to the host. The primary pathogenic groups of worms are large and small strongyles (cyathostomes), and most programs are aimed at their control. The majority of anthelmintics are effective against the adult stages of these worms; however, in recent years, resistance of cyathostomes to BZDs, with the exception of OBZ, has been recognized.

BZD resistance should be suspected if fecal egg counts remain high 1–2 weeks after the administration of a BZD anthelmintic, when counts should be less than 50 eggs/g (epg).

Significance of Egg Counts

Egg counts are a useful guide to the degree of infection of an animal or group of animals. Individual variations in egg count occur at similar levels of infection, depending on the immune status of the host. The consistency and volume of feces also influence the epg. In general, less than 500 epg indicates mild infection, while more than 1,500 epg indicates severe parasitism.

Control Programs

1. All animals should be treated on arrival at the farm and isolated for a minimum of 48 h before gaining access to pasture.

2. Mares should be treated soon after foaling, to eliminate the periparturient rise in fecal egg counts, before being placed on pasture.

3. Treat mares and foals with a broad-spectrum anthelmintic every 4 weeks, or ivermectin every 8 weeks, to prevent summer and

autumn peaks of infective larvae on pasture. Foals should be treated from 8 weeks of age.

4. Treat in late autumn with an anthelmintic effective against bot-fly larvae (e.g., organophosphates, ivermectin).

5. Pasture concentrations of infective larvae can be markedly reduced by twice-weekly collection of fecal deposits from paddocks, especially where there are high stocking rates. This may reduce the requirement for frequent administration of anthelmintics.

6. Anthelmintics should be rotated every 1–2 years to reduce selection pressure for resistant strains.

7. Foals may require treatment if clinical signs of *Strongyloides westeri* develop. Most broad-spectrum anthelmintics are effective.

8. Donkeys may be a reservoir of *Dictyocaulus arnfieldi*. To prevent clinical disease in in-contact horses, donkeys should be treated with an appropriate anthelmintic or removed from the pasture.

9. Tapeworm infections, usually due to *A. perfoliata*, may be associated with clinical disease in weanlings and young adults. Two to four times the normal dose of pyrantel pamoate is efficacious, usually administered in the fall of the first grazing season.

10. Moving horses to a clean pasture after treatment, as described for cattle, will aid significantly in parasite control. Grazing horses and ruminants on the same pasture is also practiced for a similar reason.

CATTLE

Endoparasites

Protozoa

CRYPTOSPORIDIOSIS. Common in calves.

Pathogenesis. Have been associated with diarrhea and malabsorption.

T R E A T M E N T: None currently in use. Supportive care is important. Control has depended on isolating affected calves and moving calf hutches to a clean area. Halofuginone lactate (60–125 μg/kg for 7 days) has proved effective in reducing oocyte shedding in experimentally infected calves.

COCCIDIOSIS. (*Eimeria zurnii, E. bovis*) Usually affects calves; also causes "winter coccidiosis" in housed adult cattle.

Pathogenesis. Acute onset of diarrhea, especially with large intestine involvement. Leakage of albumin leads to hypoproteinemia, weight loss, and decreased food consumption. A nervous form of coccidiosis may occur, usually in feedlot animals.

T R E A T M E N T: Oral sulfonamides, or amprolium. Control depends on environmental hygiene and prophylactic chemotherapy using amprolium, lasalocid, decoquinate, or monensin.

SARCOCYSTOSIS. (*Sarcocystis cruzi*) Spread by carnivores (e.g., dog, raccoon, fox).

Pathogenesis. Inflammation of vascular endothelium with fever, weight loss, edema, and abortion are common findings. Loss of hair at the tail tip (rat-tail) is often seen.

T R E A T M E N T: None effective. Amprolium and salinomycin have been used with limited success. Control by avoiding contamination of feed by dog feces.

BABESIOSIS. (*Babesia bigemina, B. bovis, B. divergens*) Young calves are resistant; young weanlings and adults are affected.

Pathogenesis. Fever, acute anemia with hemoglobinuria. Death may occur quickly in severe cases. "Pipe stem" diarrhea may be seen in early stages. Transmitted by ticks; the disease is seasonal.

T R E A T M E N T: Quinuronium sulfate, diminazene aceturate, imidocarb, or amicarbalide.

Roundworms (Nematodes)

Treatment of nematodiasis, cestodiasis, and trematodiasis is discussed in the section on parasite control, pp. 297–298.

OSTERTAGIA OSTERTAGI. Parasite of the abomasum.

Prepatent Period. Approximately 17 days. Can survive on pasture for 4 months.

Pathogenesis. *Type 1* ostertagiasis is manifested by diarrhea in late summer or early fall, in animals at pasture for the first time. *Type 2* is due to the emergence of hypobiotic larvae. It is manifested by acute onset of diarrhea and hypoproteinemia, in late winter or early spring (in northern temperate zones) after the animal's first grazing season. Chronic diarrhea and weight loss occur, often leading to death.

HAEMONCHUS CONTORTUS. Mainly a disease of sheep and goats. Calves may be affected.

Pathogenesis. Acute blood loss leads to anemia, hypoproteinemia, and growth retardation.

TRICHOSTRONGYLUS AXEI, T. COLUBRIFORMIS. Usually a mild infection of abomasum (*T. axei*) or anterior small intestine (*T. colubriformis*).

Pathogenesis. A mild catarrhal enteritis is the common presentation. Occasionally severe diarrhea and hypoproteinemia may occur.

COOPERIA SPP. Inhabit the small intestine and occasionally the abomasum. Presentation similar to *T. axei* infection.

BUNOSTOMUM PHLEBOTOMUM. Mainly in southern and midwestern USA, Africa, Europe.

Pathogenesis. Bloodsucking parasite. In heavy infections, diarrhea, weakness, and anemia are seen.

CHABERTIA OVINA. Inhabits the colon.

Prepatent Period. 50 days.

Pathogenesis. Larval stage may cause epithelial erosion, and animals may develop diarrhea and weight loss.

DICTYOCAULUS VIVIPARUS. Disease occurs in young calves toward the end of the first grazing season.

Pathogenesis. Adult stages develop in bronchi. Signs vary in severity from chronic dry cough to acute subcutaneous emphysema, with respiratory distress and death in severe cases.

Tapeworms (Cestodes)

MONIEZIA EXPANSA, M. BENEDENI. Inhabit the small intestine. Oribatid mites are involved in the life cycle.

Pathogenesis. Rarely cause clinical disease. Have been associated with diarrhea and ill-thrift.

CYSTICERCUS BOVIS. Cattle act as intermediate host for *Taenia saginata*, a parasite of humans. The metacestode, *C. bovis*, parasitizes skeletal and cardiac muscle.

Pathogenesis. Clinical disease does not occur in cattle. Severely affected carcasses are condemned at meat inspection.

Control. Prevent access to human sewage.

Flukes (Trematodes)

PARAMPHISTOMUM SPP. Inhabits rumen and reticulum. Snail acts as intermediate host. Adults occur in rumen and are generally nonpathogenic. Immature forms irritate duodenum, causing catarrhal or hemorrhagic enteritis.

DICROCOELIUM DENDRITICUM. Inhabits bile ducts and gallbladder. Snails and ants act as intermediate hosts. Infected ants are ingested by the final host (ruminant).

Pathogenesis. Mild infections are subclinical. Severe infections are manifested by weight loss and hypoproteinemia.

FASCIOLA HEPATICA. North America, Europe, Asia, Africa. Parasite inhabits the bile ducts and gallbladder.

Prepatent Period. More than 8 weeks.

Pathogenesis. Metacercariae develop in the snail (*Lymnaea* spp.). Cattle ingest the snail with herbage; flukes migrate from the intestine through the liver parenchyma, causing acute traumatic hepatitis, which is more severe with heavy infection. Anorexia, depression, and death may occur; Black disease (*Clostridium novyi* type B) may be precipitated by this migration. Chronic disease results from the presence of mature flukes in the bile ducts. Hypoproteinemia, emaciation, and depression occur.

Ectoparasites

Ticks

BOOPHILUS ANNULATUS. Mexico, Africa. Eradicated from USA. Important in transmission of *Babesia bigemina* and *Anaplasma marginale*.

IXODES RICINUS. Europe, North Africa. Three-year life cycle.

Pathogenesis. During feeding they may transmit *Babesia* spp., *A. marginale*, border disease virus, louping-ill virus (Western Europe).

DERMACENTOR ANDERSONI. Western USA. Tick may transmit anaplasmosis and several other diseases.

OTOBIUS MEGNINI. The spinose ear tick. Widespread in USA. Larvae attach to skin, engorge, and migrate to ear, where they molt and develop to adult form. Chronic irritation may result, leading to head shaking and occasionally secondary otitis externa.

Mites

SARCOPTES SCABIEI VAR. BOVIS. Rare in cattle. May cause hair loss over neck region and head.

PSOROPTES BOVIS. Uncommon.

CHORIOPTES BOVIS. Causes foot and tail mange. Scaliness and alopecia may develop on the tail and hindlegs.

DEMODEX BOVIS. Inhabits hair follicles. Hair loss and development of pustules, with nodular thickening of the skin. Pruritus is rare.

Lice

BOVICOLA BOVIS. Biting louse. Infestation occurs by direct contact with infected animals. Disease is usually noticed in winter, and poorly nourished cattle are most severely affected. Signs include hair loss over the head, shoulders, and tail region, with excessive rubbing and licking of affected areas.

HAEMATOPINUS EURYSTERNUS. Sucking louse. See *Bovicola bovis*.

SOLENOPOTES CAPILLATUS. Sucking louse. See *Bovicola bovis*.

LINOGNATHUS VITULI. Sucking louse. See *Bovicola bovis*.

Warbles

HYPODERMA LINEATUM. Adult flies lay eggs on lower extremities. Larvae migrate to the esophageal submucosa. After 3 months the larvae migrate to the subcutaneous tissues of the dorsum and perforate the skin. The resulting hide damage causes severe economic loss.

H. BOVIS. See *Hypoderma lineatum*. Larvae migrate to the epidural space.

Flies

HAEMATOBIA IRRITANS. Horn fly. These flies, by causing irritation, disturb the normal grazing pattern of cattle and thus lead to weight loss.

STOMOXYS CALCITRANS. Stable fly. See *Haematobia irritans*.
TABANUS SPP. Horse fly. See *Haematobia irritans*.
SIMULIUM SPP. Black fly. See *Haematobia irritans*.

SHEEP AND GOATS

Many of the parasitic conditions described for cattle also occur in sheep and goats.

Endoparasites

Protozoa

COCCIDIOSIS. (*Eimeria* spp.) Can be a problem in animals kept under intensive management conditions. Kids are particularly susceptible.

BABESIA SPP. (*B. motasi, B. ovis*) Identified in South America, parts of Africa, and Eastern Europe. Similar presentation to disease in cattle.

Roundworms (Nematodes)

OSTERTAGIA SPP. Cause disease similar to that in cattle.
TRICHOSTRONGYLUS SPP. Cause disease similar to that in cattle.
HAEMONCHUS CONTORTUS. Barber's pole worm. Affects the abomasum. Blood loss can be severe. Adult worms and 4th-stage larvae are bloodsuckers. Anemia and hypoproteinemia may cause sudden death. Diarrhea is not a feature of haemonchosis; however, mixed infections are common (e.g., *Trichostrongylus* spp.), so diarrhea may be present.

NEMATODIRUS SPP. Cause severe diarrhea in young lambs (black scours).

Lungworms

DICTYOCAULUS FILARIA. Causes disease similar to that caused by *D. viviparus* in cattle.

MUELLERIUS CAPILLARIS. Indirect life cycle. Significance of this parasite is unclear, but clinical disease is thought to be rare.

PROTOSTRONGYLUS RUFESCENS. Indirect life cycle. Can cause disease similar to D. *filaria*. Primarily affects young animals.

Tapeworms (Cestodes)

MONIEZIA EXPANSA. Usually subclinical.

COENURUS CEREBRALIS. The sheep acts as an intermediate host for *Taenia multiceps*, a dog tapeworm. The larval stage develops into a fluid-filled cyst in the brain or spinal cord of the sheep. The clinical disease is often referred to as gid.

CYSTICERCUS TENUICOLLIS. Intermediate stage of *T. hydatigena*, a dog tapeworm. The larval form is found in the muscles of sheep.

Flukes (Trematodes)

LIVER FLUKE. (*Fasciola hepatica*) Acute, subacute, and chronic forms are recognized. Some outbreaks are complicated by Black disease. Severity of the fascioliasis is determined by the number of metacercariae ingested. Death in the acute form results from severe hemorrhage subsequent to blood vessel rupture in the liver.

STOMACH FLUKE. (*Paramphistomum* spp.) Causes disease similar to that in cattle.

DICROCOELIUM SPP. The disease is similar to that in cattle.

Ectoparasites

Ticks

Heavy infestations may cause weight loss. Major importance is their role in disease transmission. *Ixodes, Hyalomma, Rhipicephalus, Dermacentor* spp. are included.

Mites

PSOROPTES OVIS. Causes sheep scab, a notifiable disease. Severe pruritus and wool loss occur, especially over the flank.

SARCOPTES SCABIEI. Affects the face primarily. Severe pruritus and scab formation are seen.

CHORIOPTES BOVIS. Not common. Skin of the scrotum and hindlimbs becomes thickened and wrinkled.

DEMODEX OVIS. Rare. Pustules on nose, eyes, and coronet occur.

DEMODEX CAPRI. Small skin nodules are present on the face, neck, shoulders, and trunk. Nodules contain caseous material that can be easily expressed.

Flies

SHEEP KED. (*Melophagus ovinus*) A wingless fly. Bloodsucker. Causes intense irritation.

BLOW FLY. (*Phormia, Lucilia, Calliphora* spp.) Causes myiasis. Larvae develop in wet, soiled tissue. Intense pruritus. Severely affected patients may die.

HEAD FLY. (*Hydrotaea irritans*) Causes severe irritation to sheep, resulting in self-inflicted injury to the head. May predispose to fly-strike.

Louse Infestation

SHEEP
Linognathus ovillus. Sucking face louse.
L. stenopsis. Sucking goat louse.
L. pedalis. Sucking foot louse.
Damalinia ovis. Biting louse.
GOAT
L. stenopsis
D. caprae
D. limbata

Parasite Control (Ruminants)

Control and Treatment of Internal Parasitism

A combination of pasture management and the strategic administration of anthelmintics can be used to control internal parasites where intensive stocking of pasture is practiced. The ultimate aim is to reduce pasture contamination.

1. Eliminate the periparturient rise in fecal egg counts. This is of particular importance in ewes, because they are the major source of infection for lambs. Anthelmintics should be administered around the time of lambing.

2. Avoid overstocking.

3. Control access to wet areas of pasture, where buildup of parasites (e.g., liver fluke) is favored.

4. Avoid grazing young and older stock together, because older animals may act as a source of infection. Use a leader–follower system, with young animals grazing ahead of older animals.

5. Move animals to clean pasture in early to mid-summer, after deworming, to avoid reinfection.

CONTROL PROGRAM
- Spring: Deworm cows and ewes in periparturient period.
- Early to mid-summer: Deworm weanling stock and move to clean pasture.

TABLE 16–1. DRUGS USED IN TREATMENT AND CONTROL
OF ENDOPARASITISM IN RUMINANTS

Parasites	Group	Drugs
Nematodes	Benzimidazoles	Thiabendazole, mebendazole, fenbendazole, oxfendazole, albendazole
	Probenzimidazoles	Fenbantel
	Organophosphates	Dichlorvos
	Imidazothiazoles	Levamisole, tetramisole
	Tetrahydropyrimidines	Morantel, pyrantel
	Piperazines	Piperazine citrate, diethylcarbamazine
	Avermectins	Ivermectin
Cestodes	Salicylanilides	Niclosamide
	Benzimidazoles	Mebendazole
Trematodes	Salicylanilides	Oxyclozanide
	Substituted phenols	Nitroxinil, rafoxanide

Caution: It is important to remember that not all compounds are licensed for use in food-producing animals and that some are not intended for use in lactating dairy cattle and small ruminants. All compounds have specific withdrawal periods for meat and milk consumption. These warnings are marked clearly on the product data sheet.

● Late Fall-Early Winter: Deworm young stock/weanlings before housing to eliminate hypobiotic larvae and flukes.

T R E A T M E N T: Drugs used in the treatment and control of endoparasitism are shown in Table 16–1.

Control and Treatment of External Parasitism

A variety of methods are available for treatment and control of ectoparasitism. Control is facilitated by certain factors, e.g., shearing of sheep and pasture management.

The most commonly used method of ectoparasite control is the use of parasiticides. These may be applied as dips, sprays, or pour-on formulations. Parenteral administration of ivermectin is effective against most ectoparasites. *Caution:* Ivermectin is not licensed for administration to lactating animals.

Maggots, lice, and keds are susceptible to organophosphate compounds applied topically. Tail docking of lambs and removal of excess wool in the perineal region of adult sheep are effective in reducing the incidence of myiasis.

TICKS. Eradication of ticks is generally not possible because of their persistence in the environment and, in many instances, their ability to survive by parasitizing wildlife. Treatment and partial control may be achieved by the use of sprays, medicated ear tags, or dips. Ivermectin (0.2 mg/kg, s.c.) may also be effective. Other methods of control include ploughing or burning of pasture, and rotational grazing.

SHEEP SCAB. This is a notifiable disease but is believed to have been eradicated in the USA. Drugs effective against the parasite include γ-hexachlorocyclohexane, propetamphos, and diazinon. They are used as dips.

OTHER MITES. Organophosphates, applied topically, are effective against chorioptic and psoroptic mange. Two or three applications of organophosphates, 7 days apart, are often required for sarcoptic mange. In goats with demodicosis, rotenone (diluted 1:3 in surgical spirit) may be applied to affected areas or directly into affected pustules. Amitraz is effective against demodicosis and sarcoptic and psoroptic mange. Other topical dressings include 2% lime sulfur, benzyl benzoate, and 50% methoxychlor powder. Ivermectin is effective against demodectic, sarcoptic, and psoroptic mange and may be effective against chorioptic mange.

FLIES. Flies are a major source of irritation to ruminants at pasture. Control may be achieved by the use of medicated ear tags, medicated rubbing posts/ropes (animals self-medicate when rubbing against them), spraying, larvicidal feed additives, attractant intoxicants, or a growth regulator applied to insect breeding areas by aerial spraying. Moving sheep away from wooded areas may help decrease irritation caused by the head fly, *Hydrotoea irritans*. Headcaps have also been used in some areas.

LICE

Biting. Topical dressings such as organophosphates or lime sulfur are usually effective. Treatments should be repeated and should include all in-contact animals. Ivermectin (0.2 mg/kg, s.c.) may also be useful.

Sucking. Ivermectin (0.2 mg/kg, s.c.) is usually effective.

PIGS

Endoparasites

THREADWORMS. (*Strongyloides ransomi*) Affect piglets and weaners primarily.

Prepatent Period. 8–14 days.

Pathogenesis. Diarrhea, depression, anemia. Infection occurs via ingestion of colostrum, and prenatal infection has occurred in experimental settings. Free-living forms exist.

T R E A T M E N T: Improved hygiene. Thiabendazole, febantel, or ivermectin.

ROUNDWORMS. (*Ascaris suum*) Affect postweaning and growing pigs.

Prepatent Period. 6–8 weeks.

Pathogenesis. Clinical signs uncommon. Migrating larvae may cause a mild cough. Main economic losses are due to poor food conversion efficiency and the condemnation of liver (milk spots) and plucks at slaughter.

T R E A T M E N T: Ivermectin, dichlorvos, levamisole, febantel, piperazine, OBZ, or FBZ.

STOMACH WORMS. (*Hyostrongylus rubidus*) Affect sows mainly. Adult worms are located on the gastric mucosa. Sows are thin, with pale mucous membranes and skin. Probably contributes to reduced litter size and delayed return to estrus.

T R E A T M E N T: BZD, ivermectin, levamisole, febantel, or dichlorvos.

NODULAR WORMS. (*Oesophagostomum dentatum, O. quadrispinulatum*)

Prepatent Period. Approximately 45 days.

Pathogenesis. Adult worms live in the large bowel. The main effect is the reduction in weight gain. Heavy infections may cause diarrhea.

T R E A T M E N T: BZD, ivermectin, dichlorvos, levamisole, or febantel.

LUNGWORMS. (*Metastrongylus apri, M. pudendotectus, M. salmi*) Affect young animals (4–6 months) mainly; adults are usually resistant.

Prepatent Period. 20–24 days.

Pathogenesis. Common in herds with access to pasture. Earthworm is the intermediate host. Coughing and respiratory distress are the main signs.

T R E A T M E N T: Levamisole, ivermectin, FBZ, or febantel.

KIDNEY WORMS. (*Stephanurus dentatus*) Confined to tropical and subtropical climates.

Prepatent Period. 6–18 months.

Pathogenesis. Clinical signs are uncommon. Heavy infection may result in liver damage.

T R E A T M E N T: Ivermectin, levamisole, or FBZ.

WHIPWORMS. (*Trichuris suis*)

Prepatent Period. 6–12 weeks.

Pathogenesis. Adults inhabit the cecum and colon, embedded in the mucosa. Most infections are light and subclinical. Heavy infections may cause local inflammation in the large bowel, resulting in diarrhea containing blood clots.

T R E A T M E N T: FBZ, dichlorvos, ivermectin or levamisole.

TRICHINELLA SPIRALIS. The importance of *Trichinella* is its zoonotic (transmission from animals to humans) aspect.

Pathogenesis. In pigs, infection is generally light and clinical signs are absent. Humans become infected by ingesting raw or inadequately cooked pork or pork by-products. The disease in humans is marked by fever, myositis, myocarditis.

MISCELLANEOUS. (*Fasciola hepatica, Cysticercus cellulosae*) These parasites rarely cause clinical disease.

Ectoparasites

Mites

SARCOPTIC MANGE. (*Sarcoptes scabei* var. *suis*) Common in pig herds.

Pathogenesis. Sucking louse. Pruritus results from the burrowing and feeding activities of the lice. Excoriation of the skin results in serum loss and eventual hyperkeratinization of the skin. Secondary bacterial infection may develop.

Clinical Signs. Pruritus, skin erythema on localized areas.

T R E A T M E N T: Topical dressings such as γ-benzene hexachloride (BHC), bromocyclen, diazinon, amitraz, or ivermectin (0.3 mg/kg, s.c.).

DEMODICOSIS. (*Demodex phylloides*) Follicular mite. Relatively unimportant clinically.

Clinical Signs. Small reddened areas on the snout, around the eyelids, on the medial aspect of thighs, and along the abdomen.

T R E A T M E N T: Difficult to eradicate. Topical dressings such as amitraz and rotenone have been used successfully in other species.

Louse Infestation

HAEMATOPINUS SUIS. Sucking louse; the only louse that infests pigs. Rarely causes clinical problems, except when infestation is heavy. The louse is thought to be a vector for *Eperythrozoon suis* and the viruses of swine pox and African swine fever.

T R E A T M E N T: Ivermectin, organophosphates (pour-on solution), γ-BHC, or amitraz.

Parasite Control

Control of Endoparasitism in Pigs

Endoparasitism is unlikely to be a problem in pigs kept indoors on concrete floors. In extensive management systems, where pigs have access to pasture, helminth infections can be a problem.

The principles outlined for horses and ruminants, i.e., elimination of periparturient rise and prevention of pasture contamination, apply to the control of internal parasites in pigs.

Control Program for Extensive Management Systems

1. Treat breeding females with a broad-spectrum anthelmintic, e.g., TBZ (50 mg/kg) before breeding and again about 7 days before farrowing.
2. Move animals to clean pasture after treatment; if this is not possible, repeat treatment at 4–6-week intervals.
3. If lungworms are suspected, treat with levamisole, ivermectin, or FBZ.
4. Boars should be treated twice yearly.

Control Program for Pigs Kept Indoors

1. Treat breeding females before farrowing and again at weaning.
2. Treat weaners before entering fattening house and 8 weeks later.
3. Treat boars twice yearly.
4. Wash sow's udder before farrowing to remove threadworm larvae from skin.

NEW WORLD CAMELIDS

Specific information for parasite control in New World Camelids is not generally available. General principles should be applied. The information supplied for ruminants can be extrapolated to New World Camelids, which share many of the parasitic conditions. In areas where the white-tailed deer worm (*Parelaphostrongylus tenuis*) is a problem, ivermectin administration at 4-week intervals from May to September may be protective.

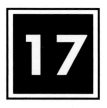

Vaccination Programs

HORSES

Tetanus *(Clostridium tetani)*

An alum-precipitated toxoid is available. Foals are vaccinated at 6–8 weeks of age, and again at 3 months and 6 months, to overcome interference by residual maternal antibody. Adults should receive an annual booster. Pregnant mares require a booster in late gestation to optimize colostral antibody concentration.

Influenza (Influenza viruses)

Killed vaccines are most commonly used and contain subtypes A1 and A2 of the virus.

Foals

Although there appears to be a poor response to vaccination in foals under 6 months because of maternal antibody, vaccination may be advisable from 6 months of age in open herds. This primary vaccination should be boosted within 90 days. Boosters every 4–6 months are recommended up to 3 years of age, due to the short-lived immunity provided by the vaccines.

Adults

Annual boosters are recommended. Animals at high risk (show horses, brood mares) should be vaccinated two or three times annually.

Equine Viral Rhinopneumonitis (herpesvirus)

Recent information has confirmed that EHV-4 (formerly EHV-1 subtype 2) is the type associated with respiratory disease. An EHV-4 killed vaccine is now available in combination with a trivalent influenza vaccine. In foals, the vaccine is given at 2 months of age and is boosted 4–6 weeks later. Boosters every 6 months are advised. EHV-1 (formerly EHV-1 subtype 1) is now regarded as the type causing abortions. Genotypes 1p and 1b are considered to be primarily associated with abortions. A killed inactivated vaccine and a modified live vaccine are available. Pregnant mares should receive killed vaccines, and boosters are required at 5, 7, and 9 months' gestation.

Equine Viral Arteritis (togavirus)

A modified live vaccine has been developed and is used to control outbreaks of disease.

Eastern/Western/Venezuelan Equine Encephalitis (alphavirus, family togaviridae)

These are mosquito-borne viruses with the peak incidence of disease during mosquito season. Vaccines are available containing Eastern and Western encephalitis viruses or all three. Some vaccines are available as a combination of the encephalitis viruses and tetanus toxoid or influenza. Foals are vaccinated at 2–3 months of age and boosted 2–4 weeks later. Annual boosters are recommended before the mosquito season.

Rabies (rhabdovirus)

An inactivated virus vaccine is available. Foals may be vaccinated at 2–3 months of age and boosted 2–4 weeks later. Annual boosters are recommended subsequently.

Strangles (Streptococcus equi)

Several different vaccines are available. Vaccination may be helpful in limiting the incidence of disease on farms with enzootic strangles. Postvaccinal swelling at the injection site and abscessation are encountered. The efficacy of the vaccines has been questioned.

Potomac Fever (Ehrlichia risticii)

A killed vaccine is available. It is administered as an initial course of two injections and boosted once or twice yearly in enzootic areas.

Botulism (Clostridium botulinum)

Vaccination is not commonly practiced, but a toxoid is available to decrease incidence of disease in outbreak situations. Annual vaccination of adults, with vaccination of mares before foaling, is advised in problem areas.

Salmonellosis *(Salmonella typhimurium, S. enteritidis)*

Killed vaccines containing S. *typhimurium* or a combination of S. *typhimurium* and S. *enteritidis* have been used, but their efficacy under field conditions remains questionable.

CATTLE

Infectious Bovine Rhinotracheitis (bovine herpesvirus type 1)

Vaccines available for infectious bovine rhinotracheitis (IBR) include modified live and inactivated types.

Modified Live Vaccines

Two types of modified live vaccines (MLVs) are available, a parenteral (intramuscular) and an intranasal vaccine. Parenteral MLV has been implicated in abortions. Intranasal MLV is considered safe. Beef calves are vaccinated before weaning and again 1 month before shipping. Heifers should be vaccinated before the first breeding, preferably receiving a primary dose at 6–8 weeks and a secondary dose at 2–3 weeks before breeding.

Inactivated Vaccines

Inactivated vaccines for IBR are administered intramuscularly. They are safe for use in pregnant animals but are expensive and fail to produce a solid, long-lasting immunity.

Bovine Viral Diarrhea (pestivirus)

Vaccination is aimed at controlling mucosal disease. MLV and inactivated vaccines are available. The MLV is not recommended for use in pregnant animals. Initial vaccination of all females should be carried out 3–6 weeks before breeding, and in subsequent years maiden heifers should be vaccinated before breeding.

Parainfluenza Virus Type 3

Vaccines consist of attenuated or killed virus and are often combined with IBR and/or respiratory syncytial virus vaccines. Vaccine is delivered intranasally.

Respiratory Syncytial Virus (paramyxovirus)

Inactivated and MLV vaccines are available. Efficacy trials are inconclusive.

Pasteurellosis *(Pasteurella hemolytica)*

Vaccination against *Pasteurella hemolytica*, using killed bacterins or live vaccines, has had limited success. However, the use of leukotoxin-based vaccines has had considerable success in reducing the severity of lung lesions on experimental challenge. Its efficacy in field disease outbreaks is unproven.

Leptospirosis *(Leptospira* spp.)

Monovalent and polyvalent formalin-inactivated bacterins are commonly used in problem herds. Calves should be vaccinated at 4–6 months of age, with a booster 2–4 weeks after the primary injection and annual boosters thereafter. Because cross-immunity between *Leptospira* spp. is poor, polyvalent vaccines are more efficacious.

Haemophilus somnus

A killed bacterin is available. It is administered to calves 3–4 weeks before weaning and again 2–4 weeks later.

Moraxella bovis

Killed vaccine is available and is introduced intramuscularly, given three times at 2-week intervals before the fly season begins. A number of other vaccines have been used. All vaccines have had variable efficacy in the field.

Salmonellosis *(Salmonella typhimurium, S. dublin)*

Live attenuated or killed vaccines are available. Live attenuated vaccines have had considerable success in the UK. Killed vaccines appear to be less successful. Cows should be vaccinated in late pregnancy to ensure adequate colostral antibodies.

Brucellosis *(Brucella abortus)*

Strain 19 (S-19) and S-45/20 vaccines are available. S-19 is a live vaccine and is administered at 4–8 months of age. The use of vaccines is dictated by regional control programs, with supervision by state or federal regulatory bodies.

Escherichia coli

Killed bacterins for parenteral use are available for control of *E. coli* K99–induced diarrhea in newborn calves. Pregnant animals should be vaccinated at 6 and 3 weeks before calving to provide high colostral antibody concentrations. Monoclonal antibody may be administered to calves within 6–10 h of birth to protect against *E. coli* K99–induced diarrhea.

Coronavirus and Rotavirus

Parenterally administered killed vaccines have been used to immunize pregnant animals 6 and 3 weeks before parturition, to achieve high colostral antibody concentrations. Oral vaccines for administration to calves within a few hours of birth are also available. Both types of vaccines are of questionable efficacy in the field.

Clostridium spp.

Polyvalent, killed, adjuvanted vaccines containing combinations of *Clostridium chauvoei*, *C. septicum*, *C. novyi* types *B* and *D*, and *C. perfringens* are available. They are administered to young stock once maternal antibody has waned (at 4–6 months). The initial vaccination consists of two injections 2–4 weeks apart; annual boosters are recommended.

Vaccination for *C. botulinum* may be recommended in certain areas. Two injections of toxoid 2–4 weeks apart are administered, with boosters every 2 years.

Rabies (rhabdovirus)

This inactivated virus vaccine is administered subcutaneously or intramuscularly to cattle over 3 months of age. It is used only in enzootic areas (e.g., South America, parts of the USA). It is cost effective only in valuable animals.

Anthrax (Bacillus anthracis)

An avirulent nonencapsulated spore vaccine is administered immediately before the grazing season in endemic areas. Two vaccinations, 2–4 weeks apart, are recommended.

Anaplasma Marginale

Inactivated and MLVs are available. Animals at risk should be vaccinated 6 weeks before exposure.

Campylobacter fetus

An oil-adjuvanted bacterin, administered 1–6 months before breeding. A single dose gives long-lasting immunity.

Dictyocaulus viviparus

A vaccine containing inactivated larvae is available for calves. It is administered orally at 8 weeks of age and again 4 weeks later. Calves must remain indoors during the vaccination period and for 2 weeks after the second dose.

SHEEP AND GOATS

Clostridium spp.

A primary course of two injections of bivalent vaccines containing *Clostridium perfringens* types C and D administered 2–4 weeks apart is recommended in lambs and kids over 2 months of age. Annual boosters should be given.

C. tetani vaccine is also recommended, with a similar course of injections as for *C. perfringens* types C and D. Vaccination for *C. tetani* is usually only used in individual cases (e.g., retained placenta or after surgery). The toxoid is administered intramuscularly.

Orf (parapoxvirus)

Maternal antibody is not protective. Vaccination of young stock within the first week of life may be performed.

Pasteurellosis (Pasteurella haemolytica)

Killed bacterins are available, containing *P. haemolytica*. Vaccination with the bacterin parenterally, combined with PI_3, nasally or parenterally, has been practiced.

Foot Rot (Bacteroides nodosus)

Vaccines have been used in sheep in the UK and Australia to control foot rot. The available vaccines vary in the serotypes of *B. nodosus*; several different adjuvants have been used in an attempt to avoid abscess formation or tissue reaction at injection sites. Because the duration of immunity is short (12 weeks), vaccination should be timed to coincide with the expected period of susceptibility. Frequent boosters (every 3–4 months) may be required in outbreak situations.

Corynebacterium pseudotuberculosis

Vaccination has been attempted in sheep and goats using autogenous vaccine or commercially available killed bacterins. Efficacy is generally poor.

Blue Tongue (orbiovirus)

An MLV vaccine containing only one of the five serotypes is available in the USA for control of blue tongue. Other vaccines are being developed that contain several serotypes.

Rabies (rhabdovirus)

An inactivated vaccine is available for use in sheep and goats at high risk of rabies.

Chlamydial Abortion (Chlamydia psittaci)

An inactivated vaccine that may prevent abortion, but not infection, is available. It should be administered a few weeks before breeding.

Campylobacter fetus

Vaccination of sheep appears to be effective. Two injections are administered 2–4 weeks apart before breeding, or in the first half of pregnancy. Outbreaks of abortion may be controlled if early diagnosis is immediately followed by vaccination.

SWINE

Erysipelothrix rhusiopathiae

Vaccination of gilts, sows, and boars with E. rhusiopathiae vaccine is recommended. A primary course is two injections a few weeks apart (depending on individual vaccines). Not all vaccines are safe for use in pregnant animals. Fattening stock are usually not vaccinated unless an outbreak of disease is expected.

Atrophic Rhinitis (Bordetella bronchiseptica)

Several vaccines are available, all containing B. bronchiseptica, some in combination with strains of Pasteurella multocida. Recommendations vary with the type of vaccine. Some vaccines are recommended for use in breeding sows to achieve high colostral antibody concentrations. Other vaccines may be used in piglets. Because atrophic rhinitis is a multifactorial disease, vaccine efficacy is variable.

Colibacillosis

Escherichia coli vaccines are aimed at protecting the neonate from acute diarrhea. Various vaccines and programs are used. A combination of oral and parenteral vaccination of sows has been successful in preventing disease in piglets.

Intestinal Clostridiosis *(Clostridium perfringens type C)*

C. perfringens type C vaccine is administered to sows twice during gestation, generally at 6 and 2 weeks before farrowing.

Leptospirosis *(Leptospira spp.)*

Formalinized bacterins (usually bivalent with *Leptospira pomona, L. interrogans)* are used. Vaccination of gilts and sows before breeding is recommended and is aimed at decreasing the incidence of abortion.

Salmonellosis *(Salmonella cholerae suis)*

Vaccination of sows with live attenuated *S. cholerae suis* has been used in problem herds to protect newborn piglets from the disease. The degree of benefit is debated.

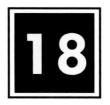

Tests of Liver and Kidney Function

LIVER FUNCTION TESTS

The functions of the liver are diverse, and no single test is sufficient to evaluate liver function. The available liver function tests may be classified on the following basis.

1. Serum activity of liver-derived enzymes (e.g., alkaline phosphatase and sorbitol dehydrogenase)

2. Tests of hepatic secretion and excretion (e.g., bromosulphthalein clearance)

3. Tests of liver metabolic function (e.g., protein metabolism).

Serum Enzymes

Liver-Specific Enzymes

SORBITOL DEHYDROGENASE (SD). SD is specific for acute hepatocellular damage. It has a short half-life in serum (24–48 h). Assay must be conducted on fresh serum.

GLUTAMINE DEHYDROGENASE (GD) AND ORNITHINE CARBAMYL TRANSFERASE (OCT). GD and OCT are liver-specific enzymes that are less frequently measured.

Non-Liver-Specific Enzymes

These enzymes also exist in high concentrations in other organs

ASPARTATE AMINOTRANSFERASE (AST). High activity of AST in skeletal and cardiac muscle, liver, intestinal mucosa, and erythrocytes. AST is present in the cytosol and is bound to mitochondria. Increases in AST activity are indicative of tissue damage; however, taken in isolation, an increased AST activity is not specific for any tissue.

To differentiate between AST of liver and AST of muscle origin, serum creatine kinase (CK) should be measured simultaneously with AST. AST has a prolonged serum half-life (2–3 days) relative to CK (peaks at 6 h). Concurrent increases in AST and CK indicate muscle disease or the simultaneous existence of liver and muscle disease. An increase in AST in association with a normal CK indicates hepatocellular disease.

ALANINE AMINOTRANSFERASE (ALT). ALT originates from muscle and liver.

ALKALINE PHOSPHATASE (ALP). Isoenzymes of ALP exist in liver, bone, intestine, renal tubular cells, and placenta. Corticosteroids induce a specific isoenzyme of ALP. Increased serum activity occurs in association with bile duct obstruction. An increased serum ALP activity can be normal in young animals.

γ-GLUTAMYL TRANSFERASE (GGT). GGT occurs in high concentrations in liver and kidney. Increased serum activity of GGT usually implies liver damage, because renal GGT is released into the urine by brush border cells of the tubules. It exists in high concentrations in biliary tissue and is considered to be a good indicator of cholestasis. GGT is not stable at room temperature.

ARGINASE (ARG). ARG, a mitochondrial-bound enzyme, is present in many body tissues. ARG increases in serum after acute hepatocyte damage. ARG is not routinely measured.

LACTATE DEHYDROGENASE (LDH). LDH is widely distributed in skeletal and cardiac muscle, liver, kidney, lung, and erythrocyte. Because of LDH's long half-life, activity of this enzyme remains increased for several days.

Tests of Secretion and Excretion

BROMOSULPHTHALEIN (BSP) CLEARANCE. Hepatic anion transport is tested by determining the rate of BSP clearance. The clearance half-life is the time taken for the BSP concentration in the plasma to be halved. In states of reduced liver perfusion (e.g., congestive cardiac disease), BSP clearance is prolonged.

Clearance of BSP is affected by bilirubin, and for this reason the test is not accurate in jaundiced patients.

INDOCYANINE GREEN CLEARANCE. This test can be used in place of BSP clearance.

BILIRUBIN. In the horse, most (approximately 70%) of the bilirubin is unconjugated (indirect). Increases in serum bilirubin occur with fasting, gastrointestinal stasis, intravascular hemolysis, biliary obstruction, and liver disease. Fasting hyperbilirubinemia is unique to the horse.

BILE ACIDS. Bile acids are synthesized in the liver and secreted in the bile; they may enter the circulation via the hepatic or portal system.

Increases in "fasting" bile acids have been demonstrated in a variety of liver diseases. At present, increased serum bile acid concentrations are specific for detecting the presence of chronic liver disease in the horse. They do not aid in determining the type of liver disease. In cattle, bile acids are sensitive and specific for hepatic disease, and the test is sensitive enough that fasting the animal is unnecessary.

Liver Metabolism

Plasma Proteins

ALBUMIN. Albumin is synthesized in the liver, and hypoalbuminemia may result from liver disease. Hypoalbuminemia from liver disease must be differentiated from other causes, which include excessive loss of albumin—for example, through the kidney, intestines (e.g., parasitism), or hemorrhage—and decrease in protein synthesis (e.g., dietary deficiency or malabsorption).

GLOBULINS. Globulins consist of alpha, beta, and gamma fractions. The alpha and beta globulins are synthesized primarily by the liver and, to a lesser degree, in intestinal mucosal cells. The gamma globulins (IgG, IgM, IgE, and IgA) are produced by plasma cells in response to antigenic stimulation.

Decreases in the alpha and beta fractions (in large animals) are not commonly the result of liver disease.

MISCELLANEOUS. Other parameters that may be evaluated include fibrinogen and clotting factors.

Other Tests to Evaluate the Liver

Liver Biopsy

A liver biopsy is performed when difficulties are encountered in determining the nature and extent of the pathologic changes. Localized lesions may be missed, because the amount of tissue sampled is small.

A liver biopsy has the disadvantage of being invasive.

Ultrasonography

The liver's size, shape, and architecture can be evaluated using ultrasonography.

RENAL FUNCTION TESTS

Urinalysis

SPECIFIC GRAVITY (SG). SG reflects the degree of tubular reabsorption of water. The normal SG ranges from 1.015 to 1.045 and depends on the degree of hydration, although single samples collected randomly may vary considerably.

Low urine SG is associated with diuresis, excessive fluid administration, renal disease, diabetes insipidus, and Cushing's disease.

High urine SG occurs during dehydration and fever (transient increase).

OSMOLALITY. Osmolality reflects the urine-concentrating ability of the kidney. The urine:plasma osmolality ratio is a method of calculating the concentrating ability of the renal tubules. The ratio can be used in diagnosis of prerenal azotemia and renal tubular disease.

pH. The pH is normally alkaline (7.4–8.4) in herbivores. Aciduria is a normal finding in suckling calves and foals. Acidity is increased in states of prolonged exercise.

PROTEIN. Urine generally does not contain detectable amounts of protein. Protein that is filtered at the glomerulus is reabsorbed in the tubules, and proteinuria is considered abnormal, except in neonates and periparturient animals. Proteinuria must be assessed in conjunction with the urine specific gravity.

Transient proteinuria may follow the excessive ingestion of a protein-rich feed or severe exercise.

Renal diseases such as glomerulonephritis, amyloidosis, and pyelonephritis result in a marked proteinuria.

Infections (e.g., cystitis and vaginitis) of the urinary tract result in postrenal proteinuria.

Blood (hemoglobin) and myoglobin can cause a positive reaction for protein.

BLOOD. Hemoglobinuria, hematuria, and myoglobinuria will give a positive reaction on the test strips. It is not possible to differentiate blood or hemoglobin from myoglobin using commercial test strips. Red blood cells may be differentiated from hemoglobin only when a small quantity of either is present; hemoglobin causes a uniform color change, whereas red cells produce stippling of the strip. This method of differentiation does not work when a large amount of either is present. The appearance of the serum sample will aid in differentiation; e.g., if hemolysis is severe, the serum will have a reddish tinge.

Centrifugation of the urine sample will cause sedimentation of red cells, leaving a clear supernatant. Myoglobin and hemoglobin can sometimes be differentiated using the ammonium sulfate test (2.8 g of ammonium sulfate and 5 ml of urine are mixed and then centrifuged); a dark supernatant indicates myoglobin.

KETONES. Ketones are present in the urine when the plasma concentration is high. Conditions associated with ketonuria include bovine ketosis and pregnancy toxemia of ewes and does (twin-lamb disease).

GLUCOSE. Glucose is not present in normal urine. Its presence in urine indicates a high plasma glucose concentration. The latter is a transient finding in animals treated with xylazine, detomidine, or corticosteroids. Glucosuria is associated with diabetes mellitus, hyperadrenocorticism, and enterotoxemia (*Clostridium perfringens* type D).

URINE SEDIMENT. Urine sediment may be examined for the presence of epithelial cells, leukocytes, erythrocytes, parasites, microorganisms, tubular casts, and crystals.

URINE CULTURE. If bacterial infection of the urinary tract is suspected, urine culture should be performed. Cystitis and pyelonephritis are relatively rare in horses but occur with greater frequency in cattle. Samples collected by urinary catheter are generally not contaminated; samples collected during voiding are frequently contaminated. In cattle, pyelonephritis is frequently associated with *Corynebacterium renale* or coliforms.

ENZYMURIA. Enzymuria is not commonly measured in large animals. γ-Glutamyltransferase (GGT) is present in high concentrations in the tubular epithelial cells and is released into the urine after tubular damage. Increased GGT is an early indicator of renal tubular damage.

The urine GGT:creatinine ratio may also be used to assess renal function.

In general, enzymuria tests are not practical or indicated under clinical conditions.

Serum Analysis

BLOOD UREA. Blood urea is a nitrogenous waste product of protein metabolism; it is formed in the liver and excreted by the kidneys.

Increases in plasma urea concentrations occur in reduced renal perfusion (e.g., dehydration), obstruction to urine outflow (e.g., urethral calculus), and extensive muscle catabolism.

The blood urea concentration may vary with fluctuations in the dietary protein and in association with tissue trauma, fever, and infection.

CREATININE. Because its production is constant and it is excreted by glomerular filtration, serum creatinine concentration can be used as an index of glomerular filtration. Increases in serum creatinine are associated with reduced renal perfusion (e.g., dehydration) and obstruction to urine outflow.

ELECTROLYTES. Increases in serum K^+ are associated with marked decreases in renal perfusion (e.g., during severe dehydration) and obstruction to urinary outflow.

Tests of Renal Clearance

Renal clearance (ml/min) of a substance x (C_x) gives an estimate of the kidney's ability to remove the substance from plasma.

C_x can be expressed by the equation

$$C_x = \frac{U_x}{S_x} \times V_u$$

where U_x is the urine concentration and S_x is the serum concentration of substance x, and V_u is the volume of urine in ml/min.

Fractional Clearance of Electrolytes

This index of tubular function relates the clearance of the electrolyte to the clearance of creatinine. The fractional clearance of substance x (FC_x) is expressed by the equation

$$FC_x = (U_x/S_x)/(U_{cr}/S_{cr})$$

where U_x is the urine concentration and S_x is the serum concentration of substance x, and U_{cr} is the urine concentration and S_{cr} is the serum concentration of creatinine.

Other Tests to Evaluate Renal Function

ULTRASONOGRAPHY. Kidney size and architecture can be evaluated and renal (and cystic) calculi detected using ultrasonography.

RENAL BIOPSY. In small ruminants, particularly goats, the left kidney is generally palpable through the body wall and can be immobilized sufficiently to allow a percutaneous biopsy to be performed. In horses, ultrasound-guided biopsies render the procedure easier and safer. In cattle, per rectum manipulation and stabilization of the left kidney may aid biopsy.

Appendix I*

NORMAL HEMATOLOGY VALUES

	Units	Bovine	Equine	Porcine	Ovine
Hemoglobin (HgB)	g/L	80–150	110–190	100–160	80–160
Hematocrit (Hct)	L/L	0.24–0.46	0.32–0.52	0.32–0.50	0.24–0.50
Red blood cell (RBC) count	$\times 10^{12}$/L	5.0–10.0	6.5–12.5	5.0–8.0	8.0–16.0
Mean corpuscular volume (MCV)	fL	40–60	34–58	50–68	23–48
Mean corpuscular hemoglobin (MCH)	pg	11–17	11–19	16.6–22.0	9.0–12.0
Mean corpuscular hemoglobin concentration (MCHC)	g/L	300–360	310–370	300–340	310–380
Reticulocytes	%	0%	0%	0–1%	0%
White blood cell (WBC) count	$\times 10^9$/L	4.0–12.0	5.5–12.5	11.0–22.0	4.0–12.0
Segmented	$\times 10^9$/L	0.6–4.0	2.7–6.7	3.08–10.4	0.7–6.0
	%	15–45%	30–65%	28–47%	10–50%
Bands	$\times 10^9$/L	0.0–0.12	0.0–0.1	0.0–0.88	Rare
	%	0–2%	0–2%	0–4%	Rare
Eosinophils	$\times 10^9$/L	0.0–2.4	0–0.93	0.06–2.42	0–1.0
	%	2–20%	0–4%	0–11%	0–10%
Basophils	$\times 10^9$/L	0–0.2	0–0.17	0–0.44	0–0.3
	%	0–2%	0–3%	0–2%	0–3%
Lymphocytes	$\times 10^9$/L	2.5–7.5	1.5–5.5	4.29–13.6	2.0–9.0
	%	45–75%	25–70%	39–62%	40–75%
Monocytes	$\times 10^9$/L	0.03–0.84	0–0.8	0.22–2.2	0–0.75
	%	2–7%	0–7%	2–10%	0–6%
Platelets	$\times 10^9$/L	100–800	100–600	310–510	250–750

*Data derived from a population of healthy animals tested at the Atlantic Veterinary College, Charlottetown, Prince Edward Island, Canada.

Appendix II*

NORMAL CLINICAL CHEMISTRY VALUES

	Units	Bovine	Equine	Porcine	Ovine
Sodium	mmol/L	135–151	135–148	140–150	143–151
Potassium	mmol/L	3.9–5.9	3.0–5.0	4.7–7.1	4.6–7.0
Chloride	mmol/L	96–110	98–110	100–105	102–116
Calcium	mmol/L	2.11–2.75	2.80–3.44	1.80–2.90	2.30–2.86
Phosphorus	mmol/L	1.08–2.76	1.00–1.80	1.30–3.55	0.82–2.66
Magnesium	mmol/L	0.80–1.32	0.74–1.02	0.78–1.60	0.9–1.26
Urea	mmol/L	3.0–7.5	3.5–7.0	3.0–8.5	2.0–10.0
Creatinine	μmol/L	67–175	110–170	90–240	69–105
Glucose	mmol/L	1.8–3.8	3.6–5.6	3.6–5.3	1.2–3.6
Cholesterol	mmol/L	–	1.20–4.60	–	–
Total bilirubin	μmol/L	0–30	4–102	0–4	0–5

Appendix continued on following page

	Units	Bovine	Equine	Porcine	Ovine
Direct bilirubin	μmol/L	0–3	0–7	0–4	0–5
Alkaline phosphatase	I.U./L	121	95–233	10–400	66–158
Creatine kinase (CK)	I.U./L	<350	<500	<500	<350
Aspartate amino-transferase (AST)	I.U./L	46–118	197–429	25–57	48–128
Alanine amino-transferase (ALT)	I.U./L	–	10–23	34–58	–
γ-Glutamyl transferase (GGT)	I.U./L	<31	<25	<25	<70
Total protein	g/L	66–78	60–77	34–60	61–81
Globulin	g/L	35–43	35–41	16–38	34–42
Albumin	g/L	23–43	25–36	18–22	27–39
A/G ratio	—	0.66–1.30	0.60–1.50	0.60–1.50	0.54–1.22
Iron	μmol/L	14.5–29	14.5–25	14.5–36	29–40
Total iron-binding capacity (TIBC)	μmol/L	44.8–62.7	44.8–62.7	44.8–62.7	44.8–62.7
Bromsulphalein (BSP)	minutes	ALL SPECIES		T ½ = < 2.5	
Ammonia	μmol/L	10–82	10–82	10–82	10–82
Osmolality	mosm/kg	285–315	285–315	285–315	285–315
Cerebrospinal fluid (CSF) protein	g/L	0.16–0.33	0.29–0.72	0.24–0.40	0.08–0.70
Fibrinogen	g/L	< 6.0	< 5.0	< 4.0	< 5.0
Prothrombin time (PT) mean		11.0	9.0	11.0	NA
range	seconds	10–12	7–11	9.5–12.0	NA
Partial thromboplastin time (PTT) mean		38.0	39.0	18	NA
range	seconds	30–50	30–50	13–21.0	NA

*Data derived from a population of healthy animals tested at the Atlantic Veterinary College, Charlottetown, Prince Edward Island, Canada.

Appendix III

DRUG DOSAGES

The following dose rates are approximate. In animals with reduced drug clearance, a decreased frequency of administration is advised; these animals include neonates, septicemic and dehydrated animals, and animals with hepatic or renal disease. In animals used for food, attention must be given to withholding times for milk and meat; this information is available from the package insert. Withholding times are valid only for the dose amount, route of administration, indication, and species for which the product is licensed.

Legend: BID—every 12 hours, TID—every 8 hours, QID—every 6 hours, IM—intramuscularly, IV—intravenously, PO—orally, SC—subcutaneously

Drug	Dosage/Frequency	Route of Administration
Bacterial Drugs		
Amikacin sulfate	6.5–7.5 mg/kg BID (horses)	IV, IM
Amoxicillin Na$^+$	20 mg/kg BID–QID (horses)	IM
Amoxicillin trihydrate	20 mg/kg BID (horses)	IM
	7 mg/kg TID (calves)	PO
Ampicillin Na$^+$	10–20 mg/kg QID (horses, cattle)	IM, IV
Ampicillin trihydrate	10–20 mg/kg BID (horses, cattle)	IM
Ceftiofur Na$^+$	1.1 mg/kg once daily (adult cattle, horses)	IM
Chloramphenicol Na$^+$ succinate	25 mg/kg TID (horses)	IM
	50 mg/kg QID (horses)	IV, PO
Erythromycin estolate	25 mg/kg QID (horses)	PO
Erythromycin ethylsuccinate	25 mg/kg TID (horses)	PO
Erythromycin gluceptate/ lactobionate	5–10 mg/kg TID (horses)	IV
	4–8 mg/kg BID (horses)	IV
Furazolidone	10–12 mg/kg BID (cattle)	PO
Gentamicin sulfate	2–4 mg/kg BID/TID (horses)	IM, IV
Lincomycin	10 mg/kg BID (cattle)	IM
	5–10 mg/kg once daily (pigs)	IM
Metronidazole	10–25 mg/kg TID–QID (horses)	PO
Neomycin sulfate	5–15 mg/kg BID (cattle)	PO
Oxytetracycline HCl	10–20 mg/kg BID (calves)	PO
	3–10 mg/kg BID (horses)	IV
	5–10 mg/kg BID (cattle)	IV, IM
Penicillin G (Na$^+$, K$^+$)	20–40,000 I.U./kg QID (horses, cattle)	IV, IM
Penicillin G procaine	10–20,000 I.U./kg BID (horses, cattle)	IM
Penicillin V (phenoxymethylpenicillin)	110,000 I.U./kg BID–TID (horses)	PO
Potentiated sulfonamides (trimethoprim-sulfadiazine)	12–25 mg/kg of combination BID–TID (horses)	IV, PO
	25 mg/kg once daily (cattle)	IV, IM
Rifampin	5–10 mg/kg BID (horses)	PO
Streptomycin	5–10 mg/kg BID (cattle, horses)	IM
Sulfonamides	100–200 mg/kg initially, followed by	IV
	50–100 mg/kg BID (horses, cattle)	IV

Appendix continued on following page

Drug	Dosage/Frequency	Route of Administration
Sulfonamides *Continued*	200 mg/kg once daily (horses, cattle)	PO
Tetracycline	5–10 mg/kg BID (calves)	PO
Ticarcillin	25–50 mg/kg QID (horses)	IV
	25–50 mg/kg TID (horses)	IM
Tilmicosin	10 mg/kg once, repeat in 72 h if indicated (cattle)	SC
Tylosin	5–10 mg/kg BID (cattle, pigs, horses)	IM
Anti-Inflammatory Drugs		
Acetylsalicylic acid (aspirin)	50–100 mg/kg BID (cattle)	PO
	50–100 mg/kg BID (horses)	IM, IV
Dexamethasone	0.05–1.0 mg/kg for anti-inflammatory effect, single dose (all species)	IV, IM, SC
	0.02–0.05 mg/kg once daily (long term anti-inflammatory)	IV, IM
	10–20 mg (bovine ketosis)	IV, IM
	25 mg (induce parturition in bovine)	IV, IM
Dipyrone	10–20 mg/kg (all species)	IV, IM
Flunixin meglumine	1.0 mg/kg once or twice daily (horses)	IM, IV, PO
	1–2.0 mg/kg BID (cattle, small ruminants)	IM, IV
Meclofenamic acid	2.2 mg/kg/day (horses), up to 10 days	PO
Methylprednisolone Na$^+$ succinate	0.25 mg/kg (horses)	IV
Naproxen	10 mg/kg BID (horses)	PO
	5 mg/kg (horses)	IV
Phenylbutazone	4.0 mg/kg BID first day; reduce to 2.0 mg/kg BID (horses)	PO, IV
	2–4.0 mg/kg alternate days (cattle)	PO, IV
Prednisolone acetate	0.25–1.0 mg/kg (all species)	IM
Prednisolone sodium succinate	0.25–1.0 mg/kg (all species)	IV
Prednisone tabs	0.25–1.0 mg/kg (all species)	PO
Antihistamines		
H$_1$ Blockers		
Pyrilamine	1 mg/kg BID (horses, cattle)	IV, IM, SC
Tripelennamine (H$_1$)	0.5–1.1 mg/kg, q 6–12 h (horses, cattle)	IM, IV
H$_2$ Blockers		
Cimetidine HCl (H$_2$)	6 mg/kg TID–QID (horses)	PO, IV, IM
Ranitidine HCl (H$_2$)	1–3 mg/kg BID (horses)	PO
	0.5 mg/kg BID (horses)	IV

Drug	Dosage/Frequency	Route of Administration
Sedatives and Analgesics	Dose rates vary with species and the health status of the animal. Combinations of these compounds may produce an additive effect, and doses of individual drugs must be reduced accordingly.	
Acepromazine	0.03–0.06 mg/kg (horses, cattle)	IV
	0.05–0.1 mg/kg (horses)	IM, PO
Buprenorphine	0.006 mg/kg (horses)	IV, IM
Butorphanol	0.02–0.1 mg/kg (horses, cattle)	IV, IM
Chloral hydrate	50 mg/kg (or to effect) (horses, cattle)	IV
Detomidine	0.005–0.03 mg/kg (horses)	IV, IM
Meperidine HCl	2–5 mg/kg (horses)	IM
Methadone	0.05–0.1 mg/kg (horses)	IV, IM
Pentazocine	0.3 mg/kg (horses)	IV, IM
Xylazine	0.1–1.5 mg/kg (horses)	IV, IM
	0.02–0.2 mg/kg (cattle)	
	0.02–0.05 mg/kg (small ruminants)	IV, IM
Autonomic and Cardiac System		
Atropine	0.02–0.05 mg/kg (all species)	IV, IM
Clenbuterol	0.0008 mg/kg BID (horses)	PO, IV
Dobutamine	0.0025–0.01 mg/kg/min (all species)	IV
Dopamine	0.0025–0.005 mg/kg/min (all species)	IV
Epinephrine	0.005–0.01 mg/kg (all species)	Slowly IV, SC
Glycopyrrolate	0.002–0.004 mg/kg (all species)	IV, IM
Propranolol	0.1–0.3 mg/kg BID (horses)	Slowly IV
Tolazoline	2.0 mg/kg (cattle)	IV
Yohimbine	0.1–0.2 mg/kg (all species)	IV, IM
Cardiac Drugs		
Digoxin	0.035–0.08 mg/kg/day loading (horses)	PO
	0.01–0.03 mg/kg/day maintenance (horses)	PO
	0.012–0.014 mg/kg/day loading (horses)	IV
Lidocaine	For treatment of ventricular premature beats. *Loading dose:* 1.0–1.5 mg/kg to a max of 5.0 mg/kg over 5–10 min. Followed, if necessary, by a constant infusion at 0.02–0.04 mg/kg/min	IV

Drug	Dosage/Frequency	Route of Administration
Quinidine gluconate	1.0–1.5 mg/kg as a bolus, repeat every 10–15 min until cardioversion occurs, for up to a total dose of 10–12 mg/kg, or until signs of toxicity (horses)	IV
Quinidine sulfate	20 mg/kg q 2 h until atrial fib. resolves or max of 6 doses (horses)	PO
Diuretics		
Dimethyl sulfoxide	1.0 g/kg as a 10–20% solution in 5% dextrose once or twice daily (all species)	IV
Furosemide	0.2–1.0 mg/kg, repeat as needed (all species)	IV, IM
Mannitol	0.5–2.0 g/kg bolus (all species), can be repeated 2–3 times in first 24 h	Slowly IV
Gastrointestinal		
Activated charcoal	1–3 g/kg in water, via stomach tube (all species)	PO
Bismuth subsalicylate	1–2 ml/kg q 4–6 h (calves, foals)	PO
Dioctyl sodium succinate	10–20 mg/kg in 1–2 L warm water (horses)	PO
Iodochlorhydroxyquin	1–2 mg/kg once daily initially. Reduce by half, or more, once response obtained (to treat chronic diarrhea in horses)	PO
Metoclopramide	0.2 mg/kg/h for 30 min (horses)	Slowly IV
	0.02–0.1 mg/kg TID/QID (horses, cattle)	Slowly IV, IM
Mineral oil	2–5 L (adult horses)	PO
Sucralfate	20–40 mg/kg QID (foals)	PO
Respiratory System		
Aminophylline	4–7 mg/kg TID (horses)	PO
Clenbuterol	0.0008 mg/kg BID (horses)	PO, IV
Cromolyn sodium	80 mg nebulized, daily for 4 days should give a therapeutic effect for up to 20 days (horses)	Nebulization
Theophylline	10 mg/kg BID (horses)	PO
Anticonvulsants		
Phenobarbital	10–20 mg/kg loading; then 2–10 mg/kg TID (foals)	Slowly IV
Phenytoin	1–10 mg/kg; q 8 h TID (foals)	PO
Diazepam	0.1–0.5 mg/kg (all species) as needed for seizure control	IV

Drug	Dosage/Frequency	Route of Administration
Vitamins		
Vitamin E	50 mg to adult (450 kg) (horses, cattle)	IM
Thiamine	0.5–5.0 mg/kg (horses)	IV, IM, PO
	5–10 mg/kg q 4 h for 6–8 treatments (ruminants)	IV, IM
Vitamin K	0.1 mg/kg (all species)	SC

Index

Note: Page numbers followed by the letter f refer to illustrations; page numbers followed by the letter t refer to tables.